Atlas of Neurodevelopmental Pathology

Patrick Shannon • Sumit Das • Yael Fisher

Atlas of Neurodevelopmental Pathology

Springer

Patrick Shannon
Pathology and Laboratory Medicine
Mount Sinai Hospital
Toronto, ON, Canada

Sumit Das
Laboratory Medicine and Pathology
University of Alberta and Stollery Children's Hospital
Edmonton, AB, Canada

Yael Fisher
Department of Pathology
Rambam Health Care Campus
Haifa, Haifa, Israel

ISBN 978-3-032-14147-7 ISBN 978-3-032-14148-4 (eBook)
https://doi.org/10.1007/978-3-032-14148-4

This Springer imprint is published by the registered company Springer Nature Switzerland AG
The registered company address is: Gewerbestrasse 11, 6330 Cham, Switzerland

To my wife Kayla, who has been by my side throughout both my successes and failures; to my daughter, Arya, and of course my fur children, Larry and Marshall.

Sumit Das

To my family for their support, and to all of the very many families who so generously trusted these cases to our care, and with abundant gratitude to my colleagues in Pathology, Clinical Genetics, and Radiology including S. Keating, G. Taylor, E. Morgen, A. Parks, D. Chitayat, K. Chong, and S. Blaser. I would particularly like to thank the patient and skilled eyes and hands of B. Chow, W. Tsui, N. Saito, C. Elliot, E. Almeida, E. Colovini, M. Lin, I. Sue-Chue-Lam, N. Sharif, P. Yue, S. Nacci, A. Muralanthan, A. Elliott-Benjamin, and M. Thompson, as well as many technologists, particularly M. Cooke, C. Mackinnon, and A. Wing, and my long-suffering and wholly estimable administrative assistant P. Gandhikumar. This atlas would be utterly impossible without their aid, care, and professionalism. I would also like to thank Dr. H. Sarnat for his steady encouragement and many intelligent observations through the years.

Patrick Shannon

To my mother, Deborah, who first planted the seed of curiosity in me, and to my beloved family—Gil, Iris, Ayala, and Oren—who joined me on the journey of a lifetime.

Yael Fischer

Preface

Neurodevelopment neuropathology is one of the most complex areas in the practice of neuropathology. There is a wide array of developmental anomalies that can affect the brain and spinal cord but the mechanisms behind many of these anomalies still remain unclear, although various theories have been proposed, which are discussed in this atlas. We believe post-mortem examination of brain and spinal cord anomalies begins with thorough review of pertinent clinical history and proper removal of these structures during fetopsies, which includes in situ examination. This is why Chap. 1 entails what we think is a systematic approach to brain and spinal cord removal from patients while Chap. 2 provides our thoughts regarding the overall approach to conducting fetopsies involving brain and/or spinal cord anomalies. Understanding malformations of the central nervous system (CNS) requires an understanding of normal CNS embryology along with fetal neuroanatomy and histology, which on their own are also complicated subjects. For this reason, we have included summaries of the embryology of different parts of the brain as introductions to the malformations in their respective regions. This atlas has provided us the opportunity to share the complex neuropathological findings noted in the vast number of CNS malformations we have encountered over a number of years.

In addition to neuropathological characteristics, the genetic etiologies of many of the CNS malformations discussed here are also complex, as the list of genes thought to contribute to some of these anomalies seems to be increasing. Through this atlas, we hope to share not only what we believe is known thus far in the literature regarding the different neurodevelopmental anomalies but also our experience with regard to how we approach post-mortem examinations of these complex cases.

This edition of the *Atlas of Neurodevelopmental Pathology* is intended for residents and fellows in neuropathology as well as practitioners including neuropathologists and pediatric pathologists who either by interest or necessity wish to have an illustrative reference of CNS malformations.

Toronto, ON, Canada
Edmonton, AB, Canada
Haifa, Israel

Patrick Shannon
Sumit Das
Yael Fisher

Acknowledgments

The creation of an atlas covering the large scope of neurodevelopment neuropathology is a daunting task that is certainly not possible without a dedicated team who are enthusiastic about the subject. While an atlas is typically thought of as a series of images, valuable information should be transmitted by the images as well as the written summaries of each disorder discussed in the atlas.

Our team worked tirelessly to produce this *Atlas of Neurodevelopmental Pathology*, with the goal of sharing our knowledge and experience with regard to how we approach complex cases of CNS malformations.

A special acknowledgment needs to go to co-author Dr. Shannon (neuropathologist) without whose immense collection of images of both common and rare central nervous system malformations, this atlas would not be possible. We are also indebted to our other neuropathology colleagues who were kind enough to share images of their rare and complex malformations as well as those who were supportive of us undertaking this endeavor.

We are additionally grateful to the staff at Springer for believing in our idea of a neurodevelopmental atlas, particularly Richard Lansing who saw the potential in this atlas, and to Lee Klein, whose publishing expertise and guidance ensured this project remained on track to the finish line.

Contents

1 Extraction of the Perinatal Brain and Spinal Cord During Necropsy

One of the biggest challenges in the examination of the fetal brain is its removal from the cranium. The fragile nature of the premature fetal brain makes it an absolute necessity to perform brain extraction with utmost care. The technical difficulties that come with handling of the premature brain are in part due to the high water content, the poorly developed fibrous glial framework, the lack of myelination and perivascular significant reticulin framework (van Dijk et al. 2021) and the fragile underdeveloped axonal tracts. Much of the premature brain consists of ground substance (Vasung et al. 2016), and postmortem fluid shifts further increase water content. The fragile brain parenchyma is further encased in a continuous fibrous arachnoid, such that any rupture of the arachnoid leads to herniation and distortion of the underlying contents. These aspects of fetal brain tissue along with potential postmortem delays in performing the autopsy, result in the macerated brain being more vulnerable to architectural distortion and diagnostic compromise than many systemic organs. Because of the lack of tissue support intrinsic to the fetal brain, we strongly encourage underwater dissection and removal of the brain, once the scalp is reflected and the prosector is ready to reflect the parietal and frontal calvarium. The similarities in density between fetal brain, cerebrospinal fluid and water enable the water to support the brain against gravity once the soft tissue and bone are reflected. Underwater dissection minimizes the internal fracturing of the brain that occurs during dissection, decreases the changes in tension that occur when the angle of dissection must be changed, and enables the prosector to move carefully and deliberately without having to hurry to prevent slumping and distortion due to the effects of gravity on unsupported brain. While in water, the brain can be removed after severing the cranial nerves, blood vessels, dural attachments, and upper cervical spinal cord. The brain may also be hardened prior to fixation by in situ injection of hardening fixative fixation (i.e. formalin with 5% by volume glacial acetic acid) (see below) and removing the brain the next day (Cimmino et al. 2002). To date, we have not found this process routinely practicable although some centers prefer it for handling fragile malformed brains.

1.1 Steps for Brain Removal

General examination and documentation of head and skull morphology should proceed in a systematic manner prior to brain removal. Changes in skull shape due to early stages of craniosynostosis, craniofacial defects, dysraphisms, and relevant overlying cutaneous nevi are all evident prior to 20 weeks' gestation and should be photographed or imaged as appropriate. Head circumference is routinely measured, although it should be noted that, in our experience, even severe midgestation hydrocephalus can present without a notable increase in postmortem occipitofrontal diameter due to positional effects on the unfused calvarium lacking the support of amniotic fluid.

In a term or near-term unmacerated fetus, the process of removal may be similar to that used in a neonatal or infant autopsy. A coronal scalp incision extending over the posterior fontanelle is followed by an anterior and posterior scalp reflection. The calvarium is opened by cutting with scissors along the suture lines. The squamous bones are folded outward as the petals of a flower to expose the cerebrum, whereupon the basal vascular, neural, and meningeal attachments may be severed in the usual fashion, similar to the technique employed in an adult or pediatric autopsy.

Should the fetus be preterm or macerated or the brain substantially malformed, it is often prudent to alter the dissection technique in order to minimize artifactual distortion. Because of the lack of tissue support intrinsic to the fetal brain, we strongly encourage underwater dissection and removal of the brain.

In this mode of dissection, a "question mark" scalp incision is made from behind one ear, over the posterior fontanelle to behind the other, and then continued inferiorly and medially down to the midline at the craniocervical junction

P. Shannon et al., *Atlas of Neurodevelopmental Pathology*, https://doi.org/10.1007/978-3-032-14148-4_1

is used; this incision can be continued in the midline caudally for the posterior removal of the spinal cord or column. Once the scalp is reflected, the squamous portion of the occipital bone is removed along suture lines, and the occipital arch is cut with heavy scissors or light bone shears on each side. If carefully done, this can leave the occipital dura intact, which may be necessary if the posterior dural sinuses require careful examination. On removal of the occipital dura, the posterior fossa can be seen in situ and inspected, which is of aid in evaluating Chiari malformations and the variety of posterior fossa cysts. Once such examination and photography is done, the remainder of the dissection proceeds under water. This is most easily achieved if the entire body can be submerged but can be performed by merely immersing the head.

Once submerged, the cranial dura can be opened along the sutures and separated from the falx. We encourage severing the cervical cord and the lower cranial nerve roots first, to minimize buckling and pial rupture near the obex of the fourth ventricle—a common artifact in premature fetal brains. This is followed by the reflection of the calvarium and transection of the basal attachments of the brain in the usual fashion.

Once the brain is removed from the cranium, it is important to obtain the weight, preferably prior to fixation. In such instances, the brain can be removed from the water and immediately transferred to a pre-weighed container already containing fixative, using a container or cupped hands. In extremely premature and/or macerated fetuses, the brain can be liquefied such that neuroanatomical landmarks will not be discernible. Important information may still be obtained at the microscopic level, and therefore, it is still worth the effort of extracting the brain in such cases in spite of the technical challenges. Extra care must be taken, however, when transferring the brain from the water to the prefilled and preweighed container for fixation. Detailed explanations of the different methods for preserving brain architecture are beyond the scope of this atlas, but the interested reader is encouraged to read the excellent review by Dijk et al. (2021).

Where significant scalp, soft tissue, or bone anomalies abut or affect the brain, or where there are significant encephaloceles or meningoceles, we encourage wide dissection around the affected area and en bloc removal of the area together with the brain under water, to retain the anatomical continuity of the abnormal structures and the adjacent brain. Sectioning, sampling, and further dissection can then be undertaken with the fixed specimen.

1.2 Removal of the Spinal Cord

In general, a posterior approach is recommended to allow for an adequate assessment of posterior fossa structures and the spinomedullary junction and for neural tube defects (Cohen et al. 2014). For third-trimester or neonatal spinal cords, the midline incision is extended along the length of the spine, and the skin is undermined and reflected. The paravertebral muscles are dissected and the pedicles severed with light shears or heavy scissors, and the posterior elements are removed en bloc to expose the dura. The spinal nerve roots are severed as far laterally as possible, and then the cord together with the dura is removed intact as in a pediatric or adult postmortem removal. Particularly in the setting of arthrogryposis, spinal column deformity, neural tube defect, or poorly defined central nervous system pathology, we have found that the size and intrinsic fragility of the second-trimester spinal cord, combined with the effects of postmortem autolysis, can render detailed microscopic examination of such specimens exceedingly difficult. In such cases, we encourage the removal of the vertebral column and spinal cord en bloc; after evisceration, the lateral bony and soft tissue attachments to the spinal column are severed using scissors along its length (Fig. 1.1). Prior to 24 weeks' gestation, if an acidic fixative such as Bouin's fluid or 5% glacial acetic acid/formalin is used for the brain, the vertebral column may be immersion-fixed in the same container as the brain, and it will be adequately decalcified in 10 days to 2 weeks, occasioning no additional decalcification procedures or delay. The cord can then be sampled microscopically using axial cuts of the vertebral column and embedding in situ.

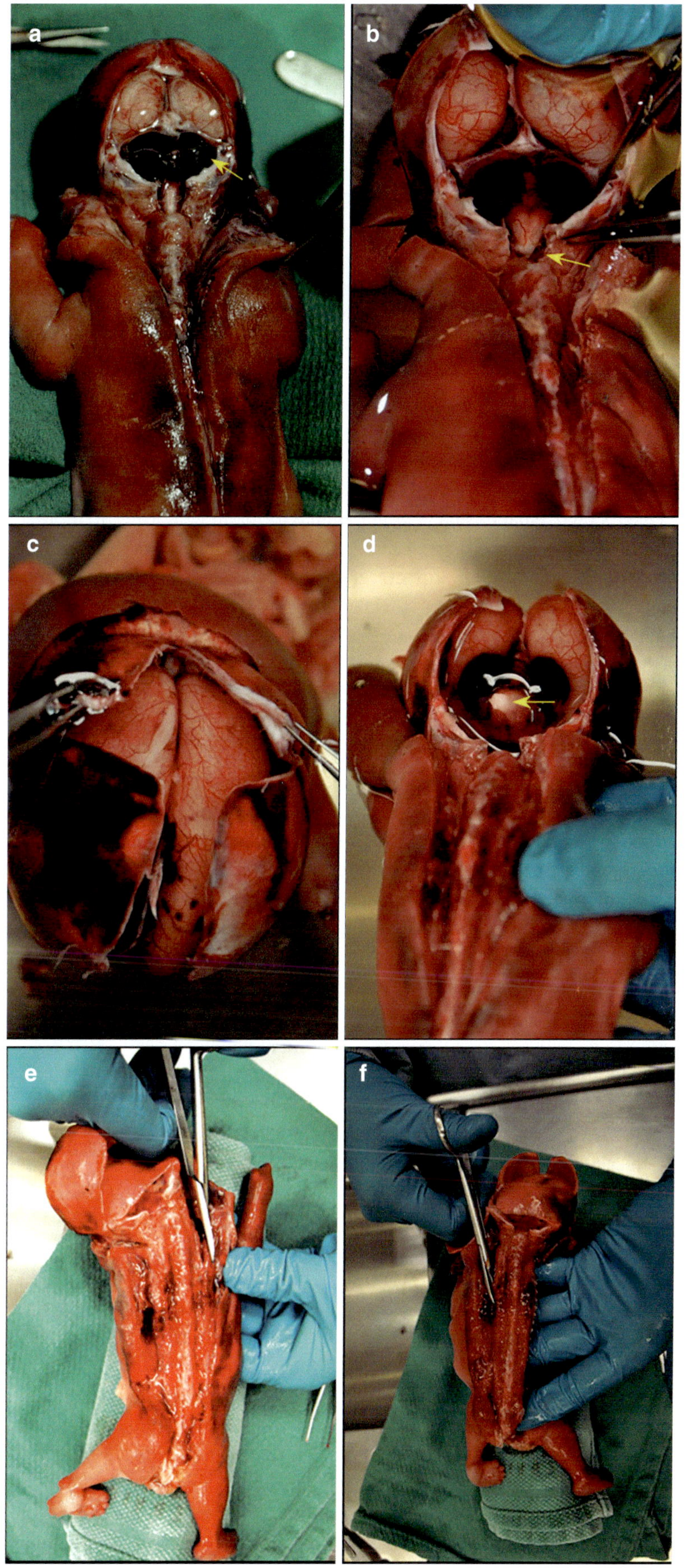

Fig. 1.1 The sequence of brain and spinal cord removal in a midgestation fetus: (**a**) The scalp has been reflected and the occipital bone and dura removed: the occipital lobes, falx and posterior fossa are exposed: in this instance there is an acute cerebellar hematoma (arrow) effacing the cerebellar hemispheres. (**b**) The upper two to three cervical laminae are cut and the posterior neural arch removed exposing the upper cervical cord: this is transected (arrows) caudal to the junction with the medulla and the lateral cervical and lower medullary nerve roots cut close to the dura. (**c**) The calvarium can then be opened along the frontal, coronal and sagittal sutures and the dura cut on either side of the falx. The squamous calvarium can then the reflected, and the attachments of the brain to the rostral cranium cut in an anterior to posterior sequence. (**d**) The head is then flexed and the posterior attachments severed. (**e**) The skin along the midline is incised and reflected, and a long paravertebral cut lateral to the transverse processes and through the sacroiliac joints can be readily made on each side of the column. (**f**) This results in an intact vertebral column with a minimally disturbed spinal cord that can be fixed and sectioned en bloc

1.3 Fixation

A variety of hardening fixatives have been used for fetal specimens. Hardening is strongly recommended at least for preterm brains. If hardening is not used, especially prior to 36 weeks, the architectural distortion that results during brain cutting renders anatomical orientation frustrating and potentiates artifactual tissue fracturing. These difficulties are of course compounded by maceration. Although hardening fixative components such as mercuric chloride and acetic acid do tend to degrade nucleic acids and may necessitate specific optimization protocols for immunohistochemistry (Paradiso et al. 2018), they also allow greater confidence in anatomical sampling and ease in blocking. If fresh tissue must be obtained, small amounts of brain tissue can be aspirated through a 20 guage needle without causing large breaches in the arachnoid.

Hardening fixatives include zinc formalin, Bouin's fluid, Zenker's fluid, ethanol, and neutral buffered formalin with 5% glacial acetic acid by volume. Ethanol has the disadvantage of producing cytological artifact, and mercuric chloride-containing fixatives require specialized disposal because of their heavy metal content. In our labs, we use the 5% glacial acetic acid/formalin mixture routinely, because it is convenient, does not discolor the tissue, and does not require any specialized handling or disposal. However, 5% glacial acetic acid/formalin mixtures need to be made fresh, immediately prior to use, in order to harden the tissue effectively. Although the tissue is stained yellow by Bouin's fluid, Bouin's has the advantage of avoiding formalin pigment deposition. We have found that if formalin pigment is troublesome, it can be eliminated by soaking the hydrated tissue section in lithium carbonate solution prior to staining. The duration of fixation should be 10 days to 3 weeks; antigenicity is decreased and the tissue becomes brittle or crumbles with prolonged hardening.

In exceptional circumstances (e.g., a family would like the brain to be returned with the body), examination may be performed after rapid (~24 h) fixation in 20% formalin + acetic acid. A method of heat-accelerated fixation with modified microwave tissue processor has been described by Barrett et al. (2004), and in one of our institutions (PS), we use a tissue processor to immersion-fix brains overnight using acetic acid/formalin warmed to a carefully controlled 50 °C under pressure if accelerated fixation is urgently required.

1.4 Dissection of the Fetal/Perinatal Brain

Ideally, the brain should have been weighed in the unfixed state, although some neuropathologists also record fixed brain weight. The brainstem and cerebellum can be removed from the cerebrum by using a scalpel to cut through the midbrain perpendicular to the long axis of the brainstem, just caudal to the mammillary bodies. If necessary, the posterior fossa contents can be weighed separately to calculate the percentage of the total brain weight. The cerebral hemispheres can be sectioned in the coronal plane at 0.5–1 cm intervals, depending on the firmness of the brain. In very fragile specimens, as can be anticipated in hydrocephalus, sectioning and photography of the specimen under water are encouraged. The brainstem is sectioned axially at 0.3–0.5 cm intervals depending on firmness. The cerebellum may be sectioned axially together with the brainstem, or in a sagittal plane with the attached brainstem depending on the cerebellar pathology. In some pathologies (e.g. Dandy Walker type malformations) it may be desirable to section the brainstem and cerebellum sagittally, and submit one half for histological examination in the sagittal plane: saggital sectioning does impair examination of nuclear architecture, so if it is desired we suggest that the other half be blocked in axial sections. The cerebellum may also be detached from the brainstem, and cut perpendicular to the folia in slight wedges; this last approach is sometimes applied to more mature (e.g., closer to term gestation) brain. For histological examination we suggest that histology and immunohistochemistry be optimised for post-mortem fetal brain in particular: adult or even pediatric control slides may not be adequate. We have found that a general panel of useful immunohistochemical stains might include neurofilament, neurofilament light chain, nestin, GFAP, CD68, Collagen 4 (or another basal lamina stain), vimentin, synaptophysin, calretinin, myelin basic protein and amyloid beta A4 precursor protein are useful: the goal of immunohistochemistry is generally not to determine the phenotype of any given cell population, but to illustrate the structure and maturation of the tissue, and estimate the abundance and distribution of its various components. Other markers (e.g. Olig 2, SATB2, Sox-10, NeuN, alpha-beta crystallin) can occasionally be useful as well.

References

Barrett C, Brett F, Grehan D, McDermott MB. Heat-accelerated fixation and rapid dissection of the pediatric brain at autopsy: a pragmatic approach to the difficulties of organ retention. Pediatr Dev Pathol. 2004;7(6):595–600.

Cimmino A, Parisi G, Mastropasqua MG, Ricco R. Una nuova procedura per la fissazione ed estrazione dell'encefalo fetale. Pathologica. 2002;94(6):320–4.

Cohen MC, Scheimberg I. The pediatric and perinatal autopsy manual. Cambridge, MA: Cambridge University Press; 2014. p. 444.

Paradiso B, Simonato M, Thiene G, Lavezzi AM. From fix to fit into the autoptic human brains. Eur J Histochem. 2018;62(3):257–65.

van Dijk MC, Kornegoor R, Mol S, Rodriguez M. Fetal and perinatal brain autopsy: useful macroscopic techniques including agar in-situ and pre-embedding methods. Pediatr Dev Pathol. 2021;24(4):299–308. https://doi.org/10.1177/10935266211000036. Epub 2021 Mar 18.

Vasung L, Lepage C, Radoš M, Pletikos M, Goldman JS, Richiardi J, Raguž M, Fischi-Gómez E, Karama S, Huppi PS, Evans AC, Kostovic I. Quantitative and qualitative analysis of transient fetal compartments during prenatal human brain development. Front Neuroanat. 2016;10:11. https://doi.org/10.3389/fnana.2016.00011

2 Postmortem Examination of Perinatal Brain and Spinal Cord Malformations

The general goal of fetal necropsy of fetusal when CNS malformation is suspected is to confirm the radiologic impression of brain and/or spinal cord malformations as well as to detect any additional anomalies that could guide further parental counseling and genetic testing, if necessary. Parents may elect to terminate pregnancy based on neuroimaging observations of CNS malformation and associated prognosis or there may be fetal death. Postmortem examination in conjunction with cytogenetic and molecular analysis is then crucial to providing an accurate diagnosis that can be used to counsel parents regarding possible future pregnancies. Because of the impact on parental counseling, one of the most important things to do in the fetal necropsy is to rule out non-genetic or low recurrence risk malformations or disruption sequences. Similarly, if genetic variants of unknown significance are discovered, the autopsy can clarify their relevance.

2.1 Approach

The steps of brain and spinal cord removal and general rules of examination are explained in Chap. 1. A thorough review of the antenatal history and imaging reports is a crucial prerequisite of an accurate postmortem examination as the information obtained from the chart review can determine the specific approach to the autopsy that would prevent unnecessary disruption of the tissue that must be collected to confirm the antenatal diagnoses. Under optimal conditions, there is generally high concordance between postmortem neuropathological observations and neuroimaging findings, especially those of the fetal MRI (Griffiths et al. 2021). The closest correlation between radiological and autopsy findings seems to occur with neural tube defects (NTDs), as some believe ultrasonographic features of NTDs tend to be more obvious than other CNS anomalies (Carroll et al. 2000). Discrepancies between neuroimaging observations and neuropathological examination seem to more commonly involve suspected agenesis or hypoplasia of the corpus callosum, some cerebellar abnormalities (e.g., hypoplasia, Dandy–Walker malformation, vermian agenesis), and mild ventriculomegaly (Griffiths et al. 2021; Carroll et al. 2000). Discrepancies of major malformations such as holoprosencephaly have been described but tend to be rare (Carroll et al. 2000). Cystic lesions could represent another group of entities that may be difficult to confirm at autopsy due to autolysis and/or the difficulties in keeping a thin fragile cyst wall intact during removal from the skull. In these scenarios an experienced prosector and in situ photography are invaluable.

Optimizing conditions for accurate postmortem examination is paramount. This includes ensuring the method of termination is appropriate for the indication and preventing prolonged fetal retention that could result in autolysis and maceration. Potassium chloride administration for termination of pregnancy has been reported (Carroll et al. 2000) to accelerate autolysis. In instances where the likelihood of autolysis and maceration is high, there are a few ways neuropathologists or perinatal pathologists could try to mitigate tissue damage. One method is to immerse the fetus in 10% formalin as one would with surgical specimens. This can be applied to very premature and small fetuses that tend to undergo hospital burial (Das et al. 2022). One may also inject formalin through the anterior fontanelle or the occiput into the ventricles to better preserve the brain tissue. Even after the brain has undergone fixation, an autolyzed brain can fragment quite easily with handling: the relevance of underwater dissection is discussed in Chapter 1 (Griffiths et al. 2021). The goal is to be able to correlate antenatal imaging and genetic diagnosis with structural findings at a very high resolution, to maximise the clinical confidence in counselling.

In cases with posterior fossa malformations (e.g., Chiari, Dandy–Walker) and neural tube defects, it is important to remove the spinal cord using the posterior approach outlined in Chap. 1 and to examine the cord in situ where en bloc removal of the spinal column is not performed. Photographs of any abnormalities observed in situ are also advisable.

P. Shannon et al., *Atlas of Neurodevelopmental Pathology*, https://doi.org/10.1007/978-3-032-14148-4_2

After fixation, and depending on the context, the brainstem and cerebellum can be cut along the sagittal plane, especially if the cerebellar vermis needs to be evaluated (Encha-Razavi 2003) and/or further evidence of cerebellar herniation below the foramen magnum is required.

More details regarding approaches to specific malformations will be discussed in their respective chapters.

2.2 Postmortem Imaging

The possibility of performing postmortem MRI has been raised by multiple authors, and while results can be contributory, they are more helpful when used in conjunction with neuropathological examination rather than as a replacement (Thayyil et al. 2013; D'Hondt et al. 2017; Kang et al. 2017; Griffiths et al. 2003). Postmortem MRI would also presumably be limited by any autolysis and distortion of the brain tissue resulting from intrauterine demise (Griffiths et al. 2021). Resource-limited centers may also be constrained by the high costs of performing postmortem MRIs as a routine test in cases of suspected CNS malformations. Given that Izzo et al. (2019) reported a high concordance rate between intrauterine fetal MRI and postmortem MRI (Izzo et al. 2019), it might be difficult to rationalize the cost of the latter if the former has been already performed.

References

Carroll SG, Porter H, Abdel-Fattah S, et al. Correlation of prenatal ultrasound diagnosis and pathologic findings in fetal brain abnormalities. Ultrasound Obstet Gynecol. 2000;16(2):149–53.

D'Hondt A, D'Haene N, Rommens J, Cassart M, Avni EF. The contribution of mid-trimester virtual autopsy with MR imaging. Pediatr Radiol. 2017;47(suppl 2):S297–421.

Das RN, Mandal B, Das M, et al. Perinatal and fetal autopsies in neuropathology: how I do it. Indian J Pathol Microbiol. 2022;65(Supplement):S207–17.

Encha-Razavi F. Identification of brain malformations: neuropathological approach. Childs Nerv Syst. 2003;19(7–8):448–54.

Griffiths PD, Jarvis D, Mooney C, et al. Post-mortem confirmation of fetal brain abnormalities: challenges highlighted by the MERIDIAN cohort study. BJOG. 2021;128(7):1174–82.

Griffiths PD, Variend D, Evans M, Jones A, Wilkinson ID, Paley MNJ, et al. Postmortem MR imaging of the fetal and stillborn central nervous system. Am J Neuroradiol. 2003;24(1):22–7.

Izzo G, Talenti G, Falanga G, Moscatelli M, Conte G, Scola E, et al. Intrauterine fetal MR versus postmortem MR imaging after therapeutic termination of pregnancy: evaluation of the concordance in the detection of brain abnormalities at early gestational stage. Eur Radiol. 2019;29(6):2740–2.

Kang X, Cannie MM, Arthurs OJ, Segers V, Fourneau C, BevilacquaE, et al. Post-mortem whole-body magnetic resonance imaging of human fetuses: a comparison of 3-T vs. 1.5-T MR imaging with classical autopsy. Eur Radiol. 2017;27(8):3542–53.

Thayyil S, Sebire NJ, Chitty LS, the MARIAS collaborative group. Post-mortem MRI versus conventional autopsy in fetuses and children: a prospective validation study. Lancet. 2013;382(9888):223–33.

3 Neural Tube Defects

In this account, we will follow O'Rahilly and Müller (2006). The human embryology differs in some details from that observed in the mouse (Greene and Copp 2014), but the cellular details are assumed to be similar. In human gastrulation, the development of the primitive streak on the discoid epiblast proceeds in caudal–cranial directions. As the streak progresses, cells at the anterior limit form the primitive (Hensen's) node (Viebahn 2001). The epiblast cells migrate near and pass through the primitive streak, leading to the formation of the three germ cell layers (Ghimire et al. 2021; Müller and O'Rahilly 2004). Eventual ingression of the primitive streak results in the formation of notochord (Schauer and Heisenberg 2021; Eagles and Gupta 2020). The thickening of the embryonic ectoderm and the formation of the neural plate are induced by the future notochord and prechordal mesoderm, resulting in the overlying ectoderm differentiating into neural plate and surface ectoderm.

Neurulation is the formation of the neural tube from the neural plate. Primary neurulation begins with the formation, apposition, and fusion of the neural folds from the neural plate. The neural plate undergoes mediolateral narrowing and rostro-caudal lengthening; this convergent extension is required for the eventual closure of the neural tube (Copp et al. 2003). The cranial two-thirds of the neural plate and tube form the future brain, while the caudal third forms the future spinal cord (Munteanu et al. 2020). Near the end of the third week, the neural plate forms the neural groove, and the lateral edges elevate to form the neural folds; indentations in the neural plate provide the boundaries of primordia of the three primary brain vesicles—the prosencephalon, mesencephalon, and rhombencephalon. The neural folds then fuse in the midline: in humans, two sites of fusion occur initially—in the rhombencephalic region near the future craniocervical junction at stage 10 and in the prosencephalon at the rostral end of the forebrain at stage 11. Fusion proceeds caudally from the prosencephalic site and both cephalad and caudad from the rhombencephalic site, leading to the closure of the cranial neuropore at roughly day 25 during stage 11. The neural canal formed in the tube forms the future ventricular system and central canal of the spinal cord (Müller and O'Rahilly 2004; O'Rahilly and Müller 2006). The caudal neuropore closes about 2 days later (~day 27), after which the entire caudal embryo is covered with the ectoderm, but secondary neurulation, which generates neural elements and the central canal caudal to S2, continues thereafter until week 6 (O'Rahilly and Müller 2006) by recruitment of multipotent cell populations in the tail bud. After canalization, this extension forms a sacro-caudal neural tube whose lumen is continuous with the lumen of the primary neural tube (Copp and Greene 2010). Following primary neurulation, the neural tube is covered with ectoderm and mesoderm, and the normal dorsal soft tissue and bony elements are induced by participation of the neural tube. Neurogenesis and gliogenesis in the spinal cord proceed from the central neuroepithelium, while ingrowth of dorsal root ganglia axons forms the dorsal columns. Descending axonal tracts arrive at variable dates: bulbospinal tracts are mostly established by the end of the embryonic period in cervical levels, and corticospinal tracts, which innervate alpha motor neurons, extend to the lumbar cord by midgestation and distal sacral levels by term. After the embryonic period, spinal cord elongation is slower than vertebral column growth, so the conus relatively ascends to the level of the third lumbar vertebra by term (O'Rahilly and Müller 2006). Clearly, spinal cord and spinal column abnormalities may be linked. Spinal cord malformations as they relate to elements of the vertebral column are discussed in a subsequent chapter.

Conceptually, neural tube defects can be classified according to whether they are defects of primary neurulation, secondary neurulation, or post-neurulation (Greene and Copp 2014), and the various forms relate mostly to the severity and location of the defect in question. Defects of primary neurulation then will include open neural tube defects, such as craniorachischisis, anencephaly, iniencephaly, exencephaly, and open spina bifida (myelocele and myelomeningocele), and defects of secondary neurulation will include some caudal

P. Shannon et al., *Atlas of Neurodevelopmental Pathology*, https://doi.org/10.1007/978-3-032-14148-4_3

spina bifida such as what may accompany terminal myelocystocele and terminal lipoma. Post-neurulation defects will include defects of the overlying soft tissue and bone such as cranial encephaloceles (Fig. 3.1). A note of terminological caution is warranted however: not all instances of acalvaria or calvarial defects need to be primarily related to an intrinsic defect in neural tube development or in the expression of signaling elements by the neural tube (Fig. 3.2). Those lesions accompanying acalvaria in amnionic rupture sequence will be discussed in Chap. 13.

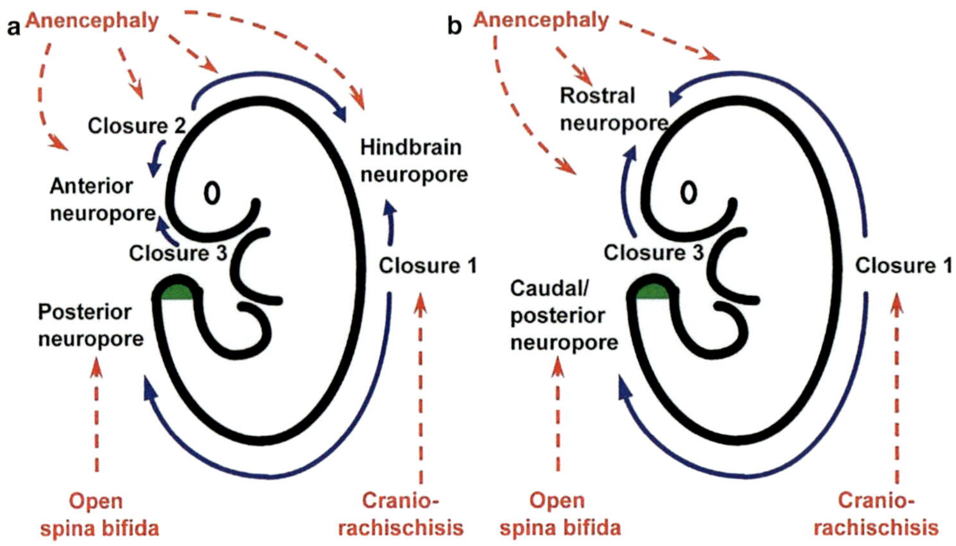

Fig. 3.1 Schematic of neural tube closure and the origin of NTDs in (A) mouse and (B) human embryos. Initiation events (closures 1, 2, and 3) and completion events (at "neuropores") are joined by unidirectional or bidirectional neural tube zippering (blue arrows). (From Copp and Greene (2010); with permission)

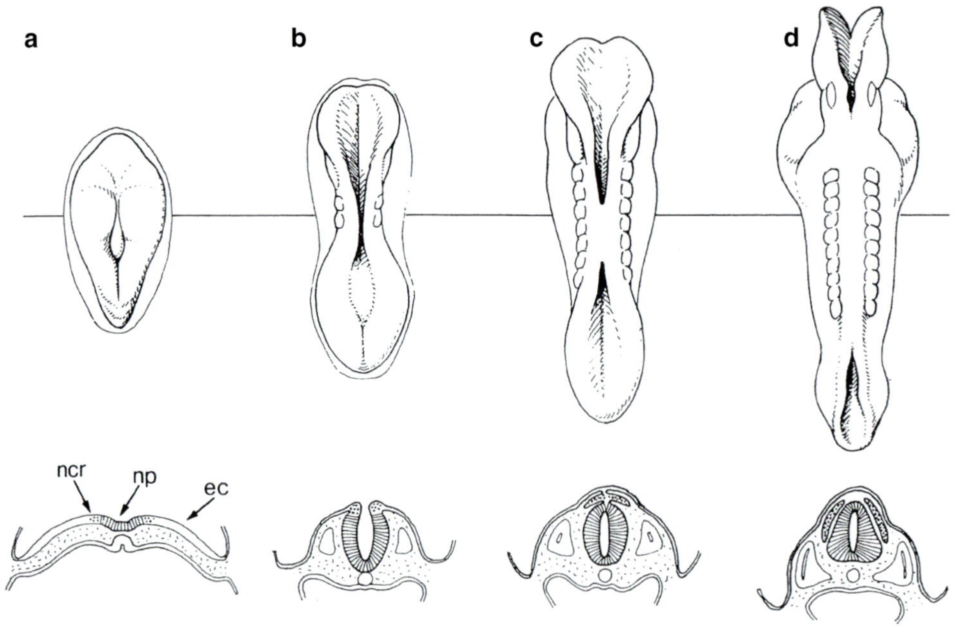

Fig. 3.2 The formation of the neural tube and neural crest. Dorsal views and transverse sections are shown for human embryos of CS 8a, CS 9b, CS 10c (seven somites), and CS 10d (ten somites). *ec* ectoderm, *ncr* neural crest, *np* neural plate. (From ten Donkelaar et al. (2023); with permission)

3.1 Exencephaly

In exencephaly, the cranial vault is generally severely hypoplastic or absent, and the brain consists of a variably organized mass sometimes partially covered with a thin membrane continuous laterally with the skin (Fig. 3.3a) often in association with a membranous defect exposing an unclosed portion of the neural tube directly to the amnionic fluid (Fig. 3.3b). Microscopically, the neural mass may contain recognizable cortical and subcortical neural elements (Fig. 3.3c), as well as choroid plexus, germinal elements, neuroepithelium, and ependymal or ependymoblastic

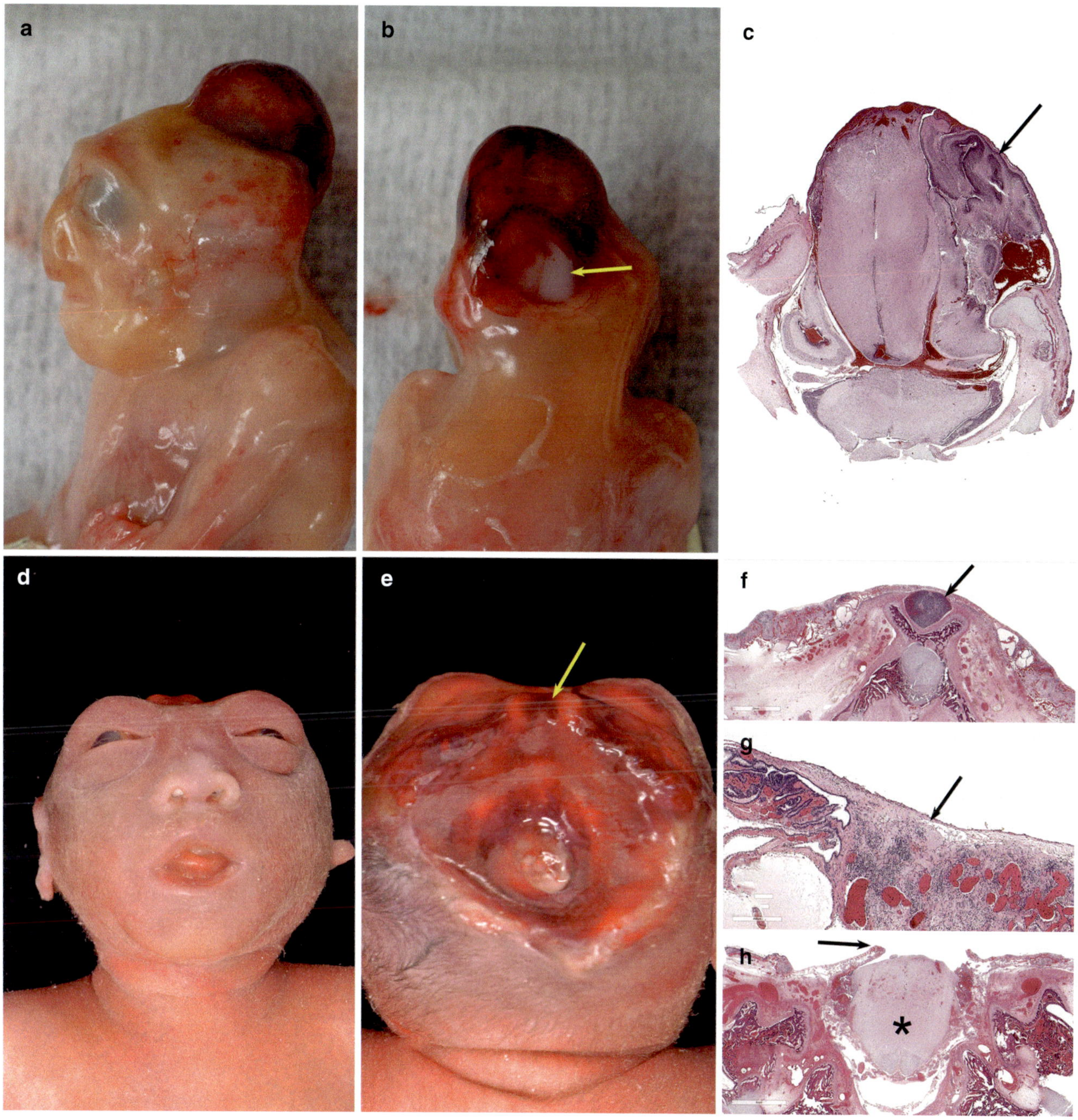

Fig. 3.3 (**a**) An 18-week-gestation fetus with absent cranial vault and exencephaly. The brain is almost entirely covered by transparent epithelialized membrane. (**b**) Posterior view demonstrating defect in membrane: the median sulcus of the fourth ventricle is visible through the defect. (**c**) The coronal section demonstrates organized brain tissue with some mechanical artifact: the major brain divisions are recognizable. (**d**) Anencephalic fetus, 24 weeks' gestation, demonstrating typical facies with absent calvarium and flat cranium. (**e**) Posterior view of **d**: the bulk of the defect is membrane covered, with effacement of the cranial fossae. The pituitary (arrow) is located in a sella, and on either side, the petrous ridges are present, and there is a membranous defect over the residual posterior fossa contents. (**f**) Section of **d** through pituitary (arrow): the brain is a flat plate on either side with cystic choroid plexus, and all is covered by epithelialized membrane. (**g**) Neural tissue and epithelialized membrane. (**h**) Section posteriorly, demonstrating the open portion of membranous covering over residual pons (asterisk): the tegmentum is disorganized

rosettes (Mittlebronn et al. 2008). Such specimens are generally best preserved in the early fetal period. By midgestation, secondary inflammatory and hemorrhagic changes may supervene, and by the early third trimester, the remaining neural elements may be limited to nests of germinal or neuroglial elements and choroid plexus, embedded in a hypervascular area covering the bony elements of the basicranium, i.e., the usual features of anencephaly with an area cerebrovasculosa (Lemire 1978). It should also be noted that intrapartum trauma to the exposed neural tissue can be very extensive, such that the residual cranial fossa is empty by the time it is received for neuropathologic examination, and the antepartum ultrasound impression of exencephaly cannot be directly confirmed. The posterior fossa is variably affected and usually hypoplastic; the cerebellum may be absent, and brainstem tegmental organization may be difficult to discern.

3.2 Anencephaly

In anencephaly, the calvarium is also severely hypoplastic or absent (Fig. 3.3d). The skull base is usually thick and flattened with shallow orbits and protruding eyes. The residual forebrain neural mass is minimal, which may be secondary to erosion and degeneration of a more prominent exencephalic mass (Wood and Smith 1984). In early gestational specimens however, the forebrain may be a disorganized open plate of neural precursors and choroid plexus variably open to the amniotic fluid and covered by a thin epithelialized membrane (Fig. 3.3e). The sella may be shallow, and the pituitary may be difficult to identify (Fig. 3.3f). The forebrain is usually replaced by an area cerebrovasculosa, which is composed of dilated thin-walled blood vessels, disorganized glial and neuronal elements, and choroid plexus, which may be strikingly cystic (Fig. 3.3g). An organized pons and cerebellum may be present, hypoplastic, or absent. Usually, the brainstem is simplified (Fig. 3.3h), and there is aplasia of corticofugal tracts. Anencephaly may also accompany partial or complete failure of the spinal neural tube to close as well (see below). The portion of the disorganized, flat neural plate connected by an epithelialized membrane is variable. In some specimens, it is a caudal opening just rostral to the neural canal (Fig. 3.1h). In others, it is almost directly over what would be the cranial axis (Fig. 3.4a, b). The area cerebrovasculosa can demonstrate frond-like masses, composed histologically of herniating choroid plexus and dilated blood vessel (Fig. 3.4d, e), but by term is usually flat and irregular, with only small nodules of neural tissues and substantial choroid plexus cysts (Fig. 3.4f, g).

Early experimental studies suggest that anencephaly can arise from foci of necrosis near the anterior neuropore (Smith and Huntington 1981). The etiopathogenesis of human neural tube defects in general is considered multifactorial (Greene and Copp 2014). Maternal folate supplementation reduces but does not eliminate the incidence, and non-genetic factors (pregestational diabetes, anti-seizure medications) are well-known risk factors. At the time of writing, OMIM records showed over 20 genetic loci associated with human anencephaly, with more linked to other severe neural tube defects or anencephaly in mice, suggesting that the list is incomplete. Occasional associations include genes linked to other well-characterized central nervous system diseases such as holoprosencephaly (e.g., ZIC2 (Dubourg et al. 2004)) or cobblestone lissencephaly (FCMD (Toda et al. 1995)), suggesting that the phenotype represents a tissue-level outcome for severe neurodevelopmental compromise with a variety of bases in cellular pathophysiology. Cytogenetic associations include trisomy 18 (Karaman et al. 2015) and del22q11.2 (Pers. Obs. PS). Anencephaly has been linked to alterations in numerous genes including MTHFR, NUAK2, TRIM36, GUBS, FOXN1, TMEM216, CC2D2A, RPGRIP1L, B3GNT1, KIF7, PDGFRA, VANGL1 and VANGL2, PAX3, CELSR1, AMT, PARD3, GLDC, SHROOM3, and PCMT1 genes (Yaliwal and Desai 2012; Bonnard et al. 2020; Singh et al. 2017; Hughes et al. 2020; Amorosi et al. 2008; Valente et al. 2010; Tallila et al. 2008; Delous et al. 2007; Shaheen et al. 2013; Putoux et al. 2011; Deshwar et al. 2020; Wang et al. 2013).

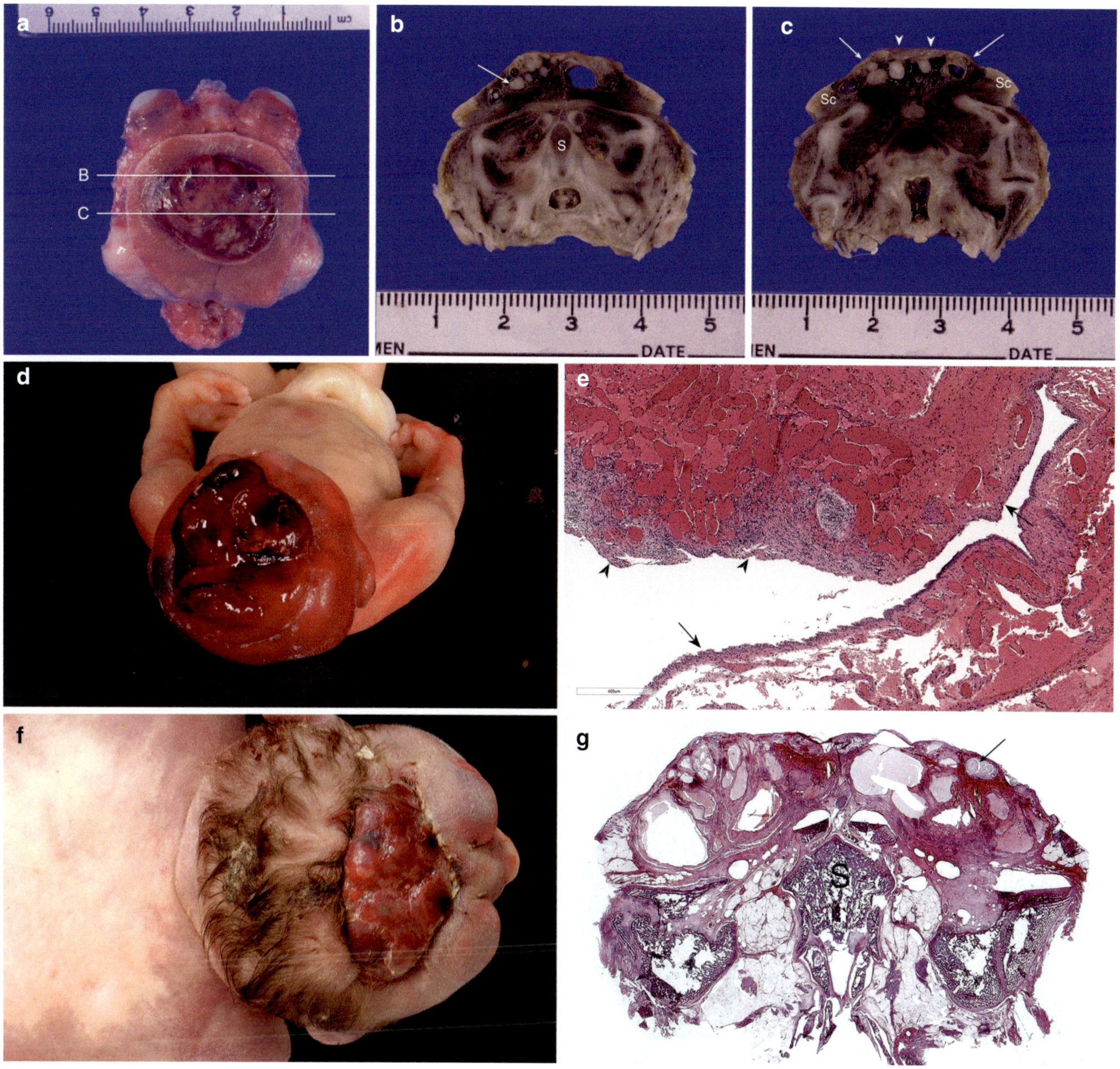

Fig. 3.4 (**a**) Superior aspect of anencephalic cranium, 21 weeks' gestation, with site of neural tube defect taken out with the surrounding skin, showing levels of coronal sections illustrated in **b** and **c**. (**b**) Epithelialized membrane covers multiple round pale nodules of disorganized brain tissue (arrow) and cystically dilated choroid plexus. "S" marks the rostral sphenoid. (**c**) Section posterior to (**b**), with central non-membrane-covered area (arrowheads) surrounded by zone of epithelialized membrane (arrows) and scalp (Sc). The pituitary is present in the midline. (**d**) Unusually exuberant area cerebrovasculosa in a 20-week-gestation fetus composed almost completely of dilated blood vessels and choroid plexus. The similarity between this morphology and that seen in some encephaloceles (see Fig. 3.6g, h below) is obvious. (**e**) Section from the lateral aspect of the area demonstrating transition from thin epithelialized membrane (arrows) to congested, non-epithelialized mass with scant neural elements and dilated thin-walled vessels. (**f**) Anencephaly at 39 weeks' gestation. The entire area cerebrovasculosa is epithelialized in this case. (**g**) The same case as (**f**): the coronal section demonstrates small nodules of brain tissue (arrows), and the large cysts are lined with choroid plexus-type epithelium. S marks the anterior sphenoid

3.3 Iniencephaly

Iniencephaly is a neural tube defect involving the craniocervical junction in which there is fixed retroflexion of the head. It has three major features (Dogan et al. 1996):

1. Occipital bone defect with an enlargement of the foramen magnum.
2. Partial or total absence of cervical vertebrae.
3. Fetal retroflexion.

In our experience, it often accompanies a rostral open neural tube defect such as exencephaly (Fig. 3.5a) or large encephalocele, but this is not invariable. There are four types: (1) isolated iniencephaly, (2) iniencephaly with encephalocele, (3) iniencephaly with spina bifida (Fig. 3.5b, c), and (4)

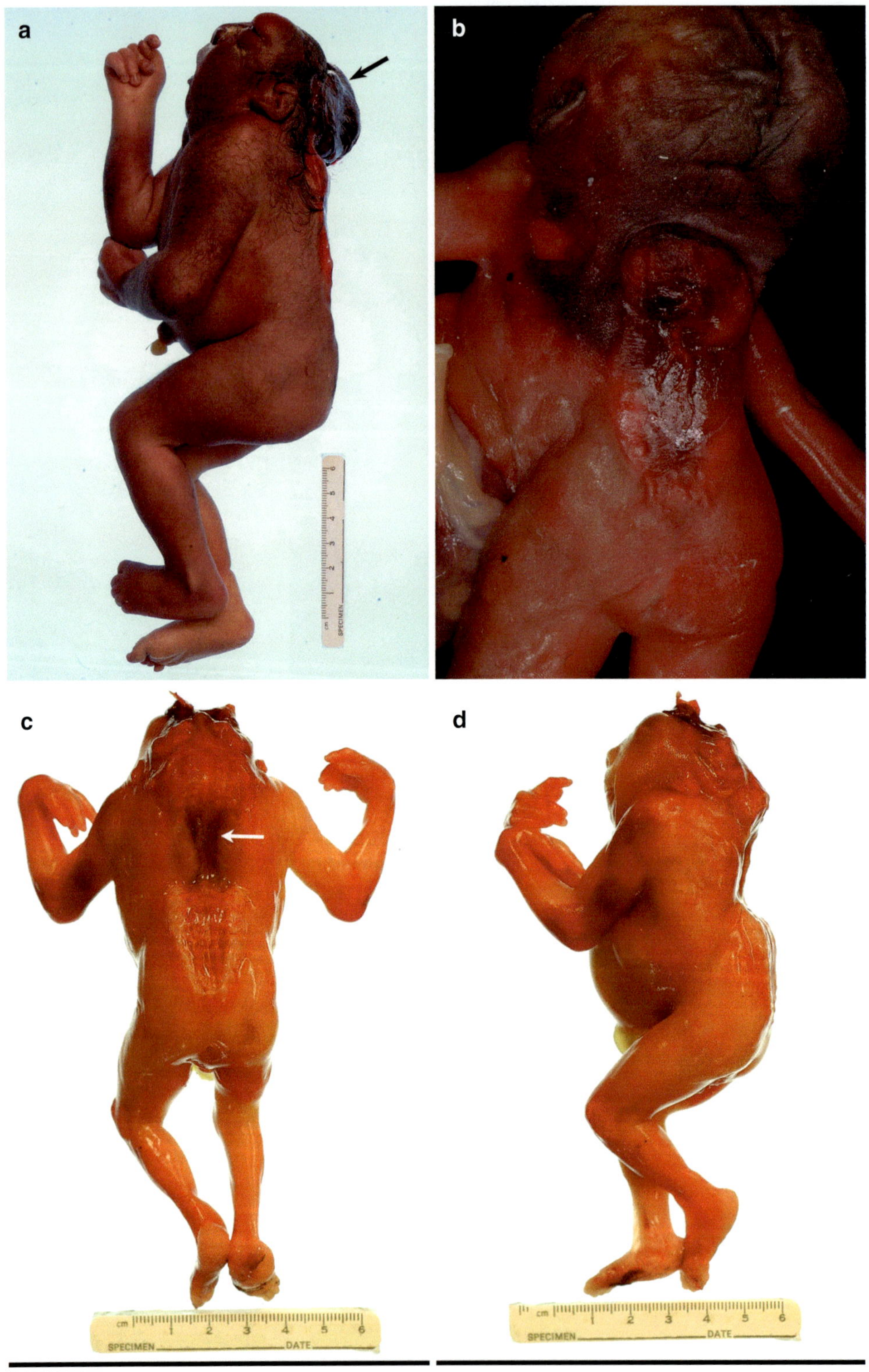

Fig. 3.5 (**a**) Iniencephaly with exencephaly (arrow) and spina bifida. (**b**) Iniencephaly in trisomy 18 with cervicothoracic spina bifida. (**c**, **d**) Anencephaly with rachischisis: the cervical spine is fixed in retroflexion. Myeloschisis (arrow) is apparent in the opened neural groove

iniencephaly with encephalocele and spina bifida (Moore et al. 1997). Iniencephaly may be associated with anencephaly, lissencephaly, holoprosencephaly, a flattened and broad medulla, cerebellar hypoplasia, and hyperextended cervical spinal cord (Saldarriaga et al. 2014); an enlarged cervical canal, segmentation errors of the cervical and thoracic spine, spinal rachischisis (see below), and myelomeningocele (Holmes et al. 2018); and duplications of the central canal of the spinal cord (Scherrer et al. 1992). The pathogenesis of the cervical abnormality is unclear but may involve an arrest of embryonic physiological retroflexion that should occur in the third week of gestation (Moore 1982).

In common with anencephaly, iniencephaly is conceived of as a neural tube defect and shares a multifactorial etiopathogenesis. Environmental risk factors include low socioeconomic level, low parity, folic acid deficiency, obesity, and drugs such as sulfonamides, tetracyclines, and antitumoral agents. It has been recorded in trisomy 18, trisomy 13, monosomy X, partial monosomy 6p, and partial trisomy 11q (Tanriverdi et al. 2015; Chen 2007) and a single report of MTHFR mutation (Balci et al. 2001).

3.4 Encephalocele

An encephalocele is the herniation of the brain tissue during development through a bony defect in the skull. The large majority of these in our population are occipital (Fig. 3.6a, b), but they can be frontal, parietal, temporal, or ethmoid. Occipital encephaloceles are often connected by a narrow neck to the underlying central nervous system and contain distorted brain tissue and are covered with skin. The impression given is that of the brain drawn into and entrapped within the encephalocele by pressure differentials; the contained tissue often demonstrates extensive secondary change, with gliosis, infarction, and old hemorrhage, and often with choroid plexus as the only recognizably organized tissue—unusual histologic findings of dilated vascular sinusoids or collagen intermixed with ependyma may result (Wang et al. 2021). Occasionally, one encounters an encephalocele externally covered by an epithelialized membrane overlying the occiput (Fig. 3.6c, d). After ruling out amnionic rupture sequence, terming such a malformation an occipital encephalocele or a variant of exencephaly is possibly a matter of preference; the key feature is that the underlying brain is not degraded by trauma or inflammation.

Cranial meningoceles contain herniated leptomeninges, but no brain elements (Fig. 3.6e, f). Occasionally, a clinically identified occipital meningocele will contain choroid plexus but no other brain tissue; this finding is usually associated with apparent traction-related distortion of the cerebellum or a Joubert malformation of the cerebellum and brainstem. Apparently, closed encephaloceles may sometimes demonstrate small openings in communication with the ventricles of the developing brain. These are demonstrable by careful sectioning of the encephalocele, which may demonstrate nodules of neural tissue intermixed with vernix and an inflammatory response (Fig. 3.6g, h).

Frontonasal encephaloceles are similar in many respects to occipital encephaloceles and may exhibit dramatic traction effects on their intracranial components (Fig. 3.6a, b). Vertex encephaloceles seem to be heterogeneous. Occasionally, they can be seen in association with amnionic rupture sequence; the site of amnionic adherence to the scalp may be minute and requires careful search to identify. We have encountered a closed encephalocele where the underlying brain clearly herniated through a bony defect, but the involved cortical mantle was replaced by a dramatic transmantle neuronal migration abnormality (Fig. 3.6d–f).

Frontoethmoidal encephaloceles may be similarly complex. Although some appear to be local defects without obvious pervasive malformations of development (Fig. 3.7g, h), we have encountered similar encephaloceles associated with extensive basal prosencephalic disorganization and containing brain with heterotopic retinal tissue.

The central nervous system malformations associated with encephaloceles are very numerous. The remaining intracranial brain may show extensive secondary change as well as primary abnormalities such as type 2 lissencephaly, polymicrogyria, Joubert syndrome, micrencephaly, pachygyria, leptomeningeal and subcortical heterotopias, ventriculomegaly, cerebellar atrophy (Inan et al. 2018), Chiari malformation, Dandy–Walker malformation, agenesis of the corpus callosum, holoprosencephaly, arhinencephaly, neuronal migration disorders, abnormal confluens sinuum, and falcine venous sinus (Weichert et al. 2017; Thompson 2009), which have all been encountered.

Clinical syndromic associations are similarly numerous and certainly beyond the scope of a brief chapter, but important associations include the Meckel–Gruber syndrome, which as originally delineated includes occipital encephalocele, renal cystic dysplasia, and hepatic fibrosis and often includes polydactyly. Currently, 14 different genetic syndromes are denoted as Meckel syndrome (MKS) in OMIM (Meckel syndrome types 1–14), though several are single-family associations, and MKS 7 and MKS 12 have not been associated with occipital encephaloceles, but instead are associated with the Dandy–Walker syndrome and complex intracranial abnormalities, respectively. Other important and associations include Walker–Warburg syndrome and the Goldenhar syndrome (facial or hemifacial microsomia).

The number of genetic abnormalities associated with encephaloceles is also very large. At the time of writing, more than 100 genes have been associated with encephalocele formation in humans; many are associated with other types of neural tube defects as well, but others are most

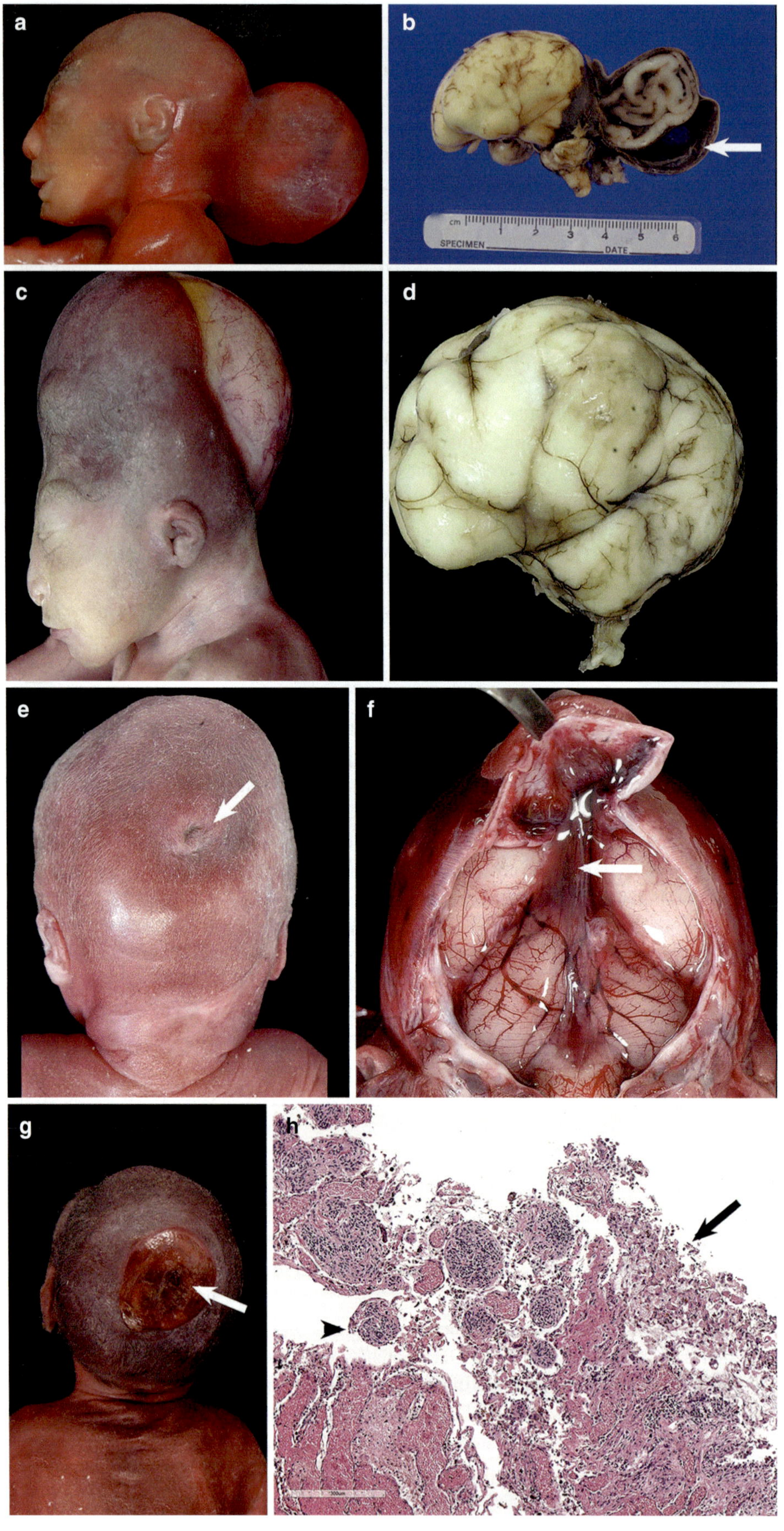

Fig. 3.6 (**a**) A large otherwise isolated occipital encephalocele, entirely covered by hair scalp. Note that the remainder of the cranial vault is hypoplastic. (**b**) The same case as (**a**). The encephalocele and occipital bone have been removed with the brain and cut sagittally, demonstrating a convoluted and curled cortical mantle with contained ventricular space herniating into the sac. A large fluid space forms part of the encephalocele as well (arrow). (**c**) A large encephalocele covered by transparent epithelialized membrane; the entire posterior occipital bone is absent, so one might call this partial acalvaria or exencephaly. (**d**) Brain in the same case as in **c**. There is little degenerative injury. The brain showed aqueduct and third ventricular fusion, but as is typical of cases with aqueduct occlusion and large encephalocele, no hydrocephalus. (**e**) Occipital meningocele marked externally only by a small redundancy of the skin. (**f**) Leptomeninges and choroid plexus extending into and trapped inside meningocele (arrow). (**g**) Occipital encephalocele with thin glabrous membranous covering and central irregularity (arrow). (**h**) Section of the central portion of the occipital encephalocele in (**g**) demonstrating innumerable small nodules of neural tissue as well as vernix with reaction (arrow). Vernix was also present in the lateral ventricles of the brain

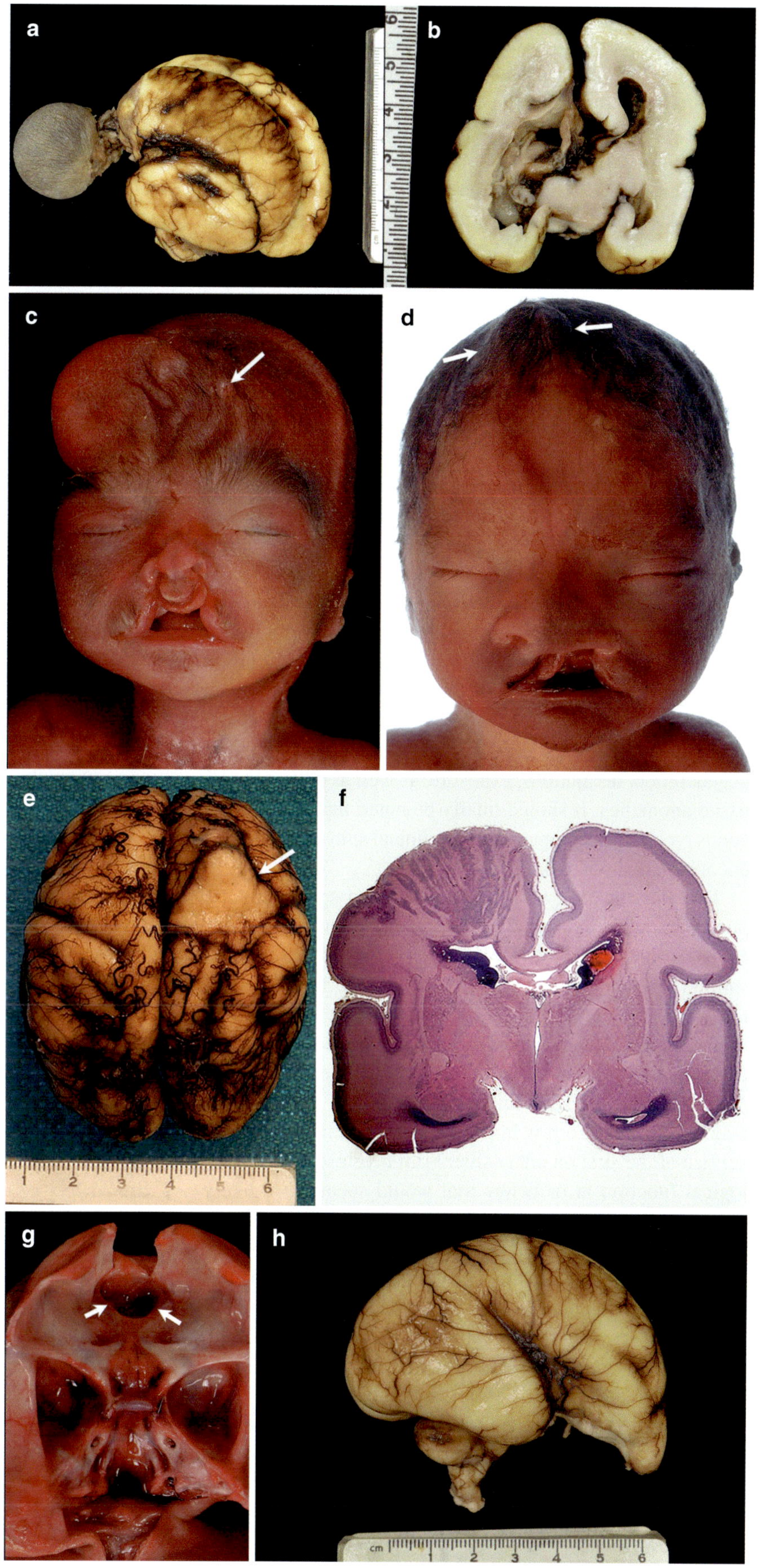

Fig. 3.7 (**a**) A narrow necked frontonasal encephalocele, covered with skin and hair, with narrow necked pedicel predominantly attached to the left cerebral hemisphere and markedly smaller left cerebral hemisphere than right. (**b**) The same case as (**a**) with left ventriculomegaly, distortion, and numerous periventricular heterotopias. The impression is that traction effects have caused disruption to the left. (**c**) Right frontal encephalocele associated with facial clefts and hypertelorism in the case with typical amputations of amnionic rupture sequence. A small point of adhesion of amnion is only obvious with careful search. (**d**) Right frontal encephalocele (arrows) with broad base associated with cleft lip and palate and hypertelorism but otherwise no anomalies. (**e**) The same case as **d** with hypovascular, abnormal brain contained subjacent to the encephalocele. (**f**) The same case as **d**, whole mounted with a convexity migration disorder extending the full thickness of the cerebral mantle. (**g**) Large defect in the cribriform plate at the site of encephalocele herniation. (**h**) In this case, the encephalocele is entirely covered by leptomeninges and mostly demonstrates mechanical distortion in the underlying brain

strongly associated with craniosynostosis or skeletal dysplasias (e.g., Li et al. 2009; Arikawa-Hirasawa 2001), indicating that the defect may not be in the neural tube or its signaling apparatus itself. Similarly, congenital cranial defects in the bone and soft tissue such as those encountered in amnionic rupture sequence or dyssegmental dysplasia (Rieubland et al. 2010; Shannon 2020) may reflect acquired or intrinsic defects in the formation of the tissues being induced, rather than in the development or function of the neural tube per se.

3.5 Spinal Dysraphism

Spinal dysraphism describes various degrees and types of failure of the spinal neural tube to close and/or induce dorsal mesenchymal elements appropriately. In all dysraphisms, the spinous processes of the vertebrae fail to arch medially to form a complete dorsal arch, i.e., spina bifida. The resulting defect in the neural arch may be covered over by skin and soft tissue (a closed defect: spina bifida occulta) or form part of a communication between the central canal of the neural tube and the amnionic space (an open defect: spina bifida aperta); the array of cord pathologies associated with spina bifida mostly reflect the size, location, and severity of the defect of closure, as well as changes resulting from neural degeneration, herniations, exposure, as well as bone and soft tissue anomalies. It should finally be noted that a low-lying conus typically accompanies most clinical spinal dysraphism encountered at postmortem.

The classification of anomalies in open spina bifida is poorly standardized in the literature, with conflicting clinical and pathological terminology. According to one classification (Schindelmann et al. 2021), which we generally use, the defects are classified according to the most severe defect in neurulation and dorsal induction encountered. In myeloschisis, some portion of the spinal cord is opened as a flat plate (Fig. 3.8a, b), and the ependyma of the central canal extends laterally, so it is in topographic continuity with the surface of the skin on either side. With myeloschisis, neurological function at or below that would seem more likely disturbed than that with a closed neural tube, as the chance for in utero or intrapartum injury would seem to be elevated. In a myelomeningocele, the herniation entails both meninges and a closed spinal cord (Fig. 3.8c, d), and in a meningocele, only the dorsal meningeal elements herniate through the defect (Fig. 3.8d, e). In our practice, we routinely embed the entire spinal column for examination in cases of clinically identified neural tube defects or Chiari malformations (see later), and myeloschisis at some level is overwhelmingly the most common morphology, possibly related to sampling intensity (Schindelmann et al. 2021).

According to other usages, the distinction between myelomeningocele and myelocele is that in a myelomeningocele, the herniated elements (cord and leptomeninges) are raised above the level of the skin, whereas in a myelocele, the herniated neural elements are at or below the level of the skin (Tortori-Donati et al. 2000; Ben-Sira et al. 2013), and myeloschisis can presumably accompany either. Given that postmortem/ex utero fluid shifts can cause an apparent deflation of the membranous elements seen on imaging, the distinction at fetal autopsy may be difficult to assert, although redundancy of the skin and membranes at the defect is suggestive.

Rachischisis is generally an open neural tube (i.e., myeloschisis) with spina bifida extending the length of the vertebral column; when associated with anencephaly, it is described as craniorachischisis and is ascribed to a total failure of neurulation and may be due to a failure of convergent extension in the neural tube (Lesko et al. 2021); it has also been described with exencephaly (Guerrero et al. 2021). With prolonged exposure to amnionic fluid and with the trauma of labor and delivery, there is often a marked destruction of the exposed residual neural tissue (Limaiem and Dimassi 2022). In rachischisis or with any spina bifida extending over many vertebral levels there is often a lumbosacral kyphosis immediately caudal to a very sharp lordosis at or near the thoracolumbar junction, and the column may show segmentation anomalies and scoliosis.

3.5.1 Closed Spina Bifida

In closed spina bifida, the abnormality may be apparent only radiologically, or there may be an overlying swelling, cyst or subcutaneous lipoma. If there is a herniating component, it may be a lipoma admixed with meningeal elements (lipomeningocele), a dorsal dural sac (meningocele), or a swelling of the spinal cord, caused by a dilated extension of the central canal (myelocystocele). In myelocystocele the dorsal lining of the cyst may be ependymal elements applied directly to the subdermal or dermal fibrous tissue.

Spinal meningoceles (Fig. 3.8e, f) are usually sacral or lumbosacral and can be present as a subcutaneous mass or a patch of hirsute skin or be grossly occult. They may accompany a variety of anomalies, including Chiari malformations, abnormalities in cerebral gyration, holoprosencephaly, anencephaly, microcephaly, hydrocephalus, hemispheric arachnoid cysts, encephaloceles, agenesis/hypogenesis/dysgenesis of the corpus callosum, heterotopias, aneurysms, arteriovenous fistulas, Dandy–Walker malformation, Joubert syndrome, brainstem and/or cerebellar anomalies (e.g., dysplasia, aplasia), hippocampal anomalies (e.g., intracranial lipoma), cerebral hypogenesis, wide midbrain

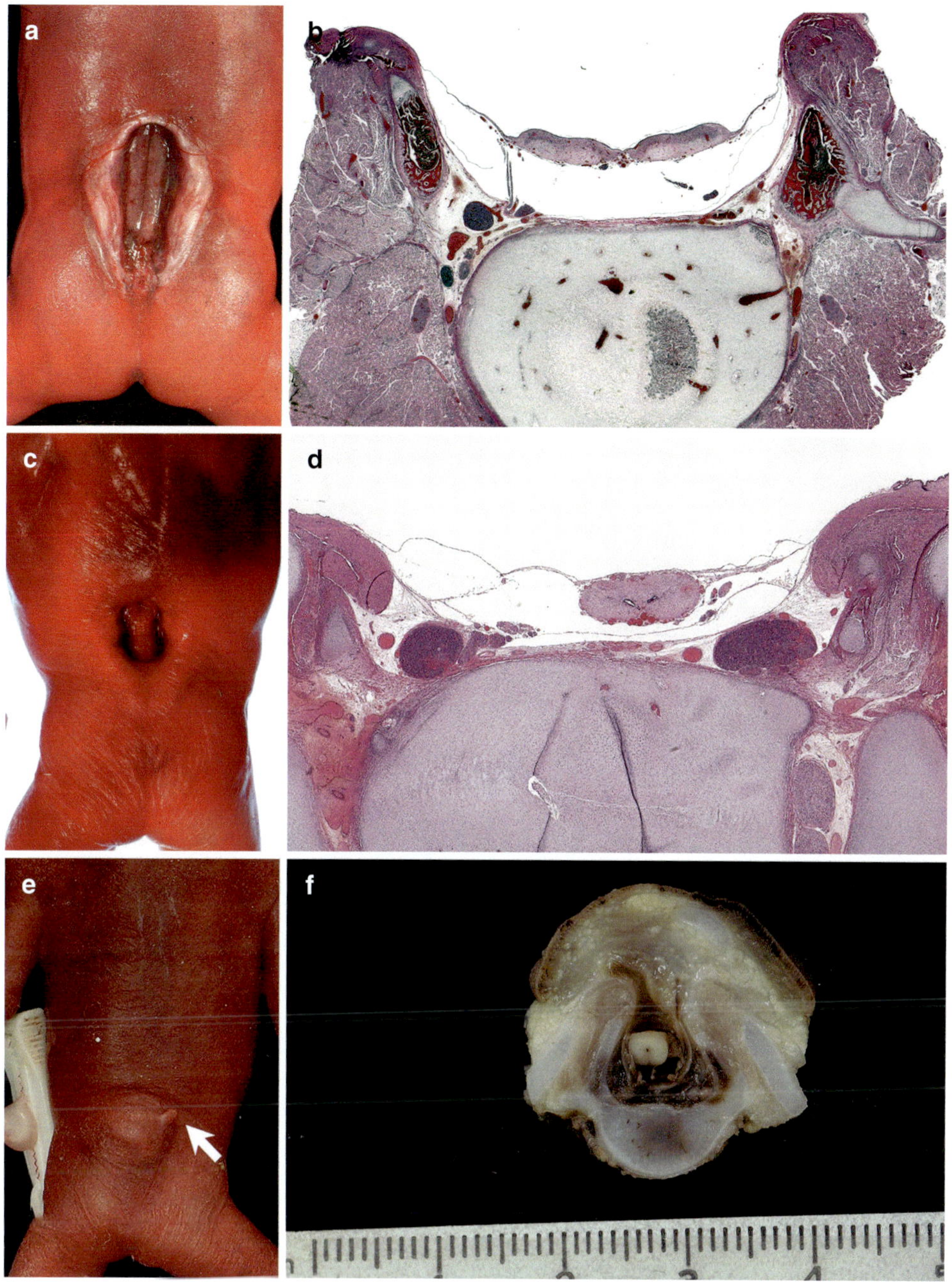

Fig. 3.8 (**a**) Myeloschisis. A large lumbosacral open defect is present, in the base of which is a clearly visible ribbon of the neural tube. (**b**) Myeloschisis. On sectioning, the cord is opened like a book, and the dorsal elements are in continuity, via fine epithelialized lateral extensions, with the skin laterally (Masson Trichrome). (**c**) Myelomeningocele. In this defect, an intact spinal cord is the herniating element: rostrally, one can see the initial stages of diplomyelia. (**d**) Similar case as (**c**), with myelomeningocele and a duplicated neural canal. (**e**) Closed neural tube defect, with meningocele marked by a lumbosacral swelling and a small cutaneous appendage (arrow). (**f**) The same case as **e** demonstrating dorsally herniating dura and arachnoid and early accumulation of dorsal subcutaneous fat

incisura, and cervicomedullary deformities (Paschereit et al. 2022; Rhodes 2020; Morais et al. 2020; Kawamura et al. 2001), although the risk of intracranial anomaly is far lower with closed than with open neural tube defects (Paschereit et al. 2022).

In a myelocystocele, the central canal of the spinal cord is variably and sometimes massively dilated. The dorsal aspect may be reduced to an ependymal lining applied directly to the dermis or subcutaneous fibrous tissue of the overlying skin (Fig. 3.9a, b). The ventral aspect of the cord is flattened and splayed dorsally in a manner reminiscent of myeloschisis, but instead of the lateral elements extending onto a membrane so that they are topographically continuous with the skin (as they do in myeloschisis), the lateral elements meet each other dorsally to surround a large subcutaneous cystic space. Usually, the caudal neural tube is involved (Fig. 3.9c–e). The cyst may be externally occult or present at autopsy as a massive, fluctuant presacral cutaneous mass, especially in the context of OEIS (omphalocele, exstrophy, imperforate anus, and sacral anomalies). Occasionally, a large myelocystocele may extend over many spinal levels in association with a Chiari malformation (Fig. 3.9f, g).

Secondary effects may be prominent in either open or closed neural tube defects. Infarction, gliosis, or hemorrhage

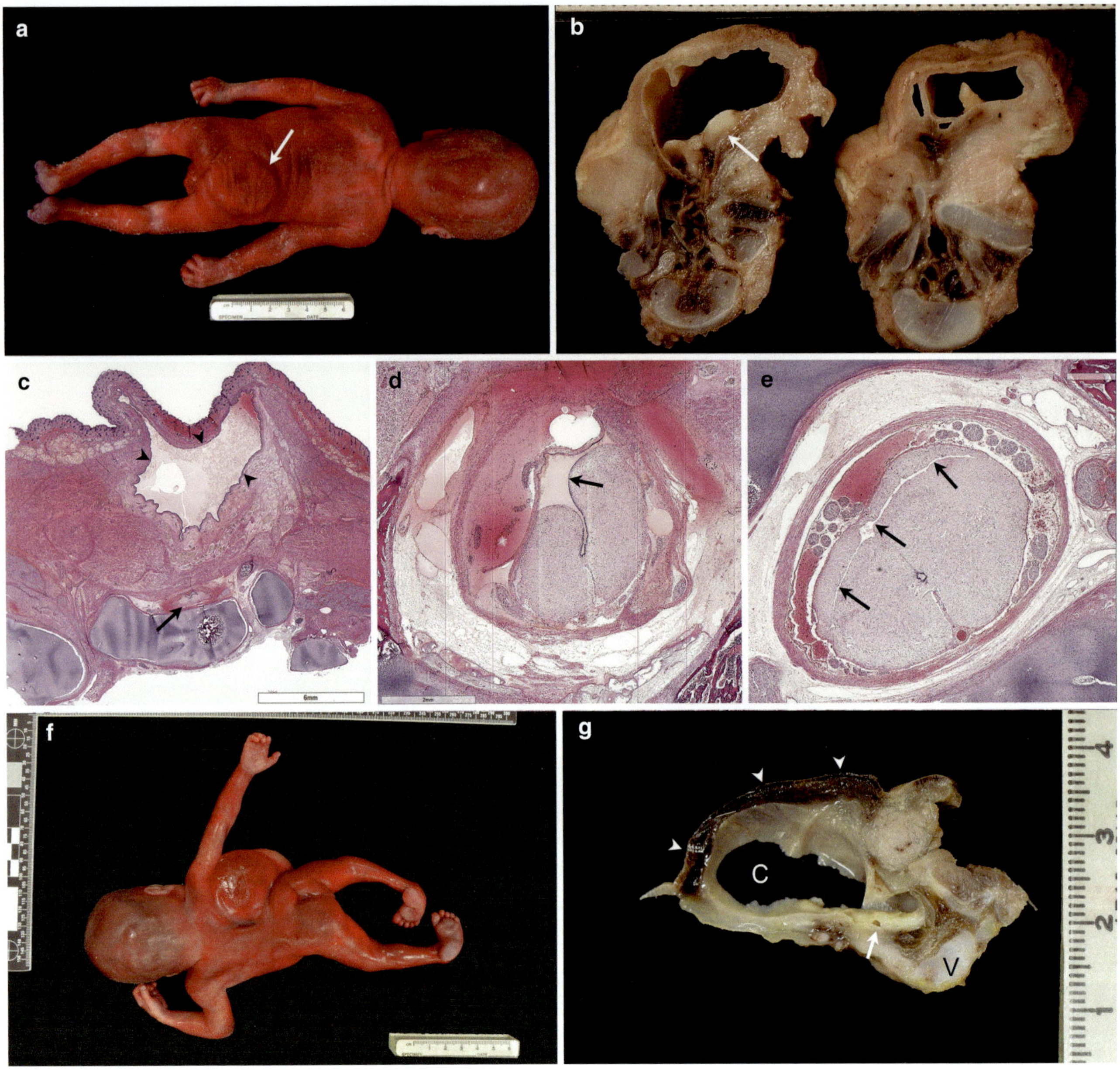

Fig. 3.9 (**a**) A 22-week-gestation fetus with OEIS, demonstrating large fluctuant soft tissue mass (arrow). (**b**) Sectioning of the spine with the attached skin demonstrates massive cystic space, the ventral aspect of which contains the spinal cord in an open-book configuration, similar to that of myeloschisis. (**c**) Similar case demonstrating massive subcutaneous cyst lined by ependyma (arrowheads). A low-lying sacral conus is present. (**d**) More rostrally, the cyst is in continuity with a dorsal cyst in the lumbar cord, lined by ependyma and clearly in continuity with the central canal. (**e**) Cervical cord from the same case as (**c**), demonstrating a slit-like space within the cord (arrow); this can be traced over multiple levels to be continuous with the cyst in (**c**) and (**d**). (**f**) A large dorsolateral myelocystocele in midgestation fetus with a Chiari type 2 malformation. (**g**) A cut through the spinal column and overlying skin (arrowheads) demonstrates a massive cyst ("c") lined by ependyma and originating from a flat opened spinal cord (arrow) that is rotated in the neural canal: "V" is a vertebral body, and there is a wide spina bifida

may occur at or near the site of herniation (Guo et al. 2014), even apart from the effects of parturition. In open neural tube defects, the amnionic vernix caseosa may access the subarachnoid space in utero (Jacobs et al. 1961) and incite a granulomatous reaction (Fig. 3.10a–d). Particularly if there is myeloschisis or a large myelocystocele, irregular syringes may extend from the cyst or central canal. These syringes are often paramedian but may branch irregularly and are sometimes lined by attenuated ependyma even when they are at a considerable distance from the central canal. Fetal syringomyelia may extend along the entire length of the cord and into the brainstem. In myeloschisis, these syringes are often

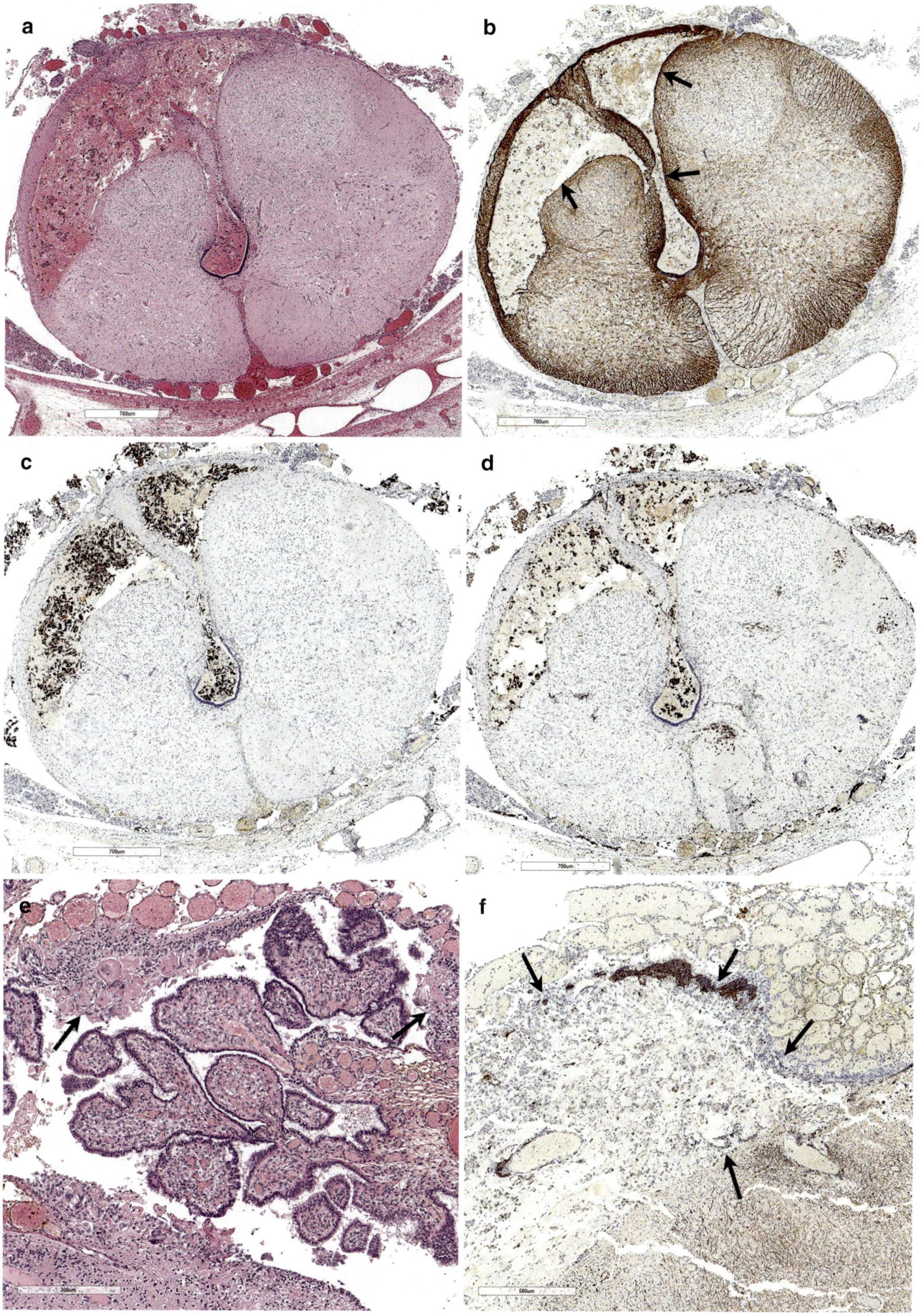

Fig. 3.10 (**a**) Cervical spinal cord of a 23-week-gestation fetus with Chiari malformation and a large myelocele with myeloschisis. At first glance, the irregular cavity may appear artifactual. (**b**) Immunohistochemistry demonstrates a thin wall lined by dense glial processes. (**c**) Immunohistochemistry for high molecular weight cytokeratin demonstrates amnionic squames in the cavity and in the subarachnoid space. (**d**) Immunohistochemistry for CD68 demonstrates a brisk reaction to the squames, as well as small aggregates within the spinal cord, suggesting injury and reaction. (**e**) Fourth ventricular choroid plexus, similar case, with brisk histiocytic reaction to amnionic squames (arrow). (**f**) The same case as **e**. Subpial dissection of vernix into lateral cerebellum, with reactive glial response (arrows, immunohistochemistry for glial fibrillary acidic protein)

accompanied by vernix (vernicomyelia) and an associated inflammatory reaction, which occasionally can reach the posterior fossa (Fig. 3.10e, f) and rarely the supratentorium. In general, fetal syringomyelia is accompanied by hydromyelia and hypoplasia of the dorsal embryonic cord, and it seems likely that the size and shape of the syrinx are affected by secondary injury as well as by the course of ascending and descending axonal tracts as they grow within the walls of the syringes (see Guo et al. (2014) for a review).

3.5.2 Lipomyelomeningocele and Lipomyelocele

In lipomyelocele and lipomeningocele, the lipomatous tissue forms part of the tissue herniating from the neural canal; this has been proposed to be a defect of secondary neurulation, with failure of the caudal neural tube to separate from the adjacent mesenchymal mass and subsequent abnormal proliferation (Greene and Copp 2014). The lipomatous tissue is generally mature adipose tissue that may be in lobules and containing brown fat, fibrous bands or tracts, peripheral nerve, skeletal or smooth muscle, or cartilage and bone (Rhodes 2020) (see Chap. 10).

References

Amorosi S, D'Armiento M, Calcagno G, Russo I, Adriani M, Christiano AM, Weiner L, Brissette JL, Pignata C. FOXN1 homozygous mutation associated with anencephaly and severe neural tube defect in human athymic Nude/SCID fetus. Clin Genet. 2008;73:380–4. [PubMed: 18339010, related citations] [Full Text].

Arikawa-Hirasawa E, Wilcox WR, Le AH, Silverman N, Govindraj P, Hassell JR, Yamada Y. Dyssegmental dysplasia, Silverman-Handmaker type, is caused by functional null mutations of the perlecan gene. Nature Genet. 2001;27:431–434.

Balci S, Aypar E, Altinok G, et al. Prenatal diagnosis in three cases of iniencephaly with unusual postmortem findings. Prenat Diagn. 2001;21(7):558–62.

Ben-Sira L, Garel C, Malinger G, et al. Prenatal diagnosis of spinal dysraphism. Childs Nerv Syst. 2013;29(9):1541–52.

Bonnard C, Navaratnam N, Ghosh K, Chan PW, Tan TT, Pomp O, Ng AYJ, Tohari S, Changede R, Carling D, Venkatesh B, Altunoglu U, Kayserili H, Reversade B. A loss-of-function NUAK2 mutation in humans causes anencephaly due to impaired Hippo-YAP signaling. J Exp Med. 2020;217:e20191561.

Chen CP. Prenatal diagnosis of iniencephaly. Taiwan J Obstet Gynecol. 2007;46(3):199–208.

Copp AJ, Greene ND, Murdoch JN. Dishevelled: linking convergent extension with neural tube closure. Trends Neurosci. 2003;26(9):453–5.

Copp AJ, Greene ND. Genetics and development of neural tube defects. J Pathol. 2010;220(2):217–30. https://doi.org/10.1002/path.2643. PMID: 19918803; PMCID: PMC4239538.

Delous M, Baala L, Salomon R, Laclef C, Vierkotten J, Tory K, et al. The ciliary gene RPGRIP1L is mutated in cerebello-oculo-renal syndrome (Joubert syndrome type B) and Meckel syndrome. Nat Genet. 2007;39:875–81. [PubMed: 17558409, related citations] [Full Text].

Deshwar AR, Martin N, Shannon P, Chitayat D. A homozygous pathogenic variant in SHROOM3 associated with anencephaly and cleft lip and palate. Clin Genet. 2020;98(3):299–302. https://doi.org/10.1111/cge.13804. Epub 2020 Aug 3.

Dogan MM, Ekici E, Yapar EG, et al. Iniencephaly: sonographic-pathologic correlation of 19 cases. J Perinat Med. 1996;24(5): 501–11.

Dubourg C, Lazaro L, Pasquier L, Bendavid C, Blayau M, Le Duff F, Durou M-R, Odent S, David V. Molecular screening of SHH, ZIC2, SIX3, and TGIF genes in patients with features of holoprosencephaly spectrum: mutation review and genotype-phenotype correlations. Hum Mutat. 2004;24:43–51.

Duckworth T, Sharrard WJ, Lister J, Seymour N. Hemimyelocele. Dev Med Child Neurol. 1968;Suppl 16:69+.

Eagles ME, Gupta N. Embryology of spinal dysraphism and its relationship to surgical treatment. Can J Neurol Sci. 2020;47:746.

Ghimire S, Mantziou V, Moris N, Martinez AA. Human gastrulation: the embryo and its models. Dev Biol. 2021;474:100–8. https://doi.org/10.1016/j.ydbio.2021.01.006. Epub 2021 Jan 20.

Greene NDE, Copp AJ. Neural tube defects. Annu Rev Neurosci. 2014;37:221–42.

Guerrero J, Heller DS, de Leon AB. Craniorachischisis with exencephaly. Fetal Pediatr Pathol. 2021;40(5):501–4.

Guo A, Chitayat D, Blaser S, Keating S, Shannon P. 2014 fetal syringomyelia. Acta Neuropathol Commun. 2014;6(2):91.

Holmes LB, Toufaily MH, Westgate MN. Iniencephaly. Birth Defects Res. 2018;110(2):128–33.

Hughes JJ, Alkhunaizi E, Kruszka P, Pyle LC, Grange DK, Berger SI, et al. Loss-of-function variants in PPP1R12A: from isolated sex reversal to holoprosencephaly spectrum and urogenital anomalies. Am J Hum Genet. 2020;106:121–8. [PubMed: 31883643, related citations] [Full Text].

Inan C, Cenk Sayin N, et al. A large posterior encephalocele associated with severe ventriculomegaly, cerebellar atrophy and transposition of the great arteries. J Clin Ultrasound. 2018;46(9):588–90.

Jacobs EB, Landing BH, Thomas W. Vernicomyelia. Its bearing on theories of genesis of the Arnold-Chiari complex. Am J Pathol. 1961;39:345–53.

Karaman A, Aydin H, Göksu K. Concomitant omphalocele, anencephaly and arthrogryposis associated with trisomy 18. Genet Couns. 2015;26(1):77–9.

Kawamura T, Morioka T, Nishio S, et al. Cerebral abnormalities in lumbosacral neural tube closure defect: MR imaging evaluation. Childs Nerv Syst. 2001;17(7):405–10.

Lemire RJ. Anencephaly. New York: Raven Press; 1978.

Lesko AC, Keller R, Chen P, Sutherland A. Scribble mutation disrupts convergent extension and apical constriction during mammalian neural tube closure. Dev Biol. 2021;478:59–75.

Limaiem F, Dimassi K. Rare and severe neural tube defect: craniorachischisis totalis. Clin Case Rep. 2022;10(3):e05606.

Li C, Mernagh J, Bourgeois J. Novel craniofacial and extracraniofacial findings in a case of Treacher Collins syndrome with a pathogenic mutation and a missense variant in the TCOF1 gene. Clin Dysmorph. 2009;18:63–8.

Mittlebronn M, Wolburg H, Kendziorra H, et al. Ependymoblastomatous exencephaly: a unique fetal malformation. Pediatr Dev Pathol. 2008;11:397–401.

Moore CA, Li S, Li Z, et al. Elevated rates of severe neural tube defects in a high-prevalence area in northern China. Am J Med Genet. 1997;73(2):113–8.

Moore KL. The developing clinically oriented embryology. 3rd ed. Philadelphia: WB Saunders; 1982.

Morais BA, Solla DJF, Yamaki VN, et al. Brain abnormalities in myelomeningocele patients. Childs Nerv Syst. 2020;36(7):1507–13.

Müller F, O'Rahilly R. The primitive streak, the caudal eminence and related structures in staged human embryos. Cells Tissues Organs. 2004;177:2–20.

Müller F, O'Rahilly R. The embryonic human brain: an atlas of developmental stages. 3rd ed. Wiley; 2006.

Munteanu O, Cirstoiu MM, Filipoiu FM, et al. The etiopathogenic and morphological spectrum of anencephaly: a comprehensive review of literature. Romanian J Morphol Embryol. 2020;61(2):335–43.

Paschereit F, Schindelmann KH, Hummel M, et al. Cerebral abnormalities in spina bifida: a neuropathological study. Pediatr Dev Pathol. 2022;25(2):107–23.

Putoux A, Thomas S, Coene KL, Davis EE, Alanay Y, Ogur G, et al. KIF7 mutations cause fetal hydrolethalus and acrocallosal syndromes. Nat Genet. 2011;43:601–6. [PubMed: 21552264, images, related citations] [Full Text].

Rhodes RH. Congenital spinal lipomatous malformations. Part 1. Spinal lipomas, lipomyeloceles, and Lipomyelomeningoceles. Fetal Pediatr Pathol. 2020;39(3):194–245.

Rieubland C, Jacquemont S, Mittaz L, Osterheld MC, Vial Y, Superti-Furga A, et al. Phenotypic and molecular characterization of a novel case of dyssegmental dysplasia, Silverman-Handmaker type. Eur J Med Genet. 2010;53(5):294–8. https://doi.org/10.1016/j.ejmg.2010.06.005. Epub 2010 Jun 11.

Saldarriaga W, De Lourido CI, Murcia FA. Two iniencephaly cases born the same day in the same hospital of Cali, Colombia. Iniencephaly cluster? BMJ Case Rep. 2014;2014:bcr2014203933.

Schauer A, Heisenberg C. Reassembling gastrulation. Dev Biol. 2021;474:71–81.

Scherrer CC, Hammer F, Schinzel A, Briner J. Brain stem and cervical cord dysraphic lesions in iniencephaly. Pediatr Pathol. 1992;12(3):469–76.

Schindelmann KH, Paschereit F, Steege A, Stoltenburg-Didinger G, Kaindl AM. Systematic classification of spina bifida. J Neuropathol Exp Neurol. 2021;80(4):294–305.

Shaheen R, Faqeih E, Ansari S, Alkuraya FS. A truncating mutation in B3GNT1 causes severe Walker-Warburg syndrome. Neurogenetics. 2013;14:243–5. [PubMed: 23877401, related citations] [Full Text].

Shannon P. Central nervous system pathology in the amniotic rupture sequence. Clin Neuropathol. 2020;39(6):288–99. https://doi.org/10.5414/NP301266.

Singh N, Kumble Bhat V, Tiwari a, Kodaganur SG, Tontanahal SJ, Sarda A, Malini KV, Kumar A. A homozygous mutation in TRIM36 causes autosomal recessive anencephaly in an Indian family. Hum Mol Genet. 2017;26:1104–14. [PubMed: 28087737, related citations] [Full Text].

Smith MT, Huntington HW. Morphogenesis of experimental anencephaly. J Neuropathol Exp Neurol. 1981;40(1):20–31.

Tallila J, Jakkula E, Peltonen L, Salonen R, Kestila M. Identification of CC2D2A as a Meckel syndrome gene adds an important piece to the ciliopathy puzzle. Am J Hum Genet. 2008;82:1361–7. [PubMed: 18513680, images, related citations] [Full Text].

Tanriverdi EC, Delibas IB, Kamalak Z, Kamalak Z, Kadioglu BG, Bender RA. A fetus with iniencephaly delivered at the third trimester. Case Rep Med. 2015;2015:520715.

ten Donkelaar, HJ, Takakuwa T, Vasun L, Yamada S, Shiota K, vander Vliet T. Overview of the development of the human brain and spinal cord. In: ten Donkelaar HT, Lammens M, Hori A. Clinical neuroembryology development and developmental disorders of the central nervous system 3rd Cham. Springer; 2023. p 17

Thompson DN. Postnatal management and outcome for neural tube defects including spina bifida and encephalocoeles. Prenat Diagn. 2009;29(4):412–9.

Toda T, Yoshioka M, Nakahori Y, Kanazawa I, Nakamura Y, Nakagome Y. Genetic identity of Fukuyama-type congenital muscular dystrophy and Walker-Warburg syndrome. Ann Neurol. 1995;37:99–101.

Tortori-Donati P, Rossi A, Cama A. Spinal dysraphism: a review of neuroradiological features with embryological correlations and proposal for a new classification. Neuroradiology. 2000;42:471–91.

Valente EM, Logan CV, Mougou-Zerelli S, Lee JH, Silhavy JL, Brancati F, Iannicelli M, Travaglini L, Romani S, Illi B, Adams M, Szymanska K, et al. Mutations in TMEM216 perturb ciliogenesis and cause Joubert, Meckel and related syndromes. Nat Genet. 2010;42:619–25.

Viebahn C. Henson's node. Genesis. 2001;29(2):96–103.

Wang C, Zhu J, Zeng Y, et al. A rare case report of Encephalocele with numerous ependymal components: A potential diagnostic pitfall. Int J Surg Pathol. 2021;29(1):85–9.

Wang F, Wang J, Guo J, Chen X, Guan Z, Zhao H, Xie H, Liu C, Bao Y, Zou J, Niu B, Zhang T. PCMT1 gene polymorphisms, maternal folate metabolism, and neural tube defects: a case-control study in a population with relatively low folate intake. Genes Nutr. 2013;8(6):581–7.

Weichert J, Hoellen F, Krapp M, et al. Fetal cephaloceles: prenatal diagnosis and course of pregnancy in 65 consecutive cases. Arch Gynecol Obstet. 2017;296(3):455.

Wood LR, Smith MT. Generation of anencephaly: 1. Aberrant neurulation and 2. Conversion of exencephaly to anencephaly. J Neuropathol Exp Neurol. 1984;43(6):620–33.

Yaliwal LV, Desai RM. Methylenetetrahydrofolate reductase mutations, a genetic cause for familial recurrent neural tube defects. Indian J Hum Genet. 2012;18(1):122–4.

4 Malformations and Disruptions of the Cerebral Hemispheres

By stage 15, the telencephalic vesicle has given rise to two distinct swellings, and the telencephalic third ventricle is evident. The basal aspect is formed by the subpallium, which gives rise to medial and lateral ganglionic eminences; these ganglionic eminences are specialized proliferative masses, which give rise to neuronal and glial precursors and which give rise to the basal ganglia and amygdala. The dorsal pallium gives rise to the six-layered neocortex. Dorsally and on the medial aspect of the telencephalic hemisphere are the medial pallium and the adjacent cortical hem at the junction with the choroidal fold. These give rise to the hippocampal cortex and parts of the adjacent cingulate and entorhinal cortex.

The isocortex starts with proliferative neuroepithelium lining the telencephalic vesicles. By 6.5 weeks post conception, a superficial, less cellular preplate has formed, containing neurons arising by radial and tangential migration, as well as Cajal–Retzius neurons (see below) (Rakic and Zecevic 2003). The neuroepithelium gives rise to neuronal precursors, which migrate radially toward the external surface of the vesicle. By 8.5 weeks, the preplate has been replaced by a layered cortical mantle comprising a marginal zone, the cortical plate that will contain the bodies of future cortical neurons, a less cellular subplate containing early maturing subplate neurons, an intermediate zone of migrating cells and cell fibers, and a thickening ventricular zone. Bridging the cortical mantle are radial glial cells, which are a cytologically transient population of glia, many of which extend from the ventricular zone to the superficial pia limitans and classically act as guides to the migration of neuronal precursors. Also, populations of radial glia with cell bodies in the ventricular zone and the subventricular zone arise that are a major source of isocortical neuronal precursors (Hansen et al. 2010). Many differentiate into astrocytes by the late third trimester (deAzevedo et al. 2003).

The marginal zone contains Cajal–Retzius neurons, which initially arise from the cortical hem (Causeret et al. 2021) and secrete reelin, an extracellular protein that serves as a stopping signal for migrating neurons. The marginal zone will form the molecular layer of the cortex and also contains a transient subpial granular cell layer. The subpial granular cell layer originates initially from the basal periolfactory neuroepithelium at roughly 9 weeks post fertilization, spreads to cover the entire cerebral hemisphere by 12 weeks post fertilization, and eventually disappears near 30 weeks. This transient layer appears to serve as a source of the Cajal–Retzius cells in the mature brain and a network of small granular cell neurons that may function as a guide or regulator of cortical interneuron migration (Meyer and González-Gómez 2018).

The neurons of the isocortex arise in the ventricular zone and reach the cortical plate by either radial migration from the neuroepithelium or tangential migration. Radial migration is achieved by the asymmetrical division of ventricular zone elements, differentiation into migrating elements, and migration from the ventricular zone into the developing cortical plate using radial glia as guides, in an inside-out fashion, such that the earliest arriving populations eventually form the deepest cell layer. In contrast, the majority of cortical GABAergic interneurons form from the germinal eminences (clinically the germinal matrices) and migrate to the isocortex in a tangential fashion or via a ventral and rostral stream (Alzu'bi et al. 2017). Radial migration peaks around 22 weeks and tapers off sharply by the beginning of the third trimester. Tangential migration, on the other hand, possibly continues into postnatal life, albeit at a low level. The germinal matrices by midgestation eventually form massive C-shaped structures on the lateral walls of the lateral ventricles extending from the recesses of the frontal horns around to the lateral and superior walls of the temporal horns. These begin to deplete near the beginning of the third trimester, in a caudal to rostral pattern.

Subjacent to the cortical plate is the transient subplate, which is a thick layer containing early maturing neurons, which form extensive circuits involved in guiding cortical and thalamic projecting axons. This layer expands from the eight post-conception week, and the subcortical circuitry

P. Shannon et al., *Atlas of Neurodevelopmental Pathology*, https://doi.org/10.1007/978-3-032-14148-4_4

persists into early infancy. Between the subplate and the proliferative elements is the intermediate zone, which contains complex developing layers of axons along with migrating and differentiating cells. The layering of the intermediate zone varies regionally (Altman and Bayer 2002). In contrast to the isocortex, the hippocampal formations start as medial and dorsal structures adjacent to the cortical hem but grow caudally and then ventrally and rostrally to project anteriorly and ventrally as the medial temporal lobes, bringing the temporal horn of the lateral ventricle with them. As a result, rudiments of the supracommissural hippocampal formation can be found on the dorsal and medial aspect of the corpus callosum (i.e. the indusium griseum).

The median wall of the telencephalon rostral to the chiasmatic plate forms the lamina terminalis, which at 5 weeks post conception partially thickens to become the commissural plate; inferiorly, this develops into the site of the anterior commissure and superiorly into the site of the corpus callosum and posteriorly the hippocampal commissure.

The cerebral hemispheres massively enlarge throughout fetal life and obtain their distinctive patterns of cortical folding by means of local differentiation of tissue elements and relative growth. In general, one refers to a fissure as a fold in the cerebrum that involves the full thickness of the mantle. Hence, the interhemispheric, Sylvian, and parieto-occipital fissures relate to a folding of the entire cortical mantle, while the sulci and gyri refer to the convoluted surface of the mantle. Sulcation seems to arise through differential cortical growth, with regions of cortical tangential expansion and thickening coupled with biomechanical differences between the cortical plate and underlying structures. Primary and secondary gyration is complete by term, but tertiary gyration continues into the postnatal period (Llinares-Benadero and Borrell 2019; de Vareilles et al. 2023).

Clearly, the marked growth, the prolonged development, and the architectural complexity and diversity required for normal brain function require an elaborate developmental apparatus. The corresponding array of maldevelopmental conditions is similarly complex. A variety of rubrics for classifying and interpreting anomalies have been developed, usually with some attention to the age and phase of the developmental stage thought to be impaired in the genesis of the abnormalities. For the purposes of illustration, however, we will take a simplified structural approach.

4.1 Ventriculomegaly

Severe congenital ventriculomegaly is often caused by cerebrospinal fluid outflow obstruction, whether by fusion or obstructive lesions of the third ventricle, aqueductal stenosis, or fourth ventricular outflow abnormalities (see cerebellar and brainstem malformations). In the supratentorium, obstructive ventriculomegaly is marked by dilations of ventricular spaces upstream of the obstruction and is accompanied in fetal life by thinning of the cortical mantle, polygyria, septal perforation, and often an apparent fusion and/or descent of the forniceal tracts (Fig. 4.1a). There may be an unrolling of the hippocampal formation (Fig. 4.1b) such that the alveus of CA1, which normally becomes opposed to the ventricular zone of the future parahippocampal gyrus and medial temporal isocortex, is maintained separate from them and in a relatively vertical orientation. This feature is common to both obstructive and post-encephaloclastic ventriculomegaly (Fig. 4.1c, d) of early onset. This is not to be conflated with hippocampal dysplasia (Fig. 4.1d, e) where cytoarchitectural progression is absent or abnormal (also see Chap. 5). Ventriculomegaly is frequently accompanied by nodular germinal matrix excrescences and periventricular neuronal heterotopias in the ventricular lining (see below). Because fetal ventriculomegaly may also accompany conditions with impaired formation, degeneration, or injury to components of the developing cerebral mantle, it should not be the sole basis on which an interpretation of obstructive hydrocephalus rests (Fig. 4.1f).

Ventricular compression and collapse are common in the presence of a cranial encephalocele with entrapment of large parts of the cerebrum; the remaining intracranial brain is

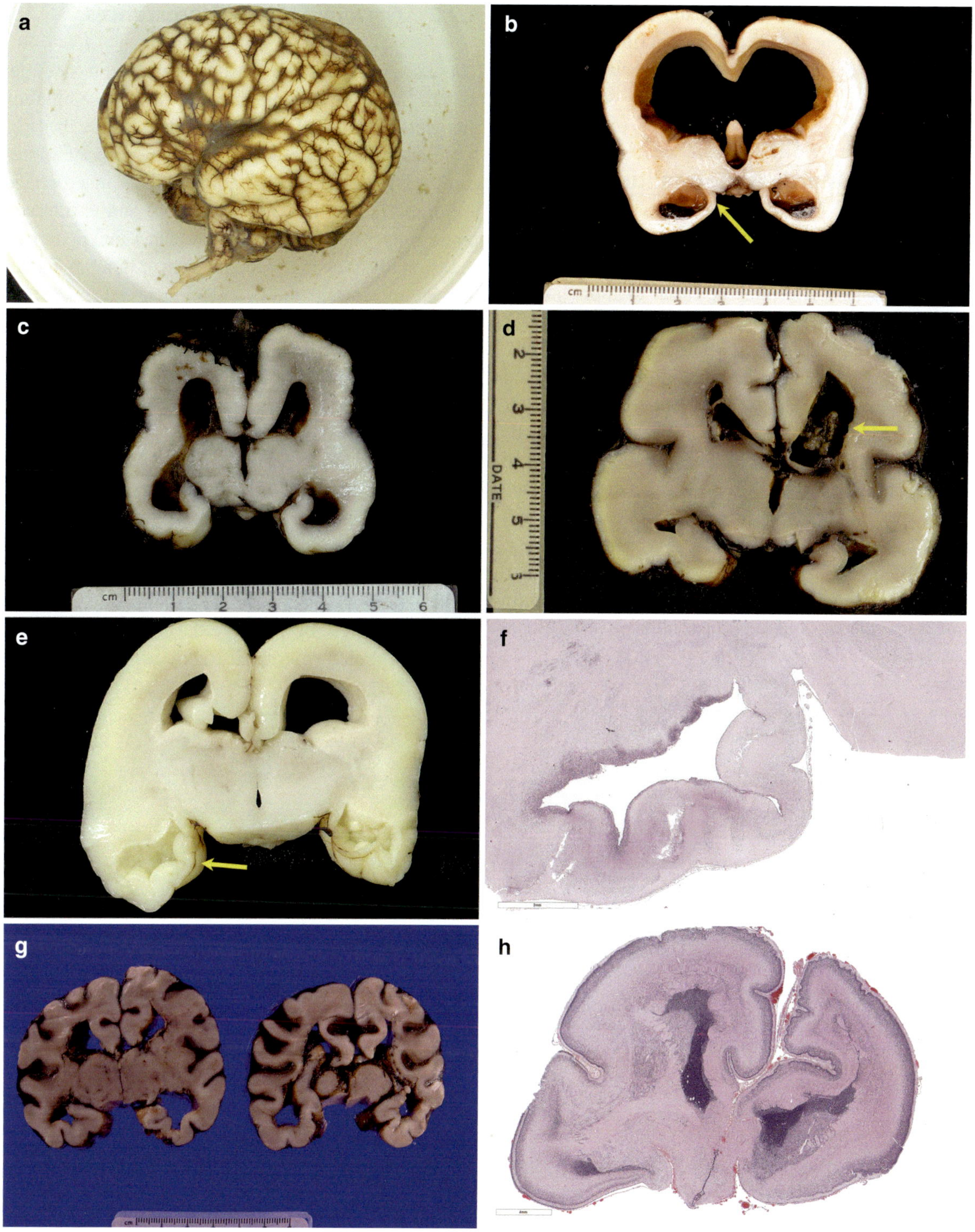

Fig. 4.1 Ventriculomegaly and ventricular collapse. (**a**) Polygyria in a 32-week-gestation fetus with hydrocephalus secondary to rhombencephalosynapsis and aqueductal stenosis. (**b**) Hydrocephalus in a 23 week gestation fetus secondary to rhombencephalosynapsis and aqueductal stenosis. Note the fusion of fornices and the absent septal leaflets. The hippocampal formations are dramatically unrolled and thinned (arrow). (**c**) Roughly symmetrical ventriculomegaly in the context of severe cytomegalovirus infection, with thinned cortical mantle and irregular cortical surface—a 30-week-gestation female. (**d**) Asymmetrical ventriculomegaly accompanying an old right-sided germinal matrix hemorrhage (arrow) with local infarction—a 28-week-gestation male. Note that the ipsilateral temporal horn is also dilated, and there is third ventricular dilation; these changes were accompanied by post-hemorrhagic aqueductal and fourth ventricular obstruction. (**e**) Ventriculomegaly of unclear origin in a short-rib polydactyly syndrome (20 weeks). Note that the temporal horns are dilated and irregular (arrow). (**f**) Whole mount of temporal lobe from (**e**) demonstrating undulating unrolled hippocampal formation. (**g**) Ventriculomegaly in a 32-week-gestation female accompanied by thinned cerebral mantle and exaggerated cortical folds and agenesis of the corpus callosum. Note the third ventricle is of normal size. This was attributed to a failure of cortical white matter development. (**h**) A 22-week-gestation male, in this case there is a with vertex encephalocele (not shown) that incorporates most of both occipital and parietal lobes and there is a hypoplastic right temporal lobe. Note that the lateral ventricles in this plane of section are almost completely fused, possibly due to the chronic alterations in cerebrospinal fluid production and circulation secondary to entrapment and destruction of the ventricular trigones and lateral ventricular choroid plexus

often collapsed with irregular slit-like and even fused lateral and third ventricles (Fig. 4.1g). Massive gyriform heterotopias can also be associated with ipsilateral ventricular obliteration (see below).

4.2 Germinal Matrix Abnormalities

4.2.1 Germinal Matrix Cysts

Small germinal matrix cysts may be easier to appreciate on ultrasound than at fetal autopsy, possibly because of the common postmortem fluid shifts, but may accompany a very wide variety of conditions, including chromosomal and metabolic disorders (Fig. 4.2a, b), rubella or cytomegalovirus infection (Fig. 4.2c), aqueductal stenosis (Fig. 4.2d), tubulinopathies (see below), and accelerated degenerative conditions (e.g., see Sect. 4.12 under extreme micrencephaly). In these conditions, at midgestation, the cyst usually is simply a space in the germinal matrix, sometimes filled or partially filled with macrophages and debris. Post-hemorrhagic cysts (Fig. 4.2e, f) may contain abundant hemosiderin and demonstrate a reactive local microvasculature.

4.2.2 Germinal Matrix Excrescences

These are pedunculated mushroom-shaped tufts of germinal matrix tissue protruding through the neuroepithelium into the ventricle (Hrabowska 1978; Friede 1989a, b) (Fig. 4.3a, b). Usually, they are accompanied by one or morecentral capillary vessels and contain microglia or macrophages with a variable amount of heme pigment and extravasated red blood cells. They are usually less than 1 mm in diameter, but occasionally, they may become 1 cm or more in diameter and appear to entrap fluid under their edges (Fig. 4.3c). Occasionally, this trapped fluid can on imaging be mistaken for a germinal matrix cyst. The excrescences usually accompany intracranial pathology and can be very numerous in obstructive hydrocephalus or following an encephaloclastic event, but are generally not in and of themselves significant. Occasionally, in the presence of massive ventriculomegaly, one sees similar structures adherent to the corpus callosum or forniceal columns (Fig. 4.3d), suggesting that the germinal matrix tissue is capable of fragmenting and settling elsewhere, which may (hypothetically) explain its occasional presence in the aqueduct (Fig. 4.3e, f). As the excrescences mature, they possibly develop into glial webs and areas of denuded ventricular lining, but this is speculative.

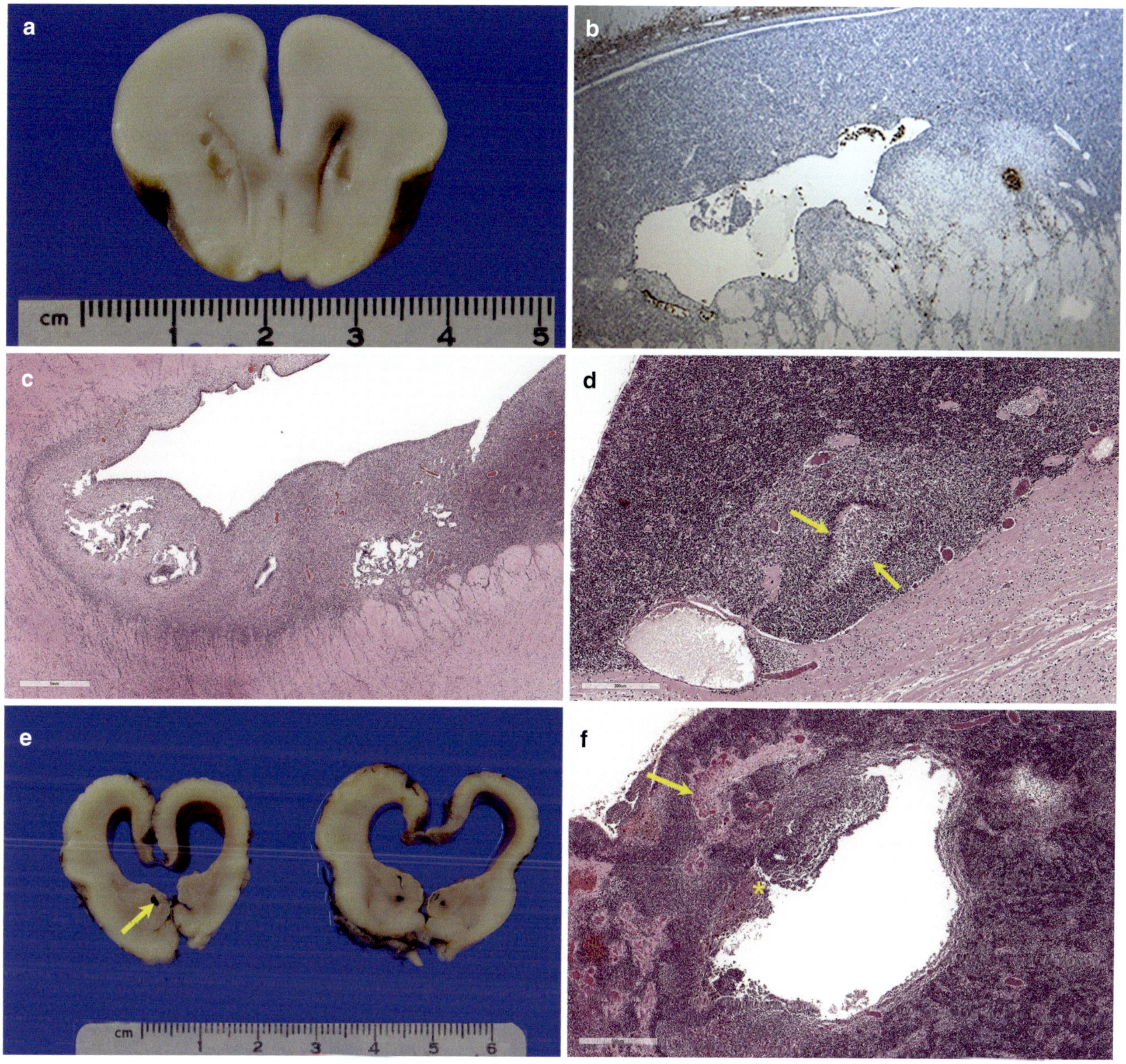

Fig. 4.2 Germinal matrix cyst. (**a**) A 23-week-gestation male with bilateral frontal cysts, cardiomegaly, and bilateral adrenal calcifications. Workup for Ras-opathies as well as mitochondrial and metabolic conditions was unrevealing. The cysts themselves are irregular germinal matrix cavities. (**b**) Staining of (**a**) demonstrates small and large aggregates of macrophages in and around cystic spaces, without pigment deposition. (**c**) A 23-week gestation with cytomegalovirus encephalitis and multiple irregular germinal matrix cysts. (**d**) A small germinal matrix cyst (arrow), almost completely filled with macrophages and debris, at 20 weeks, in a brain with aqueductal stenosis. It is difficult to rule this as an incidental finding. (**e**) Brain from a 24-week-gestation fetus with large bilateral germinal matrix cysts and post-encephaloclastic polymicrogyria and porencephaly (not shown). Here, the cysts contain abundant blood pigment (asterisks) and a fibrotic reactive microvasculature (arrow)

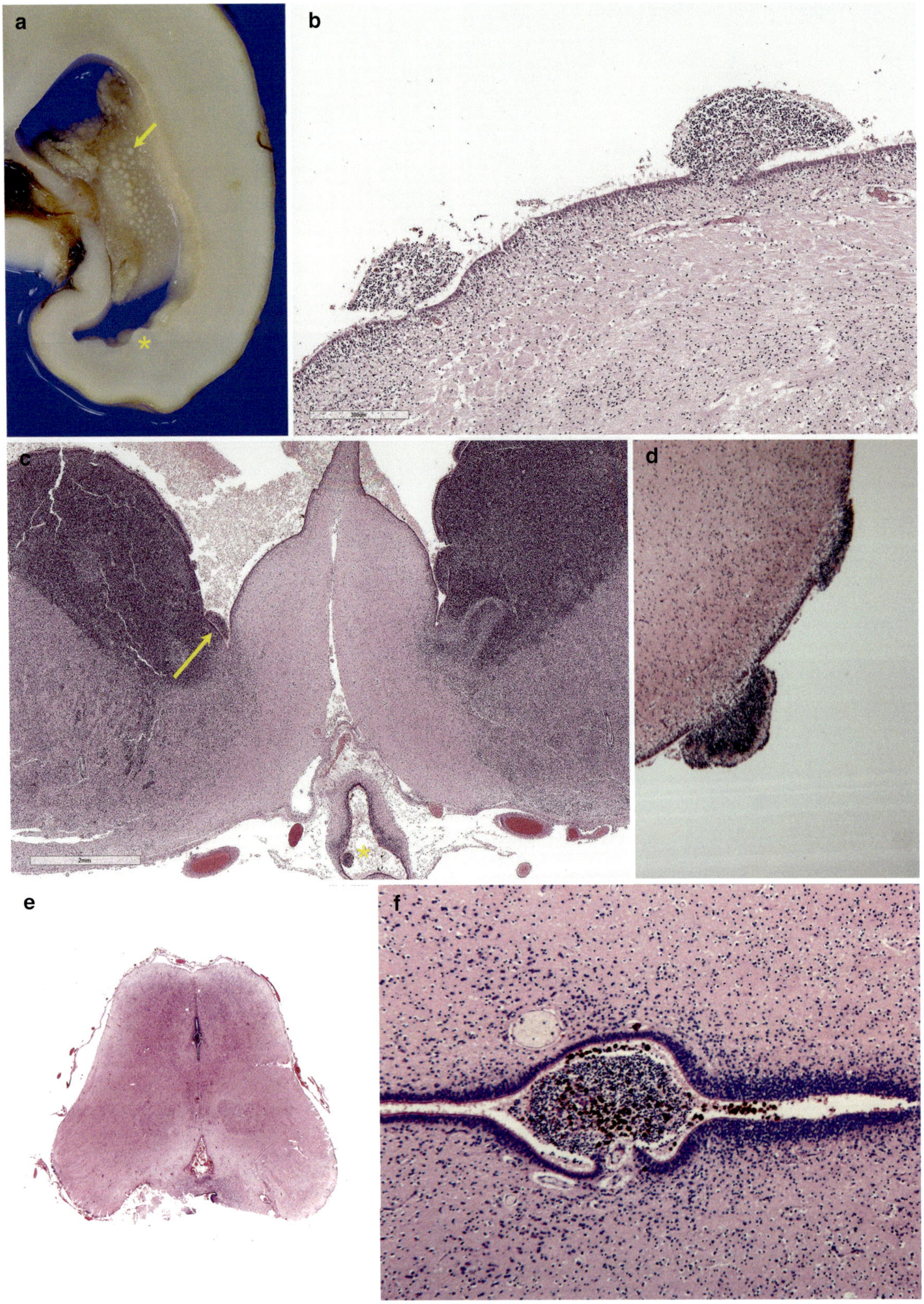

Fig. 4.3 Germinal matrix excrescences. (**a**) Trigone in a 23-week-gestation female with porencephaly. Innumerable excrescences (arrow) dot the germinal matrix. Note that these are grossly different from nodular periventricular heterotopias (asterisk). (**b**) Excrescences decorating the temporal horn in a 23-week-gestation female with in utero fetal death, massive myocardial calcifications, and germinal matrix hemorrhage. (**c**) A 22-week-gestation female with aqueductal stenosis and hydrocephalus. Here, the excrescences are large and flattened and entrap fluid beneath their edges (arrow). Also note excrescence in suprachiasmatic recess (asterisk). (**d**) Excrescences on forniceal columns, 23 weeks old, with hydrocephalus and a neuronal heterotopia obstructing aqueduct. (**e**) Aqueductal stenosis in a 23-week-gestation male. (**f**) The same case as (**e**) with excrescence in aqueduct accompanied by abundant pigmented macrophages

4.3 Periventricular Nodular Heterotopias

These are nodular aggregates of neurons located in the inner ventricular zone. In our autopsy services, by far, the most frequent association is with obstructive hydrocephalus (Fig. 4.4a), post-encephaloclastic lesions (Fig. 4.4b), Chiari type 2 malformations (see Hino-Shishikura et al. 2012), multiple migrational anomalies (Fig. 4.4c), and encephaloceles. The neurons may bear cortical markers and often demonstrate a thin capsule or associated tract of axons (Fig. 4.4d) that myelinates later in gestation; the nodules are often associated with defects in the neuroepithelium or ependyma (Fig. 4.4e). In any given case, they can range from solitary to very numerous. Occasionally, they may form masses (Fig. 4.4f) and can be associated with subcortical or transmantle heterotopias (Fig. 4.4g, h and see Sect. 4.6 "Transmantle Heterotopias"). They are thought to arise from ineffective or halted radial migration late in neurogenesis and may accompany genetic, maldevelopmental, or encephaloclastic conditions. Of those with identified genetic factors, the large majority are X linked and due to FLNA mutations (Parrini et al. 2006), in which they may be large bilateral, relatively sparing the temporal lobe, and numerous. PVNH can also accompany Ehlers–Danlos syndrome, obstructive hydrocephalus, van Maldergem syndrome (Cappello et al. 2013), and AKT3 mutation (Alcantara et al. 2017). One review (Rezazadeh et al. 2018) found an associated 37 genetic conditions including microdeletions in 17q21.31 and 22q11.2 and mutations in ARFGEF2.

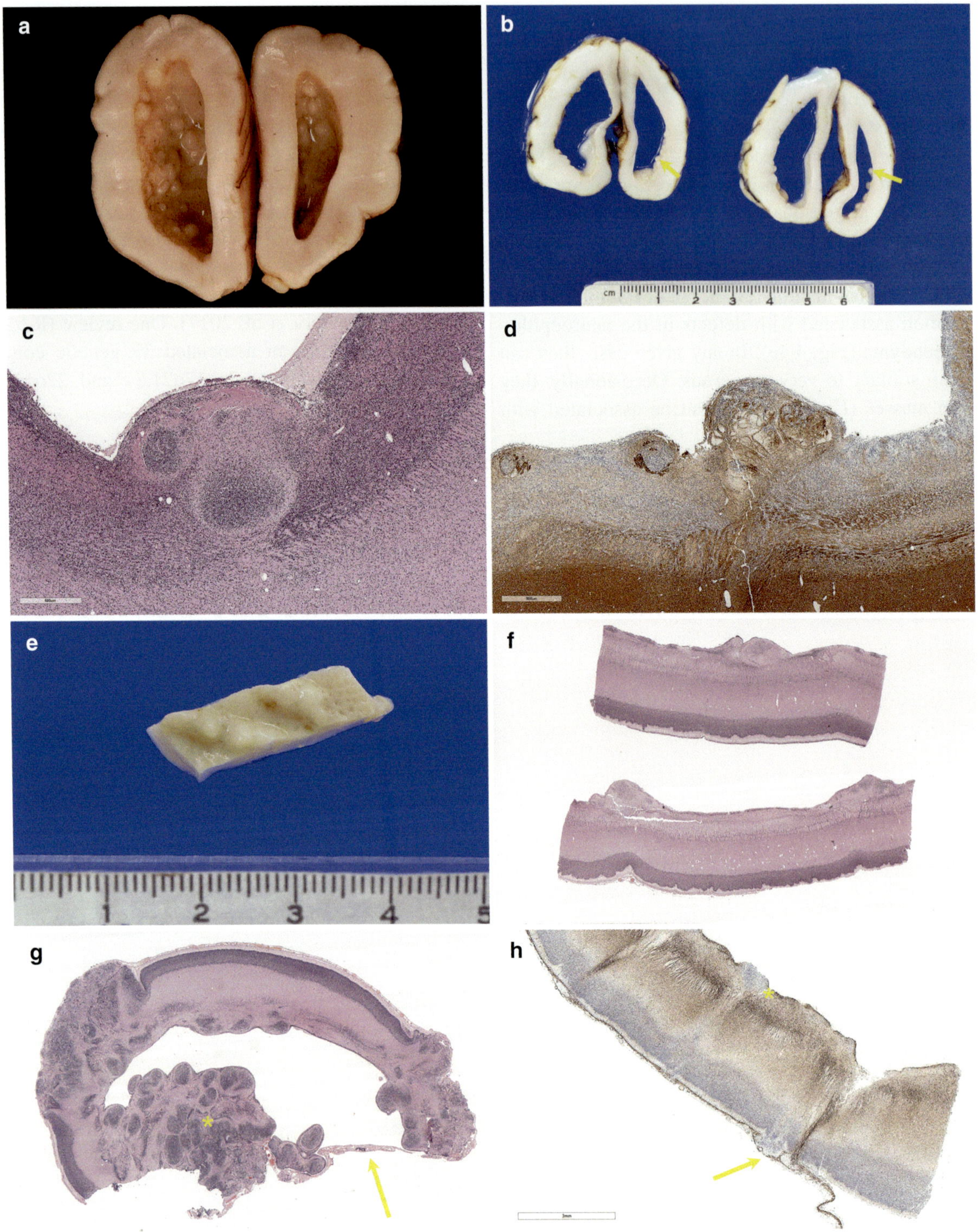

Fig. 4.4 Periventricular nodular heterotopia. (**a**) A 23-week-gestation female with aqueductal stenosis and bilateral parietal foramina. Innumerable PVNH decorate the ventricular lining, here in the frontal recess. (**b**) A 21-week-gestation male with Chiari malformation and hydrocephalus. Here, the heterotopias resemble small teeth projecting into the ventricle. Also see Fig. 4.2a. (**c**) A 20-week-gestation male fetus with arthrogryposis, leptomeningeal and periventricular heterotopias, severe placental fetal vascular malperfusion, and multiple liver calcifications. (**d**) The same case as (**c**) stained with immunohistochemistry for neurofilament light chain. Note the swirling associated axonal tracts and the subtle interruption of the deep fiber tracts. (**e**) A 22-week-gestation female, with aqueductal stenosis with rhombencephalosynapsis. Portion of parietal cortical mantle bearing PVNH arranged in ridges. (**f**) Whole mount of (**e**), demonstrating wide variation in heterotopia size and local abnormalities in fiber tract system. (**g**) Whole mount of occipital lobe, 23 weeks' gestation female, with porencephaly (arrow) covered by an arachnoid membrane, incipient polymicrogyria, and masses of nodular periventricular heterotopias (asterix) both adjacent to and opposite the porencephalic defect. (**h**) A 21-week-gestation female with porencephaly (not shown) and aqueductal stenosis and parietal lobe stained with immunohistochemistry for nestin. The periventricular heterotopias sit on thin seams of altered radial glial staining, suggesting a transmantle injury. Note the adjacent leptomeningeal heterotopia (arrow)

4.4 Subcortical Heterotopias

To simplify a complex topic (see Oegema et al. 2019), subcortical heterotopias can be categorized as band-like, nodular, radial, and transmantle. Most seem to originate as incomplete late radial migration.

Band-like heterotopias consist of subcortical ribbons or bands of neurons running parallel to the deep surface of the cortical plate. In their most dramatic form, they are characteristic of the lissencephaly that accompanies DCX mutations. However, subcortical bands of neurons can also be seen in dysplastic hemimegalencephaly (see Chap. 5), and we have seen them in an uncategorized micrencephaly with undulant cortex that have ill-defined deep borders and a paucity of radial glia and subplate neurons (Fig. 4.5a).

Nodular subcortical heterotopias (NSH) are microscopically similar to periventricular nodular heterotopias (PVNH), and the two types often coexist. Like PVNH, NSH may accompany overlying cortical abnormalities (e.g., see Zellweger syndrome in Chap. 13), or they can be adjacent to or a component of transmantle heterotopias (Fig. 4.5b).

Radial heterotopias are morphologically diverse. They may consist of small columns of subcortical neurons (Fig. 4.5c,d), aligned in the neuropil or around small blood vessels, and there is usually an accompanying cortical anomaly. We have in addition seen subcortical aggregates of nestin (+) glia intermixed with an excess of primitive-appearing precursors forming unusual masses that are difficult to classify e.g. one accompanying a minute ependymal nest superficial to the internal capsule in a case with transmantle heterotopias (Fig. 4.5e, f) and scattered irregular heterotopias marked by gliosis in a case of methotrexate embryopathy (Fig. 4.5g, h).

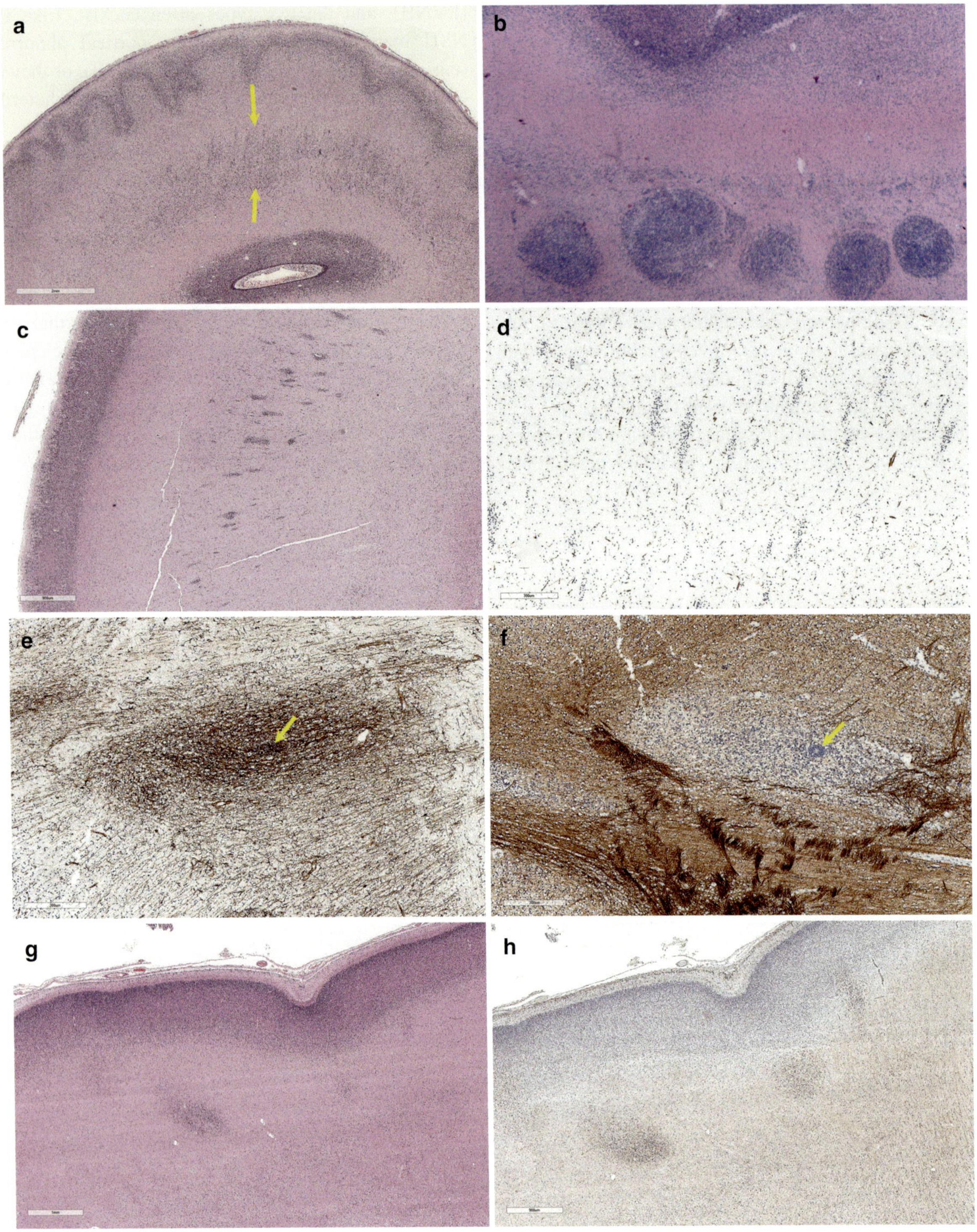

Fig. 4.5 Subcortical heterotopia. (**a**) A 23-week-gestation male with band heterotopia in the context of micrencephaly and an undulant cortex with a poorly defined deep layer and small germinal eminences (not shown). (**b**) A 30-week-gestation female. String of nodular heterotopias in the occipital lobe, ipsilateral to medial giant gyriform heterotopia (see below). (**c**) A 26-week-gestation male, with radial heterotopias and lateral peritrigonal mantle in the context of marked micrencephaly, with depleted germinal matrices. Array cytogenetics demonstrated the absence of heterozygosity encompassing more than 8% of haploid genome. (**d**) The same case as (**c**) demonstrating paucity of radially oriented glia, although tangentially oriented glia are present. (**e**) A 22-week-gestation male. Subcortical heterotopia with central ependymal rosette (arrow) and complex mass of precursors and nestin (+) glia in an outer transitional zone. Posterior opercular frontal lobe, with open occipital neural tube defect. (**f**) The same section stained with immunohistochemistry for neurofilament light chain, demonstrating central ependymal rosette and displacement of local tracts. (**g**) A 23-week-gestation female, with methotrexate embryopathy; predominantly subcortical aggregates of glia and neuronal precursors, with some involvement of cortical plate. (**h**) The same section as (**g**) with staining for nestin, highlighting aggregates

4.5 Focal Abnormalities of Cortical Organization

Leptomeningeal heterotopias: Cortical leptomeningeal heterotopias can be recognized on gross examination as circular nodules or areas of pallor (Fig. 4.6a) where the vascular pattern of the leptomeninges is obscured (Fig. 4.6b). They are characterized by discontinuity of the pia, through which glial and neuronal precursors emerge from the underlying brain into the subarachnoid space (Fig. 4.6c). These are not uncommon as isolated incidental findings, particularly along the orbitofrontal cortex, but they may be numerous. Leptomeningeal heterotopias may occasionally overlie multiple small breaches in the leptomeninges with underlying cortical abnormality (Fig. 4.6d, e); at some point, the overlap with incipient polymicrogyria is apparent. Occasionally, one encounters a number of apparently well-defined large round heterotopias that stand out from the surface of a midgestation brain (Fig. 4.6f). In such lesions, the heterotopia is an organized mushroom-shaped mass on cross section with a hypocellular cap on top of a core of radial glia and neurons; this morphology in our experience is usually associated with a transmantle heterotopia (see Sect. 4.6). The heterotopias may display a dense superficial tangential tract and may demonstrate numerous small calretinin (+) neurons and a tangential glial web. When leptomeningeal heterotopias are post-encephaloclastic, the adjacent cortex often contains scattered CD68 (+) macrophages, which is a useful marker in fetal life, as the cortical ribbon is usually devoid of macrophages until the onset of myelination.

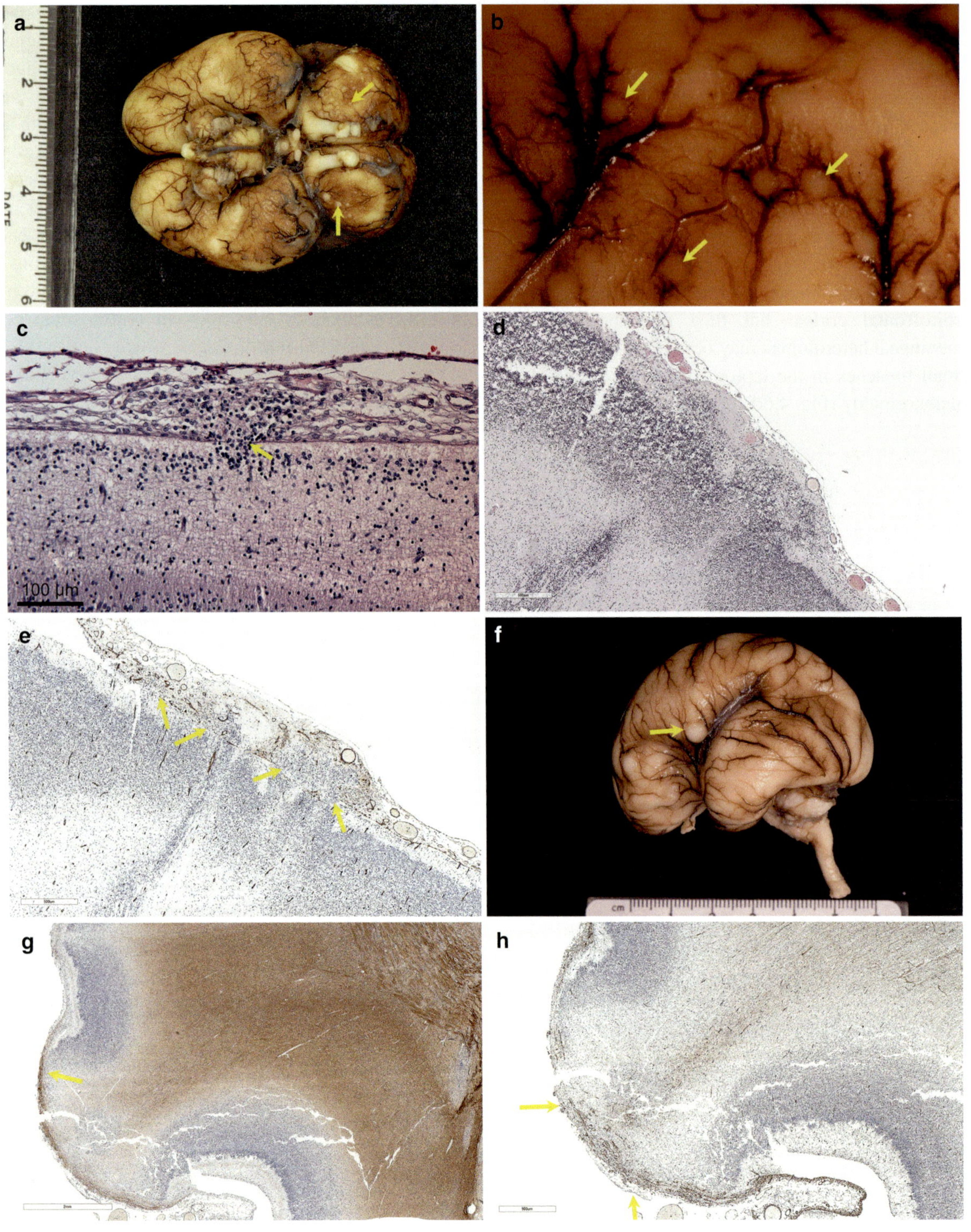

Fig. 4.6 Leptomeningeal heterotopias. (**a**) A 24-week-gestation female, with microlissencephaly and cerebellar hypoplasia, compatible with tubulinopathy, demonstrating innumerable orbitofrontal leptomeningeal heterotopias. (**b**) Frontal cortex of a 32-week-gestation male, with multiple frontal leptomeningeal heterotopias, obscuring local vascular pattern. (**c**) Small frontal leptomeningeal heterotopia with defect in pia and overgrowth of glia and small neurons into leptomeningeal space. (**d**) Male fetus, 22-week gestation, with hydrocephalus and larger irregular heterotopia with associated cortical abnormality. (**e**) The same case as (**d**) stained with immunohistochemistry for Collagen IV demonstrating multiple small breaches in the pia underlying the abnormality. (**f**) Male fetus, 23-week gestation, with hypoplastic corpus callosum (not shown) and large pale nodular frontal cortical heterotopias (arrow). (**g**) The same case as (**e**) with section stained with immunohistochemistry for neurofilament light chain, demonstrating central core of projections and dense superficial web of axons (arrow). (**h**) The same case as (**e**) with section stained with immunohistochemistry for nestin, with radial glia extending into the heterotopia with dense reduplication of superficial glial web (arrow)

4.6 Transmantle Heterotopias

These can be roughly divided into three major forms in our experience. One form is marked in near midgestation by a nodular or multinodular cortex (Fig. 4.7a); this is often but not exclusively frontal and is marked by finger-like extensions of ventricular zone-like tissue (Fig. 4.7b) into the cerebral mantle, sometimes with a central thin-walled blood vessel, in continuity with the nodular superficial masses of neurons. These may have adjacent PVNH (Fig. 4.7c), and the cortical surface is marked by a large mushroom-like leptomeningeal heterotopia (see Fig. 4.6f).

In a second form of transmantle heterotopia, PVNH and subcortical heterotopias are overlain by large or confluent leptomeningeal defects (Fig. 4.7d, e), with irregular leptomeningeal heterotopias or regions of incipient polymicrogyria. This morphology has an association with a neural tube defect (Fig. 4.7f, g) or porencephaly (Fig. 4.7h, i). The leptomeningeal and nodular periventricular heterotopias may be small and connected by a narrow seam.

The third major form of transmantle heterotopia is the giant or gyriform heterotopia, which is usually associated with ipsilateral hemimicrencephaly (Fig. 4.8a, e, f). These consist of masses of the brain where the underlying white matter is interrupted by ribbons of undulating cortex-like gray matter (Fig. 4.8b, g). The associated leptomeningeal and penetrating vasculature may be coarse and dilated with large Virchow–Robin spaces, while the adjacent cortex may show polymicrogyria, leptomeningeal heterotopias, and there may be NSH (Fig. 4.8d).

It should be added that there are numerous other combinations of dysplasia. Aicardi syndrome (OMIM #304050), for instance, can present with a particularly chaotic aggregate of disturbances of the cortical mantle (Fig. 4.8h).

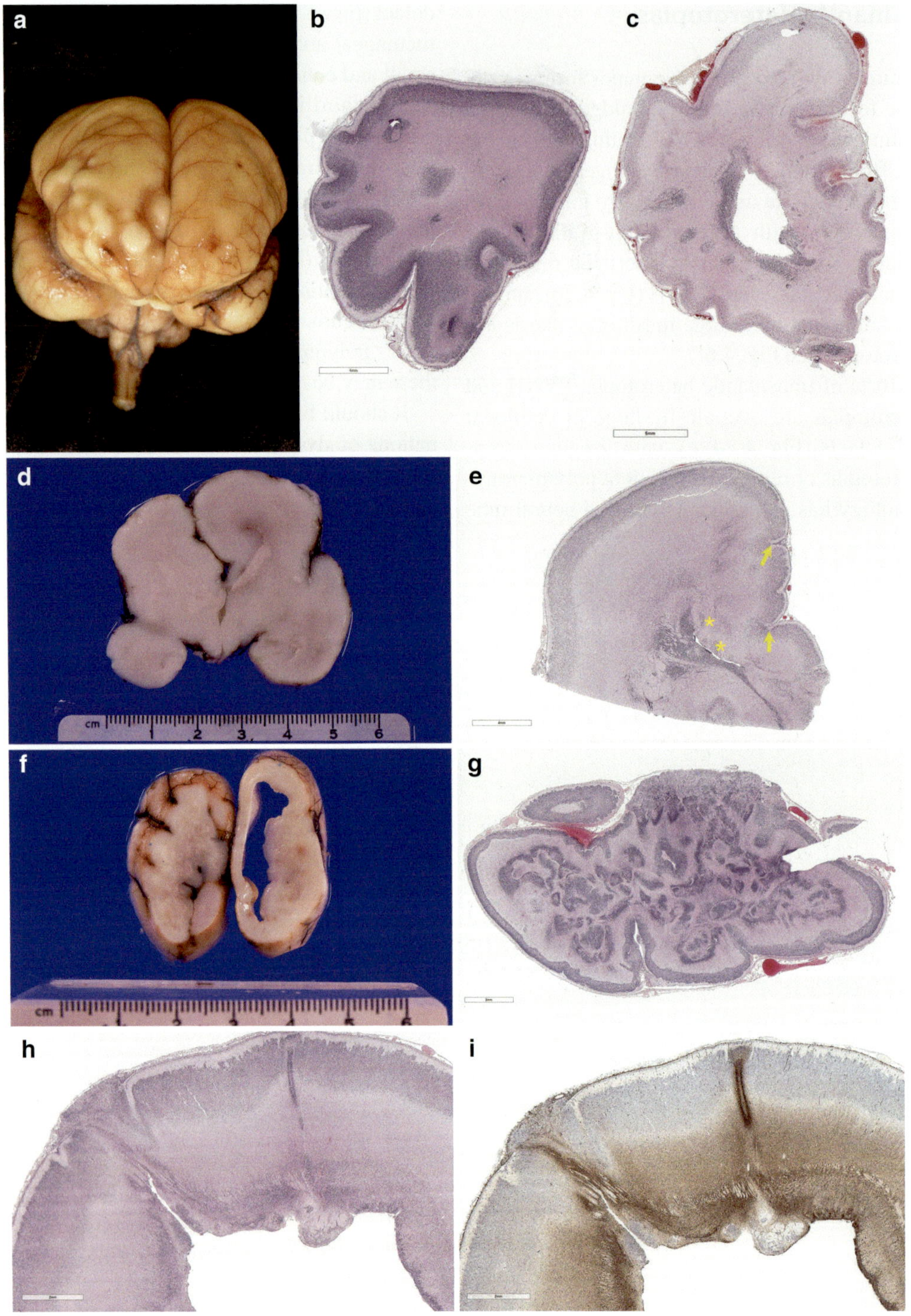

Fig. 4.7 Transmantle dysplasias. (**a**) A 23-week-gestation male, with absent corpus callosum (not shown) and nearly confluent nodules very similar to Fig. 4.6f but confined to one frontal pole. (**b**) Cross section of the frontal pole of a with extension of ventricular zone-like tissue in fingerlike projections with each nodule breaching the leptomeninges. (**c**) 30-week-gestation male, with unilateral left frontal abnormality, agenesis of the corpus callosum, interhemispheric cyst, and multiple fingerlike projections capped by a leptomeningeal breach and an underlying PVNH. (**d**) A 23-week-gestation male with agenesis of the corpus callosum, collapse of the left lateral ventricle, and hypoplastic left frontal lobe. The left olfactory bulb and tract were absent. (**e**) Frontal lobe of (**d**) with predominantly medial PVNH (asterisks), subcortical heterotopias, and cortical irregularity with small breaches of the leptomeninges and underlying cortical thinning (arrows). (**f**) A 20-week-gestation male with occipito-cervical meningocele and cerebellar hypoplasia with cortical dysplasia and aqueductal stenosis. Both occipital lobes demonstrate PVNH, and the left occipital pole is replaced with a mass of disorganized pale subcortical and cortical tissue. (**g**) Whole mount of left occipital pole with a full-thickness mass of leptomeningeal heterotopia, polymicrogyria, and nodular heterotopia. (**h**) Male fetus, 22 weeks, with left occipital porencephaly and aqueduct partially occluded by nodular neuronal heterotopia. There is a right parietal partial-thickness cleft with overlying small area of incipient polymicrogyria and an apparent transmantle glial linear scar with subjacent periventricular heterotopia. (**i**) The same section as (**h**) stained with immunohistochemistry for nestin demonstrating linear gliosis

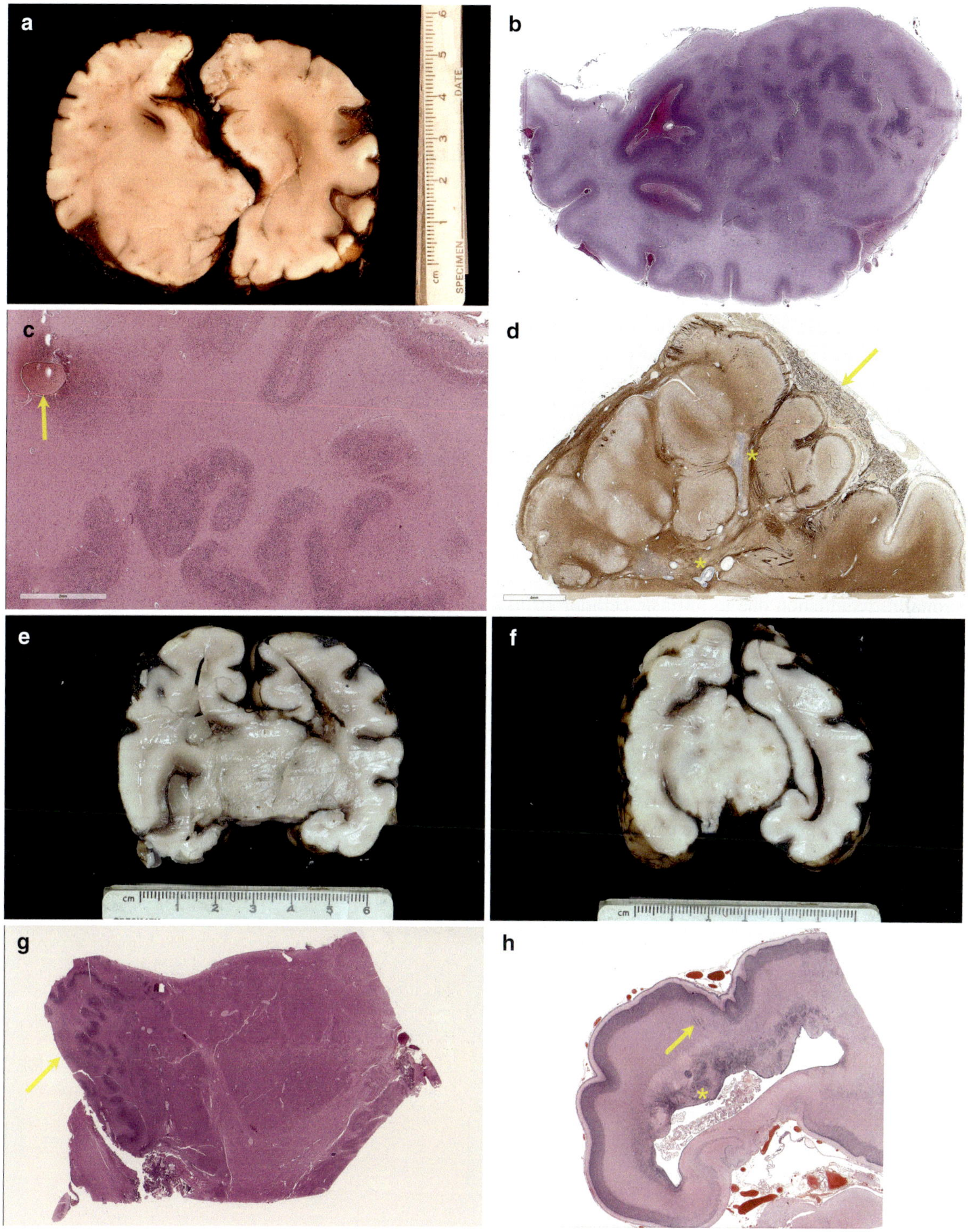

Fig. 4.8 Transmantle gyriform dysplasia. (**a**) A 36-week-gestation male, with agenesis of the corpus callosum and left frontal gyriform heterotopia distorting the inferior and medial frontal pole. (**b**) The same case, with whole mount of frontal pole, inferior on the right, demonstrating serpiginous ribbons of neurons in subcortical and deep white matter. (**c**) Serpiginous lines of unorganized cortex-like neurons with abnormally deep large blood vessel (arrows) section. (**d**) The same section stained with immunohistochemistry for neurofilament light chain, demonstrating large leptomeningeal heterotopia (arrow) and irregular extensions of ventricular zone elements into the irregular heterotopic masses (asterisks). (**e**) A 30-week-gestation female with left medial cerebral expansion superior to the left thalamus. (**f**) The same case as (**e**): mass expands into a rounded mass with associated hypoplasia of the left posterior hemisphere. (**g**) The same case as (**e**); section through the thalamus with overlying gyriform heterotopia (arrow; section rotated with inferior margin to the right); note the similarity to (**b**) and (**c**). (**h**) A 23-week-gestation female, with peritrigonal cortical mantle with nodular periventricular heterotopias, radial heterotopias (arrow), and marked cortical irregularity without leptomeningeal overgrowth. Chorioretinal lacunae, agenesis of the corpus callosum, frontal leptomeningeal overgrowth, and a large interhemispheric choroid plexus cyst were present

4.7 Polymicrogyria

Polymicrogyria describes a condition of the cerebral cortex characterized in the fully developed brain by a global or regional excess of small fused cortical gyri. During development, pial disruption in the area can usually be demonstrated (Diamandis et al. 2017; Squier and Jansen 2014; Jansen et al. 2016) with heterotopic glial and neuronal elements in the affected subarachnoid space, underlain by a cerebral cortex that is generally thinned and abnormally laminated; the number of layers does not generally predict pathogenesis. Large and aberrant bundles of axons may course through the superficial layers. The subjacent subplate may contain abnormal numbers of neurons, and these may form heterotopic masses. The morphology is similar to that observed in cobblestone lissencephaly (see Sect. 4.11.2), but in the latter, the alteration is confluent, and the leptomeningeal overgrowth tends to be the dominant feature.

Polymicrogyria may be related to encephaloclastic processes affecting the cortex (a disruption), or it may be primarily maldevelopmental, related to abnormal cell migration and neuronal differentiation due to intrinsic cellular errors. Post-encephaloclastic polymicrogyria in early fetal life presents as a local collapse and irregularity of the cortical mantle (Fig. 4.9a). Histology demonstrates an irregularly folded and laminated cortical ribbon with areas of pial disruption and leptomeningeal overgrowth as well as numerous calretinin (+) neurons in the leptomeninges, displacement of Cajal–Retzius cells, and activated intracortical microglia and macrophages. Subjacent aggregates of macrophages are common, and these tend to aggregate at the deep aspects of the subcortical ribbon or adjacent subcortical heterotopias. There may be premature synaptogenesis. At midgestation, hypertrophy and irregular branching of radial glia, microcalcifications, and hyperplasia of subplate neurons can be found (Diamandis et al. 2017). In post-hypoxic–ischemic polymicrogyria, ipsilateral or bilateral thalamic scarring is frequent, and symmetrical brainstem tegmental scarring and spinal cord injury may be present. While isolated post-hypoxic–ischemic polymicrogyria (i.e., not associated with other central nervous system injury) tends to be peri-Sylvian, anatomic distribution alone is not a reliable guide to causation, and the presence or absence of injury in deep structures, the history of the pregnancy, and the results of systemic postmortem examination, in particular those of placental examination, must be carefully investigated.

Polymicrogyria may accompany mutations in more than 20 genes (Brock et al. 2021a, b), but a distinction between genetic and post-encephaloclastic polymicrogyria cannot always be drawn. Heritable abnormalities of vascular basal lamina or endothelial cell biology (e.g., Col4a1 or Col4A2 (Shannon et al. 2021)) may result in a post encephaloclastic cortical developmental anomaly as the genetic defects precipitate endothelial dysfunction with hemorrhage and thrombosis. Purely developmental polymicrogyria (i.e. without evidence of destructive pathology) tends to be symmetrical and can be lobar or peri-Sylvian, but this on its own is not a reliable guide as it can also be focal. Some developmental polymicrogyria demonstrates florid leptomeningeal overgrowth (see "Hemimegalencephaly" in Chap. 5 and "Zellweger Spectrum" in Chap. 13), while in others, at least in our experience, this feature is not readily apparent.

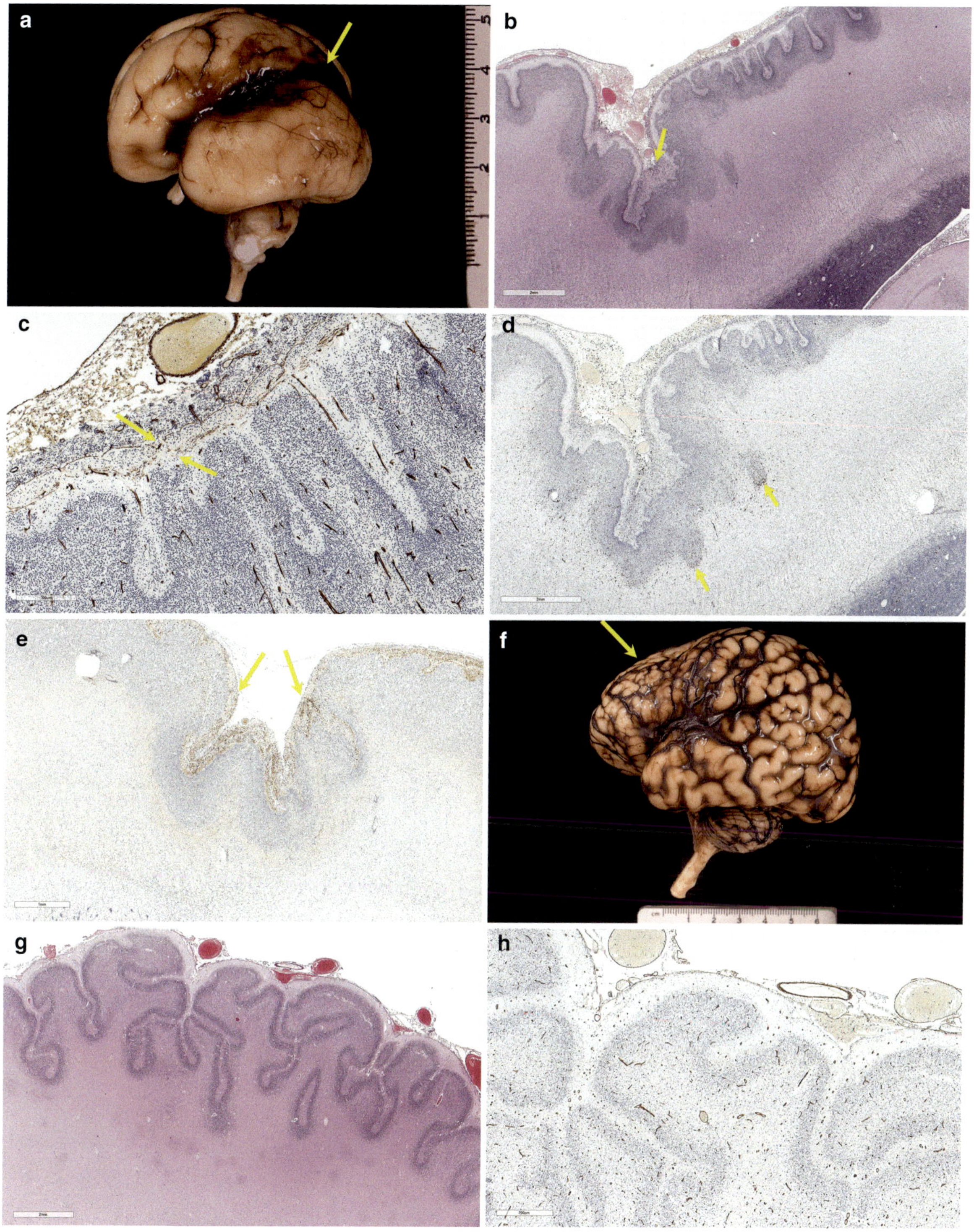

Fig. 4.9 Polymicrogyria. (**a**) A 22-week-gestation male with fetal akinesia and large stripe of dark firm cortex projecting caudally from the Sylvian fissure representing an area of incipient polymicrogyria. Thalamic and brainstem injury were also present. (**b**) The same case as (**a**); lateral peritrigonal cortex with irregular cortical ribbon and leptomeningeal overgrowth. (**c**) The same case as (**a**) stained with immunohistochemistry for Collagen IV, demonstrating breaches in the pia (arrows) with overgrowth of neural elements into the leptomeninges and an excessively folded cortical ribbon. (**d**) The same case as (**a**) stained with immunohistochemistry for CD68. The cortex and subplate contain numerous macrophages, many of which decorate the deep margin of the irregular cortical ribbon. (**e**) A 23-week-gestation female, with focal area of cortical irregularity in the right frontal operculum stained with immunohistochemistry for calretinin, demonstrating prominence of staining over an area of cortical irregularity associated with leptomeningeal overgrowth (arrows). (**f**) A 36-week-gestation female with bifrontal polymicrogyria and a known pathogenic mutation in DDX3. (**g**) The same case as (**f**) demonstrating fused gyri with a four-layer thin cortex. (**h**) The same case as (**f**) stained with immunohistochemistry for Collagen IV, without obvious pial breach

4.8 Other Fetal Cortical Dysplasias

Focal abnormalities of organization of the cortical ribbon may take the form of premature lamination or columnar organization, but care must be taken not to overinterpret regional differences in cytoarchitectural differentiation or handling artifact. We have seen extensive distinct thin hypocellular laminae in the frontal and temporal cortex at midgestation in a case of micrencephaly with multiple periventricular heterotopias, post-necrotic hepatic calcifications, and severe placental fetal vascular malperfusion (Fig. 4.10a, b), as well as in siblings with van Maldergem syndrome (Cappello et al.

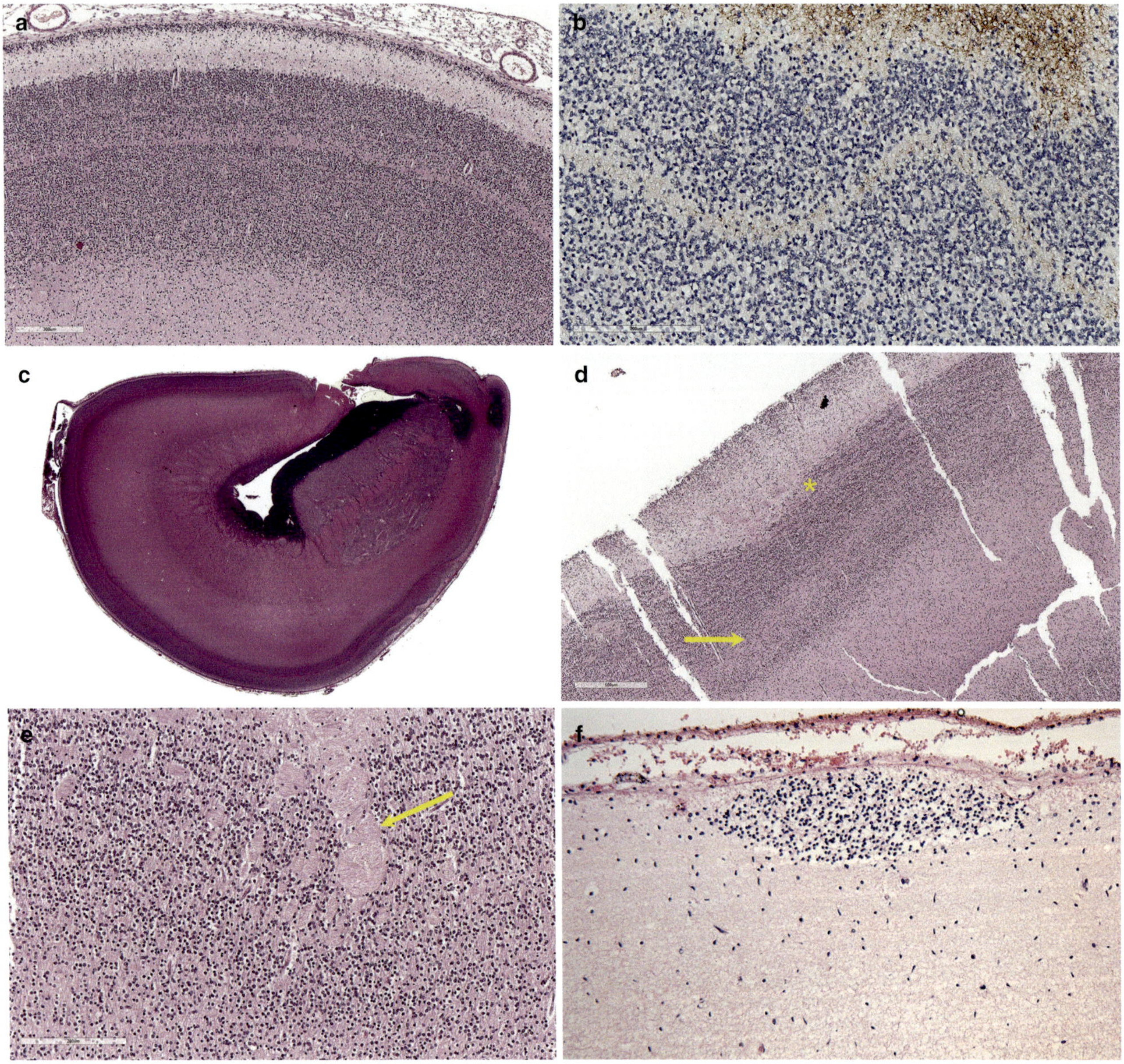

Fig. 4.10 Cortical malformations. (**a**) A 20-week-gestation female: distinct intracortical lamina (the same case as Fig. 4.4c) splitting the cortex in the context of fetal arthrogryposis, PVNH, and high-grade placental fetal vascular malperfusion. (**b**) The same case as (**a**); immunohistochemical staining for synaptophysin decorates the lamina faintly. Neither basal lamina nor bundles of axons were detected, and calretinin staining was not increased over background. (**c**) A 21-week-gestation female, coronal section of one frontal pole and a homozygous pathogenic mutation in FAT4: there is a dramatic split cortex malformation, and small periventricular heterotopias (not illustrated). (**d**) A 22-week-gestation female with hydrocephalus, aqueductal stenosis, dentato-olivary dysplasia, and severe hypoplasia of the corticospinal tracts. Lateral temporal cortex demonstrating hypocellular lamina (arrow) with exaggerated horizontal layering and irregularly thickened molecular layer (asterisks). (**e**) The same patient as (**d**) at area marked by asterisks, demonstrating invagination of the superficial cortex by heterotopic bundles of axons. (**f**) A 32-week-gestation male with hydrocephalus, aqueductal stenosis, and dentato-olivary dysplasia, with multiple small subpial heterotopias

2013). The mature morphology of this abnormality is unclear, although it might correspond to the "double-cortex-like" or "split cortex" morphology described in FAT4 mutation (also see Sprugnoli et al. 2018). Other occasional findings in other cases of multiple intracranial anomalies include areas of increased intracortical axonal tracts (Fig. 4.10d, e) and subpial aggregates of small calretinin (+) neurons.

4.9 Pachygyria

In pachygyria, the gyri are reduced in number and thickened and may display unusual patterns. In fetal specimens prior to the mid-third trimester, this is naturally a challenging judgment, but occasionally, one will see very abnormal patterns. In our experience where there is early third trimester pachygyria, one will usually see agenesis of the corpus callosum with other anomalies such as cortical heterotopias (Fig. 4.11a, b), encephalocele, areas of polymicrogyria (Fig. 4.11c, d), and one case of pachygyria associated with severe cerebral gliosis, white matter injury, cerebellar cavitating injury, and congenital heart block (Zaki et al. 2011) (Fig. 4.11e, f). The genetics of pachygyria and lissencephaly overlap considerably (e.g., Devisme et al. 2012).

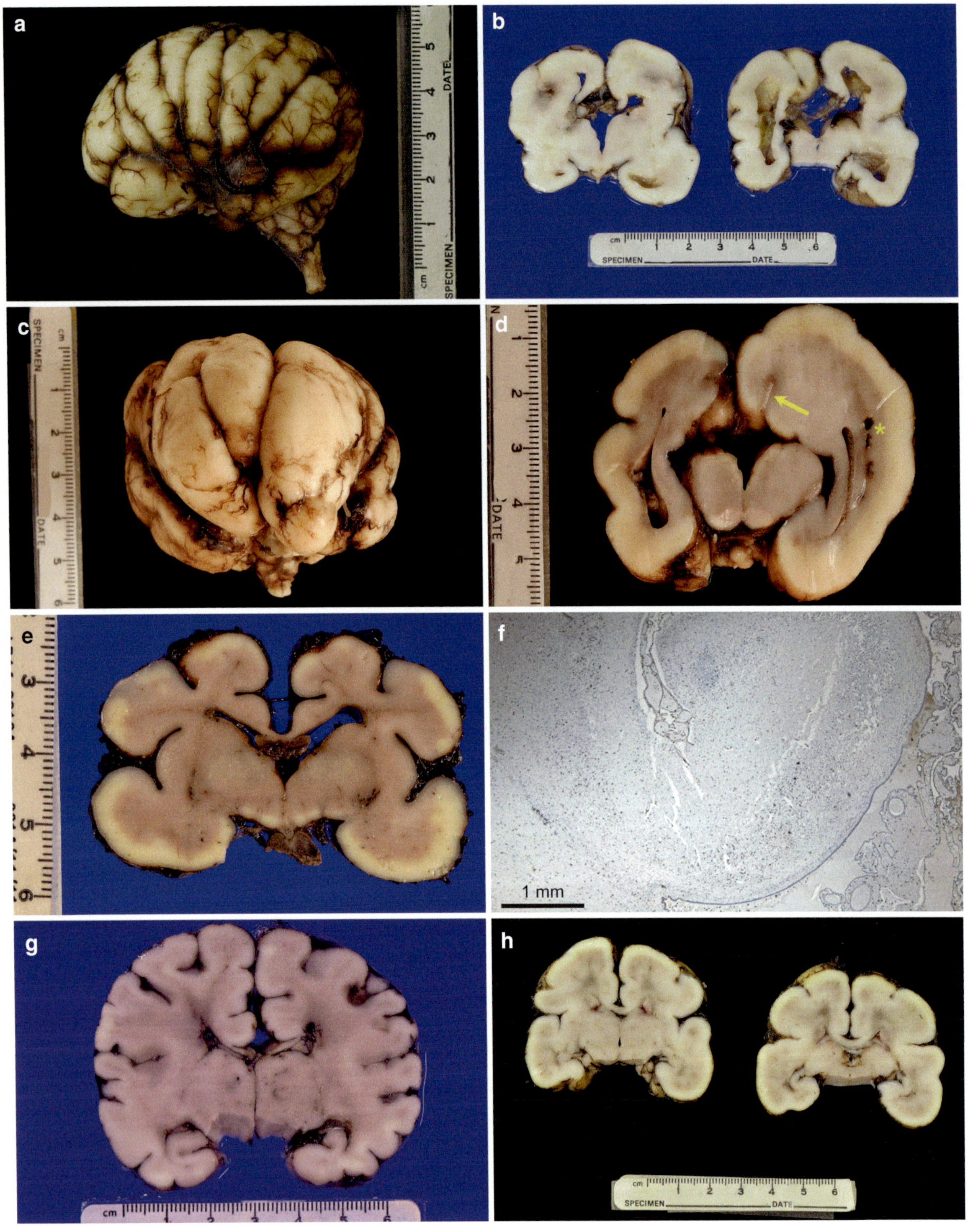

Fig. 4.11 Pachygyria and micrencephaly. (**a**) A 26-week-gestation female with coarse, vertically directed convexity gyri along with hypoplastic and dysplastic temporal lobes. (**b**) Cross section of (**a**) demonstrating agenesis of the corpus callosum, choroid plexus cysts, transmantle dysplasia, PVNH, and polymicrogyria. (**c**) A 29-week-gestation female with small frontonasal encephalocele, agenesis of the corpus callosum and pyramidal tracts, aplasia of olfactory bulbs and tracts, aplasia of the striatum, multiple subcortical infarcts, olivary dysplasia, and parietal polymicrogyria (not shown) in the setting of multiple congenital anomalies. The frontal poles in particular demonstrate thick deeply separated gyri. (**d**) The same case as (**c**) demonstrating thick gyri, subcortical infarcts (asterisks), and focus of polymicrogyria (arrow). (**e**) A 38-week-gestation male, with dramatic gyral simplification and extensive white matter gliosis with non-cavitating white matter injury, thalamic gliosis, and extensive brainstem and cerebellar gliosis in the context of a dilated cardiomyopathy with noncompaction, endocardial fibroelastosis, and second-degree heart block. (**f**) Hippocampal formation of the case in (**e**) with immunohistochemical staining for CD68 demonstrating macrophages in CA1 and subiculum, suggesting secondary neuronal injury. (**g**) Full-term male micrencephaly, thinning of the corpus callosum, and mild excess gyration on the right but without discernible abnormalities in cytoarchitecture on routine microscopy. (**h**) A 28-week-gestation male with Hb Barts and severe growth restriction with micrencephaly and delayed maturation but without gross lesions. Note the complete absence of superior temporal sulcus on the left and a very shallow indentation on the right

4.10 Isolated Micrencephaly

Micrencephaly is defined as hypoplasia of the brain, with a weight less than 3 standard deviations below the mean expected for gestational age. This may be primary or secondary. Evaluating the pathology of fetal micrencephaly may be unrewarding, as there can be minimal accompanying malformations in isolated micrencephaly (Fig. 4.11g), and the most to which one can point with confidence is hypoplasia, with an apparent delay in gross and cytoarchitectural maturation. Later in gestation, dysgyria and hypoplasia of the corpus callosum may be apparent. Autosomal recessive primary micrencephaly has been linked to more than two dozen genes, but fetal pathology is poorly reported (Rasool et al. 2020; Aslam et al. 2024). Isolated micrencephaly may also be secondary to severe growth restriction (Fig. 4.11h), so as usual, clinical context is highly relevant to interpretation.

4.11 Lissencephaly

Lissencephalies are disorders characterized by markedly reduced or absent normal cortical gyration, due to defects in radial migration. There are currently over 15 different genetically defined lissencephalies (e.g., Brock et al. 2021a, b; Gins et al. 2025), and this number will undoubtedly expand. However, the genetically defined lissencephalies tend to have distinct phenotypes (Forman et al. 2005) as might be expected.

4.11.1 Type 1 Lissencephaly

This condition is characterized by micrencephaly and in its most severe form a profound failure of gyration and opercularization (Fig. 4.12a, b). Histologically, one sees a layered cortex most dramatically abnormal in posterior cortex (Forman et al. 2005) (Fig. 4.12c). There is a rostral–caudal gradient (Fig. 4.12d) with a prominent layer of large pyramidal cells in layer 2 and a thick cortical ribbon with an indistinct delimitation of layer 4 (Fig. 4.12d–g). The primary defect seems to be both a failure of neurogenesis and of radial migration due to a failure of the protein product LIS1 to enable the assembly of dynein motors (Singh et al. 2024). Type 1 lissencephaly is characteristic of Miller–Dieker syndrome (OMIM #247200) with a deletion in chromosome 17p13.3 or as the most severe form of defect associated with a mutation in PAFAH1B1 (Dobyns et al. 1993; Leventer et al. 2001; Sheen et al. 2006; Forman et al. 2005).

4.11.2 Cobblestone (Type 2) Lissencephalies

These are a group of lissencephalies characterized grossly by an irregular finely gyrated cerebral cortex at term. In fetal specimens, there is often an effacement of the leptomeningeal pattern of blood vessels, which may range from local, particularly posteriorly (Fig. 4.13a), to a dramatic icing-like coat of the hemispheres (Fig. 4.13b). Close examination will show a fine nodular surface resembling innumerable fused leptomeningeal heterotopias. The hydrocephalus secondary to aqueductal stenosis may be striking (Fig. 4.13c), and there may be an associated occipital encephalocele. On cross section, the medial surfaces of the frontal poles may be fused (Fig. 4.13d, e) and the falx much reduced. Microscopy demonstrates extensive cortical irregularity. At low power, the cortical ribbon often seems split into two (Fig. 4.13e) with over-running of the leptomeninges by glial and neuronal elements (Fig. 4.14f). This leaves the impression of a discontinuous layer of the cerebral cortex interrupted by breaches in the pia (Fig. 4.13g) through which streams of migrating precursors have moved to invade and sometimes completely fill the subarachnoid space. The pial abnormality can be directly stained with reticulin stains or immunohistochemical stains for Collagen IV or laminin (Fig. 4.13h, i). Leptomeningeal overgrowth can almost efface the underlying cortical structure (Fig. 4.13j), and radial glia may extend through the deep former pial layer and continue in sheaves to within the overgrown leptomeninges (Fig. 4.13k). Pial discontinuity and leptomeningeal overgrowth are also a feature of the brainstem and cerebellum (see Chaps. 7 and 8). The disease is inherited as an autosomal recessive condition. Although roughly a third of cases do not have an identified mutation, those that are identified (POMT1, POMT2, POMGNT1, LARGE, FKTN and FKRP, and ISPD) seem necessary for the o-mannosylation of alpha dystroglycan. TMEM5, which has a glycosyltransferase domain, has also been implicated in cobblestone lissencephaly (Vuillaumier-Barrot et al. 2012). The cytological function of alpha dystroglycan seems to be important in establishing the relationship between the radial glia endplates and the pia limitans. Extensive genotype–phenotype correlations are available (Devisme et al. 2012; Vuillaumier-Barrot et al. 2012; Keith and Shannon 2023).

Tubulinopathies manifest themselves as brain malformations ranging from pachygyria to lissencephaly (Fallet-Bianco et al. 2014; Weber et al. 2022; Laquerriere et al. 2016; Bahi-Buisson 2014; Brock et al. 2021a, b). TUBA1A and TUBB2B mutations have presented at midgestation with a microlissencephaly with cerebellar hypoplasia (Fig. 4.14a–c). The cerebral cortex may be thinned

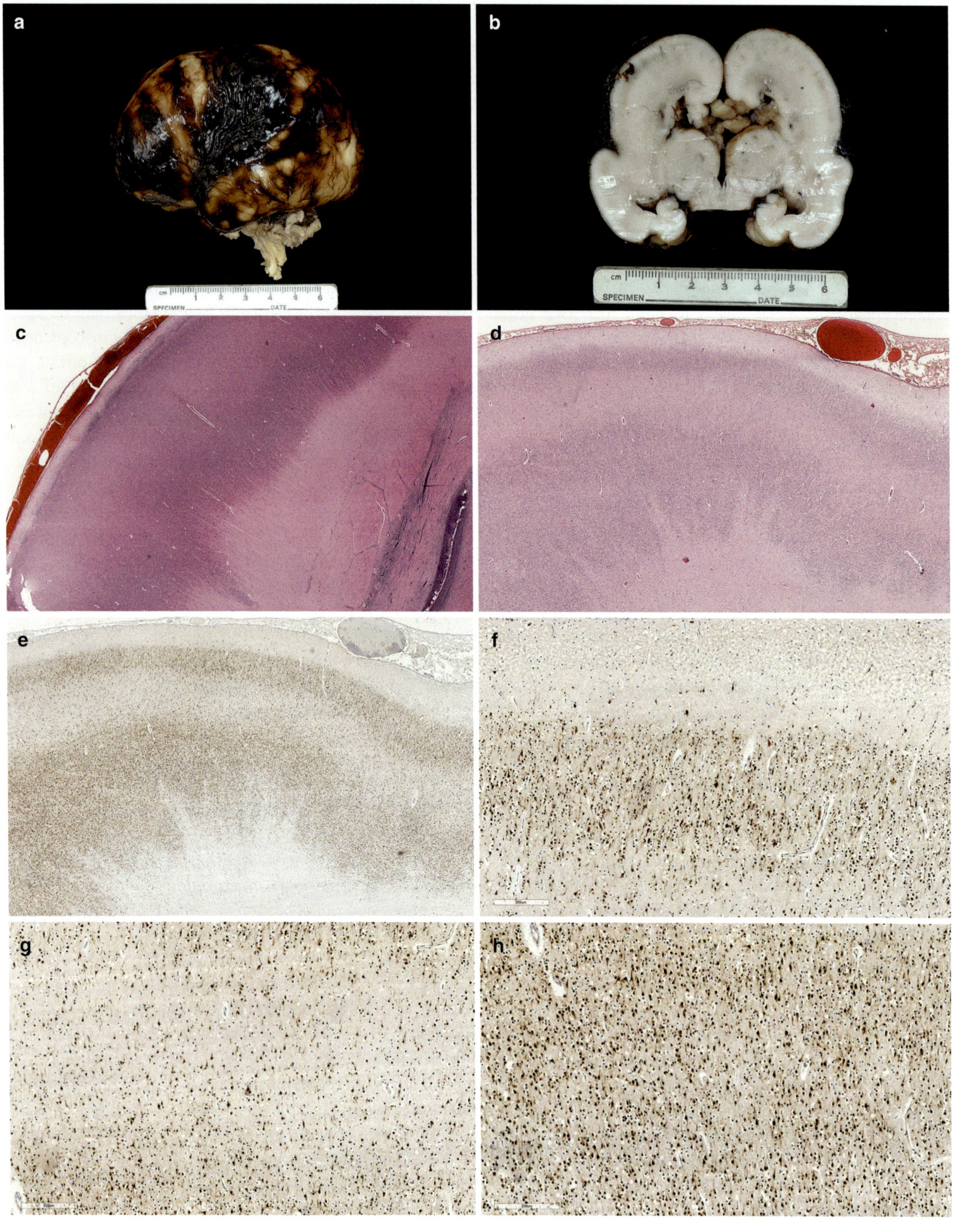

Fig. 4.12 Miller–Dieker syndrome. (**a**) A 35-week-gestation male, with interstitial deletion of chromosome 17p13.3. The lateral aspect of the brain demonstrating global cerebral hypoplasia and a smooth cortical surface. (**b**) Coronal section of (**a**) demonstrating absent convexity gyration with a thick cortical mantle and poor opercularization. (**c**) Cortex of frontal pole demonstrating thick cortical ribbon stranding irregularly into the deep white matter. (**d**) Parietal convexity cortex; note that the hypocellular layer 3 is far more distinct than in (**c**). (**e**) Section in (**d**) stained with immunohistochemistry for neurofilament light chain, showing distribution of cell bodies and a four-layered cortex. (**f**) Layers 1 and 2 demonstrating large pyramidal cells, often maloriented in layer 2. (**g**) Layer 3, with marked hypocellularity and on average smaller neurons. (**h**) Layer 4 with a mixed population of neurons, some maloriented at this magnification, stranding irregularly into the deep future white matter

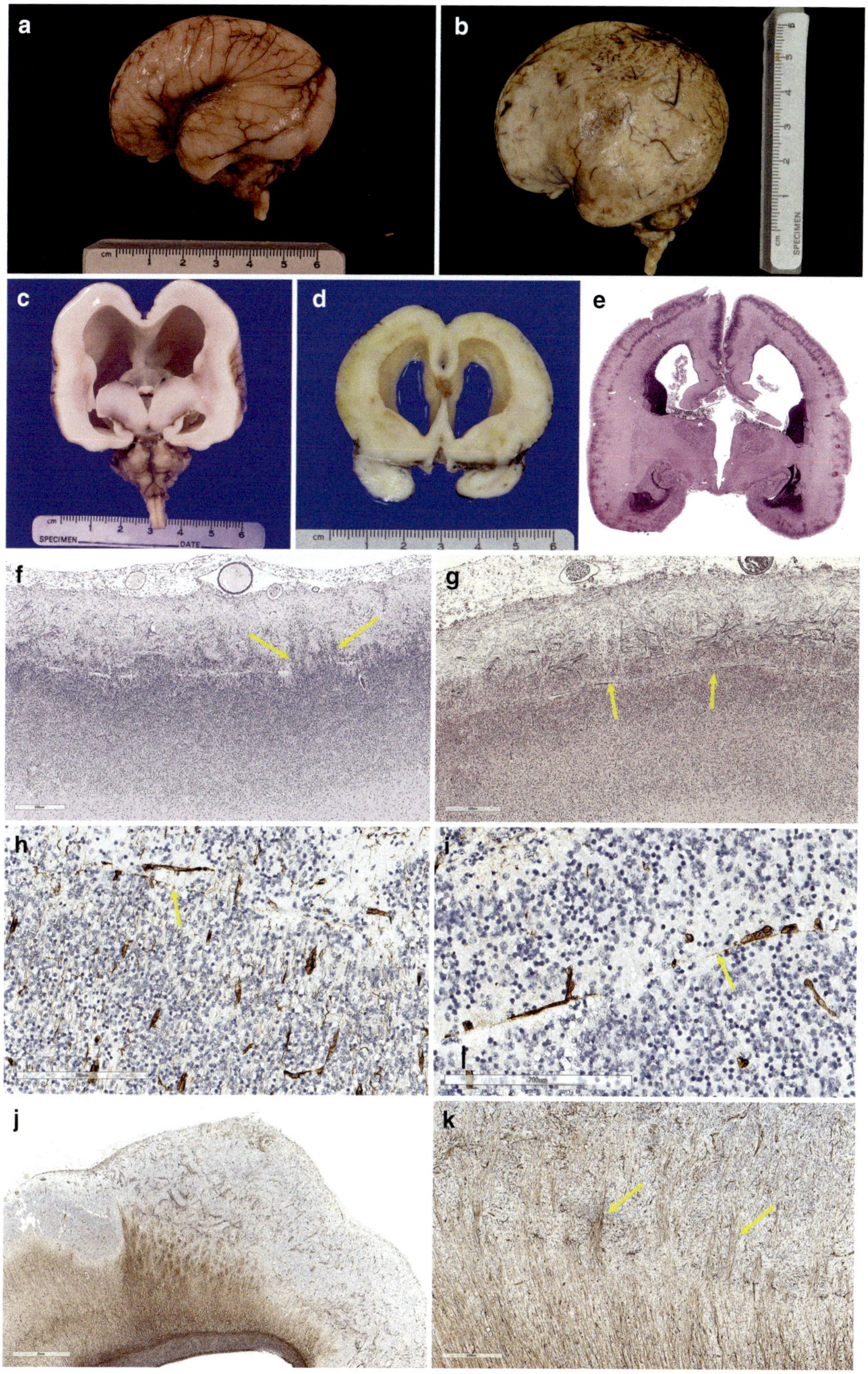

Fig. 4.13 Cobblestone lissencephaly. (**a–e**) are all different cases. (**a**) A 23-week-gestation male, with cobblestone lissencephaly with mildly pebbled surface frontally and large area of occipital effacement of vascular pattern. (**b**) A 23-week-gestation male, with cobblestone lissencephaly with global effacement of vascular pattern as well as markedly smoothed Sylvian fissure and swollen hemispheres. (**c**) A 23-week-gestation male, with cobblestone lissencephaly with marked ventriculomegaly and aqueductal obstruction by heterotopic neural mass. (**d**) A 23-week-gestation male, with cobblestone lissencephaly with fusion of interhemispheric fissure. (**e**) A 23-week-gestation male, with cobblestone lissencephaly whole mount, demonstrating deep cortical layer broken into discontinuous beaded ribbon with superficial overgrowth of leptomeninges. Note the agenesis of the corpus callosum. (**f**) A 23-week-gestation male, with cobblestone lissencephaly and frontal cortex demonstrating neural tissue streaming into leptomeninges (arrows). (**g**) The same section as (**f**) stained for reticulin, showing residual pial surface with horizontally directed blood vessels (arrows). (**h**) The same section at higher magnification with immunohistochemical staining for nestin, demonstrating residual radial glial footplates (arrow). (**i**) The same section with immunohistochemical staining for Collagen IV demonstrating residual pia limitans (arrow). (**j**) A 23-week-gestation male with massive expansion of temporal leptomeninges by heterotopic mass. (**k**) The same case as (**j**) with sheaves of radial glia extending into leptomeninges (arrows)

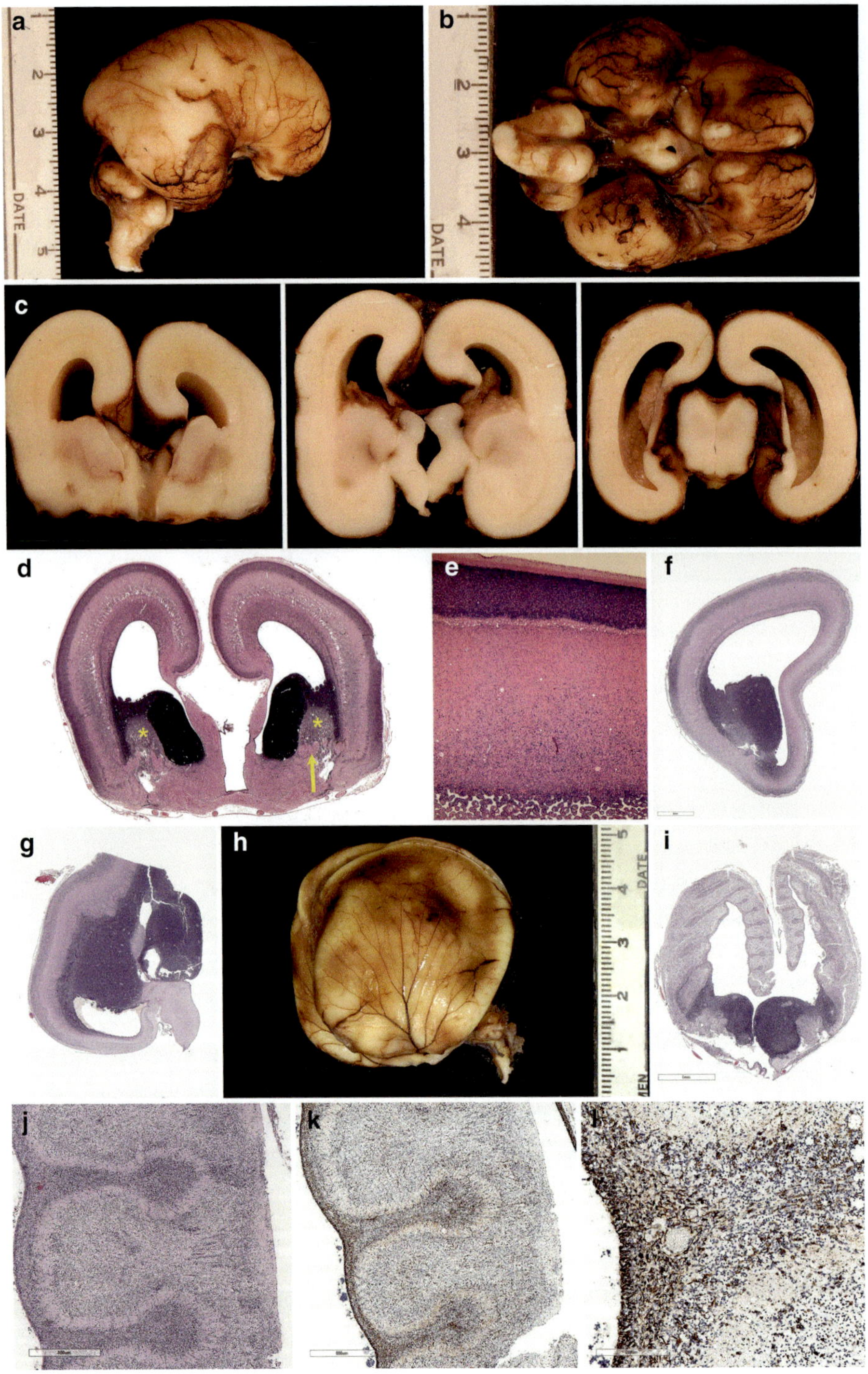

Fig. 4.14 Tubulinopathy. (**a**) A 21-week-gestation male with microlissencephaly and TUBA1A mutation: the lateral view shows marked micrencephaly and smoothed Sylvian fissure and operculum. (**b**) Basal view of (**a**) with small temporal lobes and small olfactory bulbs and tracts. (**c**) Coronal sections of (**a**) demonstrating hypoplastic deep structures, ventriculomegaly, absent corpus callosum, and indistinct small hippocampal formations. (**d**) Whole mount of frontal lobes of (**a**) with very large germinal matrices and deep large basal cysts. The corpus striatum is present (asterisks), but although there are bundles of axons resembling an internal capsule, they are essentially horizontal in orientation (arrow). There is an unusual pattern of subcortical cysts in the superficial and deep mantle. (**e**) Cortical mantle (occipital pole) demonstrating pattern of cysts in (**d**) forming distinct lines in the superficial subplate and transitional zone. One gets the impression that bundles of axonal projections are absent. The cysts are interstitial spaces containing hyaluronidase-sensitive, Alcian blue (+) ground substance (not shown). (**f**) Male fetus, 23 weeks, with TUBA1A mutation; frontal recess and basal frontal lobe with ventriculomegaly and massive germinal matrices with large cyst. (**g**) The same case as (**e**)—posterior temporal lobe with small but recognizable hippocampal formation and expansion of germinal matrices. (**h**) Microlissencephaly with cerebellar hypoplasia and TUBB2B mutation showing smooth, cockleshell-like hemispheres without obvious temporal lobes. (**i**) Frontal section of (**h**) demonstrating large cystic germinal matrix and striking undulating pattern of the cortex. (**j**) Cortical mantle with ventricular surface to the left and undulating crenellated cortical ribbon with indistinct neuronal layering. (**k**) Section of (**h**) with immunohistochemical staining for nestin, demonstrating short, thick radial glia processes without transmantle extension

and undulating, and the external granular cell layer may be thin, with few Cajal–Retzius cells and numerous small leptomeningeal heterotopias. The corpus callosum may be absent, without Probst bundles, and reliably, the corpus striatum and anterior limb of the internal capsule are poorly formed (Fig. 4.14d–f). In cases of microlissencephaly, the periolfactory stream is muted or absent (Fig. 4.14e). The germinal matrices near midgestation may be strikingly large and can display cysts. The thalami are simplified. Brainstem anomalies, which may be striking, are covered in Chap. 7. TUBB2B may have highly simplified hemispheres with unusual histology (Fig. 4.15g–j). The condition is inherited as an autosomal dominant sporadic trait and appears to arise because the mutant tubulin proteins affect the polymerization–depolymerization balance in microtubules and so affect microtubule function in neurogenesis, migration, and axonal growth.

4.12 Extreme Micrencephaly

This is a heterogeneous group of malformations, in which the brain weighs much less than the third percentile for gestational age accompanied by a marked reduction in cerebral lobation and cortical markings. The fetus generally displays the features of prolonged immobility and micrencephaly. In its most striking forms, the entire neuraxis is reduced and simplified, such that the cerebral hemispheres are small globes without commissures, while diencephalic and telencephalic nuclei are poorly delineated (Fig. 4.15a–d). The germinal matrices may be prominent, and a cerebral cortex is radically simplified or absent, without cortical divisions (Fig. 4.15e–g). Encephaloclastic or degenerate pathology is not present at midgestation. In another case of extreme microlissencephaly (see Fig. 4.5c, d), the cerebral cortex at midgestation has at least three layers, but vimentin and nestin (+) radially oriented glia are absent. In addition, radial heterotopias and increased subplate neurons are prominent, as are PVNH, and the germinal matrices are of normal size. We suspect that some of the severe microlissencephalies in this group may be tubulinopathies, but their histology is striking and as of yet unreported in relationship to genetic abnormalities elsewhere.

Seckel syndrome (primordial dwarfism with micrencephaly) is a genetically heterogeneous syndrome that may present with extreme micrencephaly (Fig. 4.15g) probably due to a globally reduced neurogenesis in the face of impaired DNA repair pathways (Fitzgerald et al. 2012). In a single case, we noted that although the hippocampal formations were present, the temporal lobes were much reduced (Fig. 4.15h, i). The neocortex showed poor cytoarchitectural maturation for gestational age, although layers 1 and 2 were distinct. Heterotopic axonal bundles could be found in the molecular layer, and particularly in the lateral temporoparietal lobes, the deep margins of the cortex blended into vague aggregates of heterotopic subcortical neurons (Fig. 4.15j). However, other published reports (McKusick et al. 1967) describe more isolated micrencephaly.

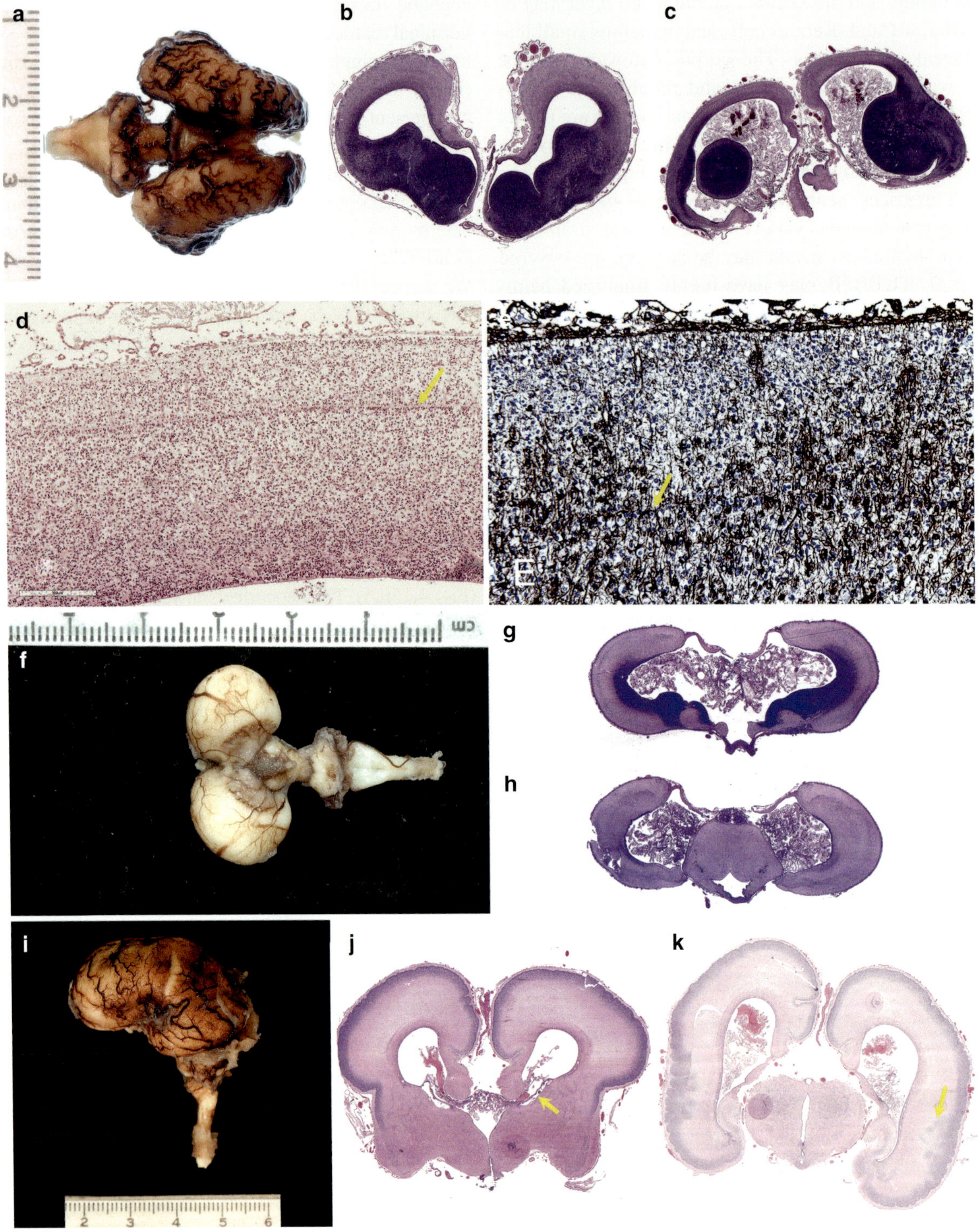

Fig. 4.15 Extreme micrencephaly. (**a**) A 23-week-gestation female with minute cerebral hemispheres, brainstem, and cerebellum. The olfactory bulbs were present. (**b**) and (**c**) Coronal sections through the hemispheres, with relatively enormous lobulated germinal matrices, absent commissural tracts and basal ganglia, reduced and minute thalami, and a very poorly differentiated cerebral mantle without obvious neuronal lamination in the cortex. (**d**) Frontal cortex, demonstrating fairly uniform cellularity other than a distinct lamina splitting the mantle. (**e**) This lamina seems to be made of neuronal cell bodies approaching a layer of glial foot processes (arrow, immunohistochemistry for nestin), although no basal lamina could be stained. (**f**) A 22-week-gestation female, similar to (**a**) with extraordinary simplification and hypoplasia of the entire brain. Note the scale. (**g**) Coronal section of frontal lobes, demonstrating similar features to (**a**) but with a C-shaped cerebral hemisphere bounded medially by choroid plexus as though there is failure of the cortical hem and the adjacent medial neuroepithelium. There are only two layers to the cerebral cortex, and the subpial granular cell layer is widely absent. (**h**) Coronal section, demonstrating hypoplastic thalamus and unusual dorsal relative thickening of diencephalon. The pineal is present. (**i**) Seckel syndrome with dramatic micrencephaly and hypoplasia of temporal lobes. (**j**) Coronal section demonstrates agenesis of the corpus callosum, poorly laminated cortex, and cystic change in the residual germinal matrices (arrow). (**k**) Further posteriorly, the cortex extends irregularly into the mantle, as though there is abortive formation of an insula (arrow)

4.13 Porencephaly and Schizencephaly

A porus is a post-encephaloclastic, full thickness defect in the cerebral mantle such that the ventricle communicates with the arachnoid (Friede 1989a, b); such defects in the fetal brain may result from hemorrhagic or hypoxic–ischemic injury, or from central nervous system infection, especially *Toxoplasma*. When such defects occur prior to the late second trimester, ventricular zone elements may come to line the subcortical walls of the porus, and the surrounding cortex demonstrates a region of incipient polymicrogyria (Fig. 4.16a, b), which may be widespread or local (Fig. 4.16c, d) (Diamandis et al. 2017). As such defects mature, they may largely be filled by the expanding adjacent cortical mantle surrounding them. We use the term schizencephaly (Yakovlev and Wadsworth 1946) if it is to be used at all, to refer to bilateral symmetrically placed pori, where by late gestation, the surrounding cortex and migrated ventricular zone elements are usually expected to at least partially line the walls of the cleft (Friede 1989a, b; Norman et al. 1995); this usage does not to denote a difference in pathogenic process from porencephaly. A fetal porus may have the walls of their clefts lined or unlined by gray matter. The clefts may be closed or open lipped, but these depend on the gestational age at which the encephaloclastic insult occurred, the lag between the injury and the pathological examination, and as well as the gestational age of the brain being examined (e.g., see Fig. 4.16c–f). From the point of view of postmortem fetal examination, the distinction of lined vs unlined seems difficult as a gray matter lining may not have had a chance to develop. Porencephalic defects may be irregularly placed, especially when due to microvascular disease (Fig. 4.16e, f), but when due to severe maternal illness or placental failure, on occasion, they may be strikingly symmetrical, falsely suggesting a primary abnormality of neural development (Fig. 4.16g, h). Both porencephaly and schizencephaly of early ischemic origin tend to demonstrate thalamic injury and at fetal autopsy may demonstrate blood pigment near the cortical lesion, as well as in the subjacent germinal matrix and in the thecal sac of the spinal cord, suggesting reperfusion injury as a component of the antecedent insult.

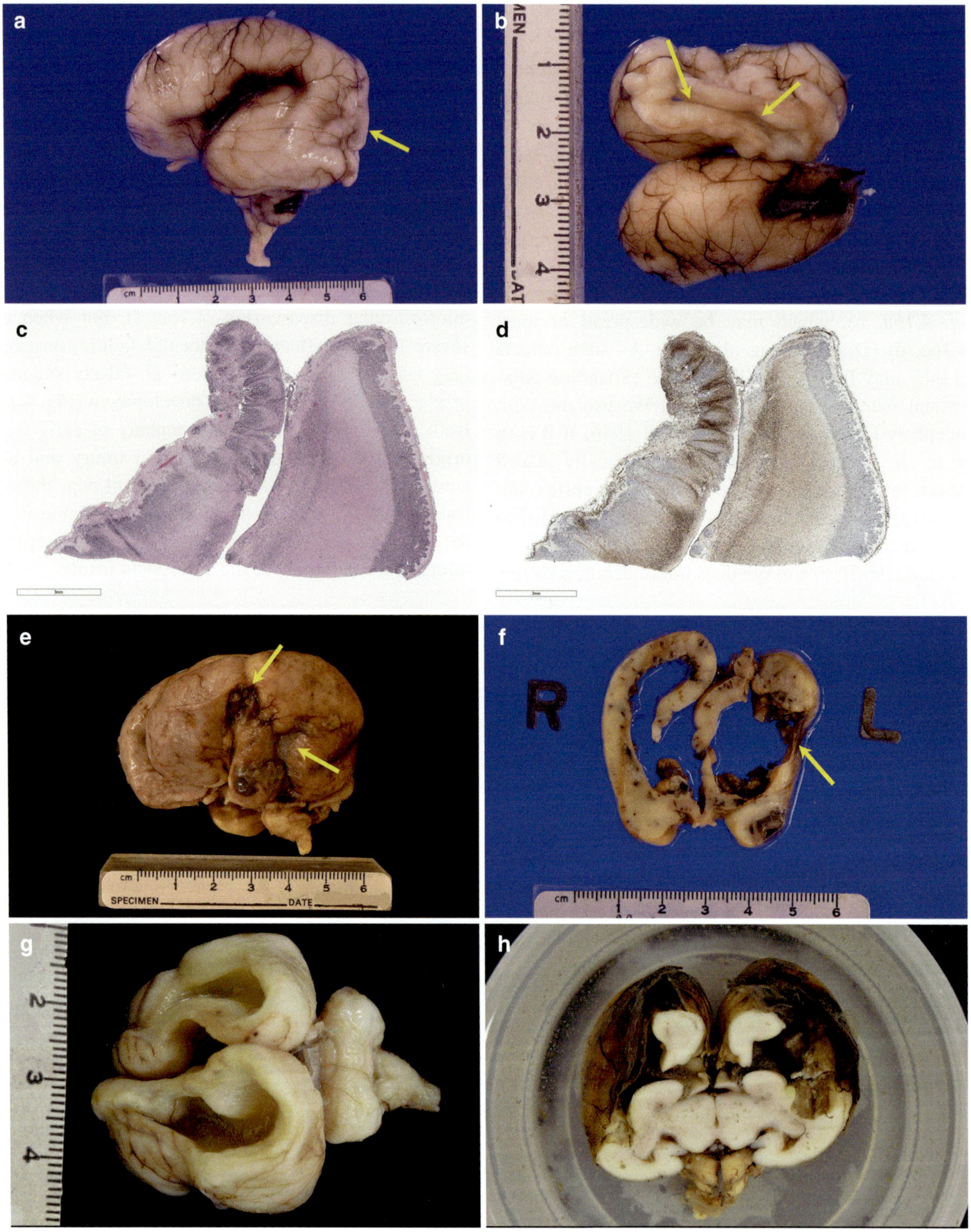

Fig. 4.16 Porencephaly and schizencephaly. (**a**) A 23-week-gestation female with occipital incipient polymicrogyria (arrow). (**b**) On one occipital pole, a membrane-covered defect (arrows) is surrounded by the lesional cortex. (**c**) Section through both sides of the defect demonstrates the porus, with both lips of the porus bearing incipient polymicrogyria, albeit to different extents. Note that while one internal wall of the porus closely abuts the incipient polymicrogyric cortex, the gray matter has not yet developed to completely line the other. (**d**) The same section as (**c**) with immunohistochemical staining for nestin, demonstrating multiple radially oriented condensations of radial glia extending from the deep surface to the overgrown leptomeninges surrounding nodules of cortical tissue. (**e**) A 22-week-gestation male with arthrogryposis; the brain is irregularly scarred and contracted with lateral membranous areas in the Sylvian fissure and lateral temporal lobe (arrows). (**f**) Coronal section demonstrating left lateral frontal porus (arrow) with necrotic and discolored intraventricular material. Microscopy demonstrated a widespread microvascular thrombotic disease. Genetic investigations including whole exome sequencing were unrevealing. (**g**) A 22-week-gestation female with bilateral symmetrical parieto-occipital pori (schizencephaly) in monochorionic twin after previous demise of twin. (**h**) A 22-week-gestation female with bilateral peri-Sylvian pori (schizencephaly) sparing the basal and paramedian cortex

4.14 Hydranencephaly

In hydranencephaly, the large majority of the cerebral mantle is destroyed or severely injured, usually by hypoxic–ischemic or viral injury. As a consequence, the ventricles are expanded, and the injured mantle is globally reduced to a fibrous or thinly gliotic membrane that may be adherent to the overlying dura (Fig. 4.17a, b), with only residual trabeculae (Fig. 4.17c), and variable sparing of basal, deep, and paramedian cortex. Brainstem, cerebellar, and spinal cord injury is common. Post-encephaloclastic hydranencephaly may also be secondary to syndromic microvascular pathologies such as Fowler disease and probably Roberts syndrome (He et al. 2023; Ekong and Rozdilsky 1978; Strasser et al. 2024).

Truncating mutations in CEPP-22, a mitotic spindle organizing protein, have been associated with an autosomal recessive malformation syndrome, in which the dorsal aspects of both cerebral hemispheres are replaced by a membrane (Fig. 4.17d, e) and the ventral parts are reduced to a flattened simplified disk without an interventricular septum (Fig. 4.17f–h) (Frosk et al. 2017) with binucleate neurons in the remaining CNS and sympathetic and dorsal root ganglia (Fig. 4.17i, j). However, the dorsal cyst in our case is lined by a continuous layer of cuboidal ciliated epithelium continuous with distinct choroid plexus. Histology suggests that hydranencephaly is secondary to an intrinsic defect in the dorsal telencephalic neuroepithelium more than injury.

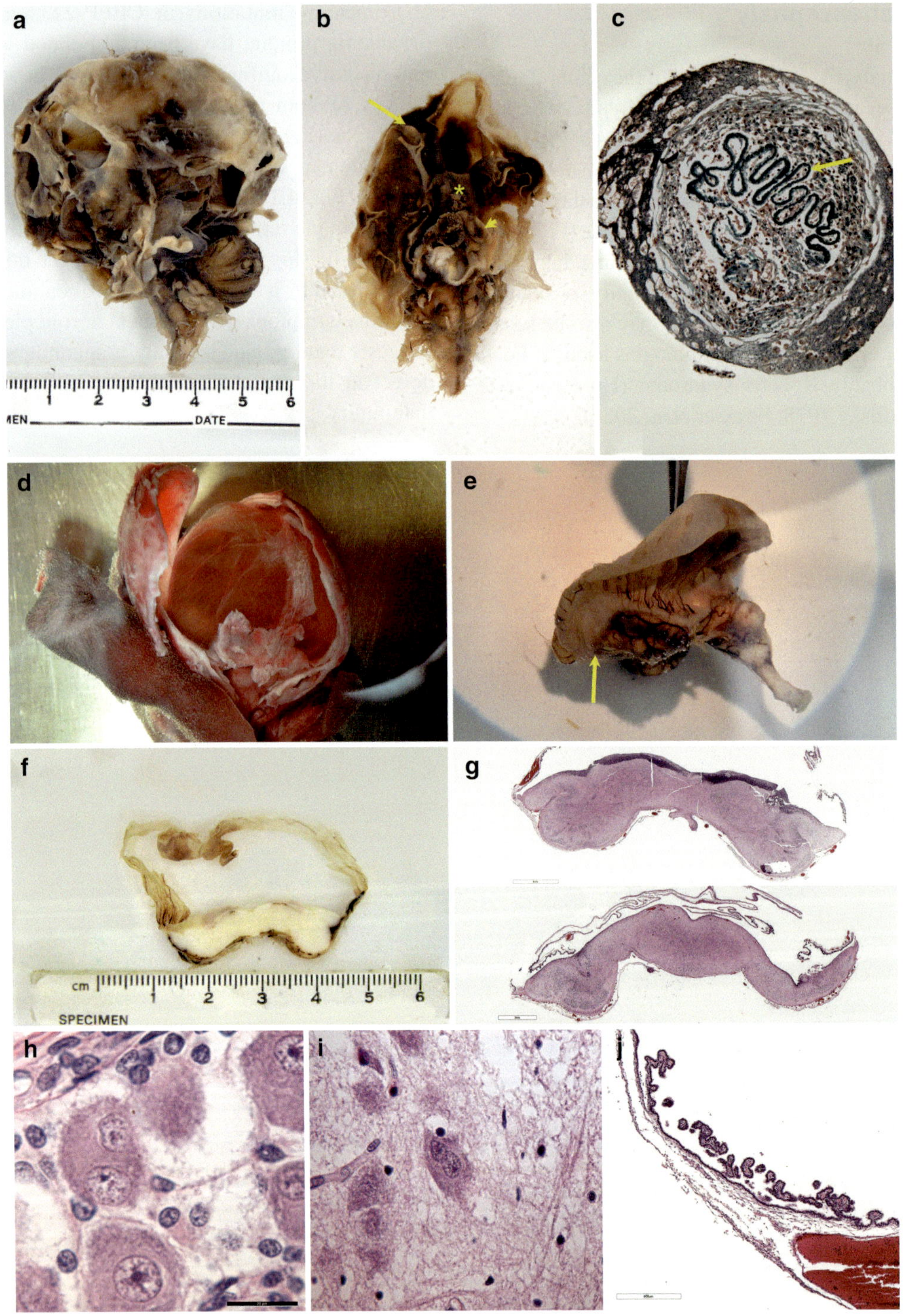

Fig. 4.17 Hydranencephaly. (**a**) A 28-week-gestation female with multiple old large placental infarcts occupying 80% of the placental disk. The cranial dura had been removed with the brainstem and cerebellum and contains cystic dilated spaces (arrow). (**b**) Coronal section through (*A*) facing posteriorly with the brainstem and cerebellum inferiorly. The brain is reduced to trabeculae crossing the large fluid-filled spaces. The falx (arrow) is intact, but the rostral brainstem ends in a shaggy mass topped by the pineal (asterisks) and a residual hematoma (arrowhead). (**c**) Section of trabeculae demonstrating residual neuroglia and macrophages coating an occluded artery with residual elastic lamina (arrow, elastic trichrome stain). (**d**) CEPP-22 mutation: A 22-week-gestation male with renal cystic dysplasia, pulmonary hypoplasia, cardiac valvular dysplasia, and features of fetal akinesia. The cerebral hemispheres dorsally are reduced to a thin-walled membrane. (**e**) The same case as (**d**). The cyst collapsed, and the basal hemispheres (arrow) are a flat disk, but the cerebellum and brainstem are intact although small. (**f**) Coronal sections demonstrate a continuous dorsal membrane attached to the basal aspect of the brain but no other ventricular structures. (**g**) Whole mounts demonstrate a single plate-like basal mass surmounted by thin germinal matrices without well-defined cortex. (**h**) and (**i**) Dorsal root ganglia and motor neurons of the spinal cord with distinct binucleation could be found. (**j**) The dorsal cerebral mantle is replaced by a membrane bearing cuboidal lining that is continuous laterally with choroid plexus epithelium

References

Alcantara D, Timms AE, Gripp K, Baker L, Park K, Collins S, Cheng C, Stewart F, Mehta SG, Saggar A, Sztriha L, Zombor M, Caluseriu O, Mesterman R, Van Allen MI, Jacquinet A, Ygberg S, Bernstein JA, Wenger AM, Guturu H, Bejerano G, Gomez-Ospina N, Lehman A, Alfei E, Pantaleoni C, Conti V, Guerrini R, Moog U, Graham JM Jr, Hevner R, Dobyns WB, O'Driscoll M, Mirzaa GM. Mutations of AKT3 are associated with a wide spectrum of developmental disorders including extreme megalencephaly. Brain. 2017;140(10):2610–2622. https://doi.org/10.1093/brain/awx203

Altman J, Bayer SA. Regional differences in the stratified transitional field and the honeycomb matrix of the developing human cerebral cortex. J Neurocytol. 2002;31(8–9):613–32. https://doi.org/10.1023/a:1025787427576. PMID: 14501203.

Alzu'bi A, Lindsay S, Kerwin J, et al. Distinct cortical and sub-cortical neurogenic domains for GABAergic interneuron precursor transcription factors NKX2.1, OLIG2 and COUP-TFII in early fetal human telencephalon. Brain Struct Funct. 2017;222:2309–28. https://doi.org/10.1007/s00429-016-1343.

Aslam K, Saeed A, Saeed HI, Bashir R, Abid H, Akhtar R, Habib N, Khan R, Asif R, Rafiq S, Asif M, Makhdoom EUH, Hussain MS, Baig SM, Anjum I. Molecular genetics, neuroimaging outcomes, and structural analyses of novel and recurrent variants of WDR62 gene in two consanguineous Pakistani families with autosomal recessive primary microcephaly. Mol Biol Rep. 2024;51(1):783. https://doi.org/10.1007/s11033-024-0972.

Bahi-Buisson N, Poirier K, Fourniol F, Saillour Y, Valence S, Lebrun N, Hully M, Bianco CF, Boddaert N, Elie C, Lascelles K, Souville I; LIS-Tubulinopathies Consortium; Beldjord C, Chelly J. The wide spectrum of tubulinopathies: what are the key features for the diagnosis? Brain. 2014;137(Pt 6):1676–700. https://doi.org/10.1093/brain/awu082. PMID: 24860126.

Brock S, Cools F, Jansen AC. Neuropathology of genetically defined malformations of cortical development-A systematic literature review. Neuropathol Appl Neurobiol 2021a;47(5):585–602. https://doi.org/10.1111/nan.12696. Epub 2021 Feb 14. PMID: 33480109; PMCID: PMC8359484.

Brock S, Vanderhasselt T, Vermaning S, Keymolen K, Régal L, Romaniello R, Wieczorek D, Storm TM, Schaeferhoff K, Hehr U, Kuechler A, Krägeloh-Mann I, Haack TB, Kasteleijn E, Schot R, Mancini GMS, Webster R, Mohammad S, Leventer RJ, Mirzaa G, Dobyns WB, Bahi-Buisson N, Meuwissen M, Jansen AC, Stouffs K. Defining the phenotypical spectrum associated with variants in TUBB2A. J Med Genet. 2021b;58(1):33–40. https://doi.org/10.1136/jmedgenet-2019-106740. Epub 2020 Jun 22. PMID: 32571897; PMCID: PMC7803914.

Cappello S, Gray MJ, Badouel C, Lange S, Einsiedler M, Srour M, Chitayat D, Hamdan FF, Jenkins ZA, Morgan T, Preitner N, Uster T, Thomas J, Shannon P, Morrison V, Di Donato N, Van Maldergem L, Neuhann T, Newbury-Ecob R, Swinkells M, Terhal P, Wilson LC, Zwijnenburg PJ, Sutherland-Smith AJ, Black MA, Markie D, Michaud JL, Simpson MA, Mansour S, McNeill H, Götz M, Robertson SP. Mutations in genes encoding the cadherin receptor-ligand pair DCHS1 and FAT4 disrupt cerebral cortical development. Nat Genet. 2013;45(11):1300–8. https://doi.org/10.1038/ng.2765. Epub 2013 Sep 22. PMID: 24056717.

Causeret F, Moreau MX, Pierani A, Blanquie O. The multiple facets of Cajal-Retzius neurons. Development. 2021;148(11):dev199409. https://doi.org/10.1242/dev.199409. Epub 2021 May 28. PMID: 34047341.

de Vareilles H, Rivière D, Mangin JF, Dubois J. Development of cortical folds in the human brain: an attempt to review biological hypotheses, early neuroimaging investigations and functional correlates. Dev Cogn Neurosci. 2023;61:101249. https://doi.org/10.1016/j.dcn.2023.101249. Epub 2023 Apr 25. PMID: 37141790; PMCID: PMC10311195.

deAzevedo LC, Fallet C, Moura-Neto V, Daumas-Duport C, Hedin-Pereira C, Lent R. Cortical radial glial cells in human fetuses: depth-correlated transformation into astrocytes. J Neurobiol. 2003;55(3):288–98. https://doi.org/10.1002/neu.10205. PMID: 12717699.

Devisme L, Bouchet C, Gonzalès M, Alanio E, Bazin A, Bessières B, Bigi N, Blanchet P, Bonneau D, Bonnières M, Bucourt M, Carles D, Clarisse B, Delahaye S, Fallet-Bianco C, Figarella-Branger D, Gaillard D, Gasser B, Delezoide AL, Guimiot F, Joubert M, Laurent N, Laquerrière A, Liprandi A, Loget P, Marcorelles P, Martinovic J, Menez F, Patrier S, Pelluard F, Perez MJ, Rouleau C, Triau S, Attié-Bitach T, Vuillaumier-Barrot S, Seta N, Encha-Razavi F. Cobblestone lissencephaly: neuropathological subtypes and correlations with genes of dystroglycanopathies. Brain. 2012;135(Pt 2):469–482. https://doi.org/10.1093/brain/awr357. Epub 2012 Feb 9. PMID: 22323514.

Diamandis P, Chitayat D, Toi A, Blaser S, Shannon P. The pathology of incipient polymicrogyria. Brain Dev. 2017;39(1):23–39. https://doi.org/10.1016/j.braindev.2016.06.005. Epub 2016 Jul 9. PMID: 27406708.

Dobyns WB, Reiner O, Carrozzo R, Ledbetter DH. Lissencephaly. A human brain malformation associated with deletion of the LIS1 gene located at chromosome 17p13. JAMA. 1993;270(23):2838–42. https://doi.org/10.1001/jama.270.23.2838. PMID: 7907669.

Ekong CE, Rozdilsky B. Hydranencephaly in association with Roberts syndrome. Can J Neurol Sci 1978 May;5(2):253–255. doi: https://doi.org/10.1017/s0317167100024628. PMID: 667753.

Fallet-Bianco C, Laquerrière A, Poirier K, Razavi F, Guimiot F, Dias P, Loeuillet L, Lascelles K, Beldjord C, Carion N, Toussaint A, Revencu N, Addor MC, Lhermitte B, Gonzales M, Martinovich J, Bessieres B, Marcy-Bonnière M, Jossic F, Marcorelles P, Loget P, Chelly J, Bahi-Buisson N. Mutations in tubulin genes are frequent causes of various foetal malformations of cortical development including microlissencephaly. Acta Neuropathol Commun. 2014;2:69. https://doi.org/10.1186/2051-5960-2-69. PMID: 25059107; PMCID: PMC4222268.

Fitzgerald B, O'Driscoll M, Chong K, Keating S, Shannon P. Neuropathology of fetal stage Seckel syndrome: a case report providing a morphological correlate for the emerging molecular mechanisms. Brain Dev. 2012;34(3):238–43. https://doi.org/10.1016/j.braindev.2011.05.007. Epub 2011 Jun 12. PMID: 21669506.

Forman MS, Squier W, Dobyns WB, Golden JA. Genotypically define lissencephalies show distinct pathologies. J Neuropathol Exp Neurol. 2005;64(10):847–57.

Friede, RL 1989a Normal development and basic reactions (pp. 11–12) In: Developmental neuropathology (Second Edition), Springer Verlag.

Friede RL. Porencephaly, hydranencephaly, multicystic encephalopathy. In: Developmental neuropathology. 2nd ed. Springer Verlag; 1989b. p. 28–43.

Frosk P, Arts HH, Philippe J, Gunn CS, Brown EL, Chodirker B, Simard L, Majewski J, Fahiminiya S, Russell C, Liu YP; FORGE Canada Consortium; Canadian Rare Diseases: Models & Mechanisms Network; Hegele R, Katsanis N, Goerz C, Del Bigio MR, Davis EE. A truncating mutation in CEP55 is the likely cause of MARCH, a novel syndrome affecting neuronal mitosis. J Med Genet. 2017;54(7):490–501. https://doi.org/10.1136/jmedgenet-2016-104296. Epub 2017 Mar 6. PMID: 28264986; PMCID: PMC5502313.

Gins C, Guimiot F, Drunat S, Prévost C, Rosenblatt J, Capri Y, Letard P, Khung-Savatovsky S, Mahi Henni MA, Elalaoui SC, Alison M, Guilmin Crepon S, Gressens P, Verloes A, Basto R, El Ghouzzi V, Passemard S. Radial microbrain (Micrencephaly) is caused by a recurrent variant in the RTTN gene. Neurol Genet. 2025;11(2):e200221. https://doi.org/10.1212/NXG.0000000000200221. PMID: 40151166; PMCID: PMC11949245. 8-7. PMID: 38926176.

Hansen DV, Lui JH, Parker PR, Kriegstein AR. Neurogenic radial glia in the outer subventricular zone of human neocortex. Nature. 2010;464(7288):554–61. https://doi.org/10.1038/nature08845. PMID: 20154730.

He S, Chen S, Li SJ, Zhang JW, Liang XL. Complex cerebrovascular diseases in Roberts syndrome caused by novel biallelic ESCO2 variations. Mol Genet Genomic Med. 2023;11(6):e2177. https://doi.org/10.1002/mgg3.2177. Epub 2023 Mar 31. PMID: 37002187; PMCID: PMC10265053.

Hino-Shishikura A, Niwa T, Aida N, Okabe T, Nagaoka T, Shibasaki J. Periventricular nodular heterotopia is related to severity of the hindbrain deformity in Chiari II malformation. Pediatr Radiol. 2012;42(10):1212–7. https://doi.org/10.1007/s00247-012-2431-1. Epub 2012 Aug 11. PMID: 22886376.

Hrabowska M. Morphogenesis of cerebral matrix ectopies in human fetus and newborn. J Hirnforsch. 1978;19(6):485–95. PMID: 225381.

Jansen AC, Robitaille Y, Honavar M, Mullatti N, Leventer RJ, Andermann E, Andermann F, Squier W. The histopathology of polymicrogyria: a series of 71 brain autopsy studies. Dev Med Child Neurol. 2016;58(1):39–48. https://doi.org/10.1111/dmcn.12840. Epub 2015 Jul 14. PMID: 26179148.

Keith J, Shannon P. Brain pathology of lissencephaly type 2 with an ISPD pathogenic variant. Neuropathol Appl Neurobiol. 2023;49(5):e12939. https://doi.org/10.1111/nan.12939. PMID: 37766395.

Laquerriere A, Gonzales M, Saillour Y, Cavallin M, Joyē N, Quēlin C, Bidat L, Dommergues M, Plessis G, Encha-Razavi F, Chelly J, Bahi-Buisson N, Poirier K. De novo TUBB2B mutation causes fetal akinesia deformation sequence with microlissencephaly: an unusual presentation of tubulinopathy. Eur J Med Genet. 2016;59(4):249–56. https://doi.org/10.1016/j.ejmg.2015.12.007.

Leventer RJ, Cardoso C, Ledbetter DH, Dobyns WB. LIS1 missense mutations cause milder lissencephaly phenotypes including a child with normal IQ. Neurology. 2001;57(3):416–422. https://doi.org/10.1212/wnl.57.3.416. PMID: 11502906.

Llinares-Benadero C, Borrell V. Deconstructing cortical folding: genetic, cellular and mechanical determinants. Nat Rev Neurosci. 2019;20:161–76. https://doi-org.myaccess.library.utoronto.ca/10.1038/s41583-018-0112-2.

McKusick VA, Mahloudji M, Abbott MH, Lindenberg R, Kepas D. Seckel's bird-headed dwarfism. N Engl J Med. 1967;277(6):279–86. https://doi.org/10.1056/NEJM196708102770602. PMID: 4378248.

Meyer G, González-Gómez M. The Subpial granular layer and transient versus persisting Cajal-Retzius neurons of the fetal human cortex. Cereb Cortex. 2018;28(6):2043–58. https://doi.org/10.1093/cercor/bhx110. PMID: 28472243.

Norman MG, McGillivray BC Kalousek DK, Hill A, Poskitt KJ with Becker LE, Cochrane DD, Muenke M. Ch. 18 Antenatal and perinatal destructive lesions (Disruptions) in congenital malformations of the brain: pathologic, embryologic, clinical, radiologic, and genetic aspects. New York: Oxford University Press; 1995. pp. 403–418.

Oegema R, Barkovich AJ, Mancini GMS, Guerrini R, Dobyns WB. Subcortical heterotopic gray matter brain malformations: Classification study of 107 individuals. Neurology. 2019;93(14):e1360–73. https://doi.org/10.1212/WNL.0000000000008200. Epub 2019 Sep 4. PMID: 31484711; PMCID: PMC6814414.

Parrini E, Ramazzotti A, Dobyns WB, Mei D, Moro F, Veggiotti P, et al. Periventricular heterotopia: phenotypic heterogeneity and correlation with Filamin A mutations. Brain. 2006;129(Pt 7):1892–906. https://doi.org/10.1093/brain/awl125. Epub 2006 May 9. PMID: 16684786.

Rakic S, Zecevic N. Emerging complexity of layer I in human cerebral cortex. Cereb Cortex. 2003;13(10):1072–1083. https://doi.org/10.1093/cercor/13.10.1072. PMID: 12967924.

Rasool S, Baig JM, Moawia A, Ahmad I, Iqbal M, Waseem SS, et al. An update of pathogenic variants in ASPM, WDR62, CDK5RAP2, STIL, CENPJ, and CEP135 underlying autosomal recessive primary microcephaly in 32 consanguineous families from Pakistan. Mol Genet Genomic Med. 2020;8(9):e1408. https://doi.org/10.1002/mgg3.1408. Epub 2020 Jul 17. PMID: 32677750; PMCID: PMC7507472.

Rezazadeh A, Bercovici E, Kiehl TR, Chow EW, Krings T, Bassett AS, Andrade DM. Periventricular nodular heterotopia in 22q11.2 deletion and frontal lobe migration. Ann Clin Transl Neurol. 2018;5(11):1314–22. https://doi.org/10.1002/acn3.641. PMID: 30480026; PMCID: PMC6243376.

Shannon P, Hum C, Parks T, Schauer GM, Chitayat D, Chong K, Shinar S, Blaser S, Moore G, Van Mieghem T. Brain and placental pathology in fetal COL4A1 related disease. Pediatr Dev Pathol. 2021;24(3):175–86. https://doi.org/10.1177/1093526620984083. Epub 2021 Jan 21. PMID: 33475042.

Sheen VL, Ferland RJ, Neal J, Harney M, Hill RS, Banham A, Brown P, Chenn A, Corbo J, Hecht J, Folkerth R, Walsh CA. Neocortical neuronal arrangement in Miller Dieker syndrome. Acta Neuropathol. 2006;111(5):489–96. https://doi.org/10.1007/s00401-005-0010-3. Epub 2006 Feb 3. PMID: 16456669.

Singh K, Lau CK, Manigrasso G, Gama JB, Gassmann R, Carter AP. Molecular mechanism of dynein-dynactin complex assembly by LIS1. Science. 2024;383(6690):eadk8544. https://doi.org/10.1126/science.adk8544. Epub 2024 Mar 29. PMID: 38547289; PMCID: PMC7615804.

Sprugnoli G, Vatti G, Rossi S, Cerase A, Renieri A, Mencarelli MA, Zara F, Rossi A, Santarnecchi E. Functional connectivity and genetic profile of a "double-cortex"-like malformation. Front Integr Neurosci. 2018;12:22. https://doi.org/10.3389/fnint.2018.00022. PMID: 29946244; PMCID: PMC6005822.

Squier W, Jansen A. Polymicrogyria: pathology, fetal origins and mechanisms. Acta Neuropathol Commun. 2014;2:80. https://doi.org/10.1186/s40478-014-0080-3. PMID: 25047116; PMCID: PMC4149230.

Strasser AS, Gonzalez-Reiche AS, Zhou X, Valdebenito-Maturana B, Ye X, Zhang B, Wu M, van Bakel H, Jabs EW. Limb reduction in an Esco2 cohesinopathy mouse model is mediated by p53-dependent apoptosis and vascular disruption. Nat Commun. 2024;15(1):7154. https://doi.org/10.1038/s41467-024-51328-3. PMID: 39168984; PMCID: PMC11339411.

Vuillaumier-Barrot S, Bouchet-Séraphin C, Chelbi M, Devisme L, Quentin S, Gazal S, Laquerrière A, Fallet-Bianco C, Loget P, Odent S, Carles D, Bazin A, Aziza J, Clemenson A, Guimiot F, Bonnière M, Monnot S, Bole-Feysot C, Bernard JP, Loeuillet L, Gonzales M, Socha K, Grandchamp B, Attié-Bitach T, Encha-Razavi F, Seta N. Identification of mutations in TMEM5 and ISPD as a cause of severe cobblestone lissencephaly. Am J Hum Genet. 2012;91(6):1135–43. https://doi.org/10.1016/j.ajhg.2012.10.009. PMID: 23217329; PMCID: PMC3516603.b;135(Pt 2):469–82. doi: 10.1093/brain/awr357. Epub 2012 Feb 9. PMID: 22323514.

Weber M, Jaber D, Encha-Razavi F, Julien E, Grevoul-Fesquet J, Steffann J, Melki J, Martinovic J. Broadening the phenotypic spectrum of TUBA1A tubulinopathy to syndromic arthrogryposis multiplex congenita. Am J Med Genet A. 2022;188(8):2331–8. https://doi.org/10.1002/ajmg.a.62866. Epub 2022 Jun 10. PMID: 35686685.

Yakovlev PI, Wadsworth RC. Schizencephalies; a study of the congenital clefts in the cerebral mantle; clefts with fused lips. J Neuropathol Exp Neurol. 1946;5:116–30. https://doi.org/10.1097/00005072-194604000-00003. PMID: 21026933.

Zaki MS, Salam GM, Saleem SN, Dobyns WB, Issa MY, Sattar S, Gleeson JG. New recessive syndrome of microcephaly, cerebellar hypoplasia, and congenital heart conduction defect. Am J Med Genet A. 2011;155A(12):3035–3041. https://doi.org/10.1002/ajmg.a.34078. Epub 2011 Oct 14. PMID: 22002884; PMCID: PMC3415795.

5 Overgrowth Syndromes

Overgrowth syndromes are characterized by a global or regional bulk increase in tissue volume. In fetal brain, these are generally characterized by a disorganized neural architecture in the affected areas. Generally, overgrowth is initiated by constitutional or somatic mutations in elements of the PIK3–AKT–mTOR pathway. These include AKT1, AKT3, DEPDC5, FGFR2 and FGFR3, MTOR, NPRL2, NPRL3, PIK3CA, PIK3R2, PTEN, TSC1, and TSC2. Poorly regulated activation of a major promitotic pathway in either the germline or as somatic mutations in pluripotent central nervous system stem cells seems to lead to an excess generation of differentiated elements.

5.1 Megalencephaly

Megalencephaly is an expansion of the brain mass by more than two times the standard deviation above the mean of brain mass for age and weight (Dobyns and Mirzaa 2019). In PIK3R2-related disease, activating mutations of the pathway result in an expanded brain with abnormal contour (Fig. 5.1a), with the cerebellum and spinal cord less strikingly affected than the cerebral hemispheres. The hemispheres may show ventriculomegaly with expanded germinal matrices (Fig. 5.1b). The cortical mantle may be expanded, but despite the gross abnormalities in contour, the low-power pathologic findings can be subtle (Fig. 5.1c). The affected cerebrum may display irregular migration anomalies with periventricular nodular heterotopias, band heterotopias, leptomeningeal heterotopias, and irregular cortical organization and premature expression of synaptophysin (Fig. 5.1d–f) (Sarnat et al. 2010). On imaging, peri-Sylvian polymicrogyria may be prominent (Mirzaa et al. 2015). We have encountered one fetal case of megalencephaly without genetic correlation that demonstrated marked pervasive abnormalities of migration and maturation involving both the cerebral hemispheres and the cerebellum (Fig. 5.2a–h). Similar features have been reported in patients with activating germline mutations in AKT3, which may be accompanied by polydactyly (Wang et al. 2025, Mirzaa et al. 2012).

P. Shannon et al., *Atlas of Neurodevelopmental Pathology*, https://doi.org/10.1007/978-3-032-14148-4_5

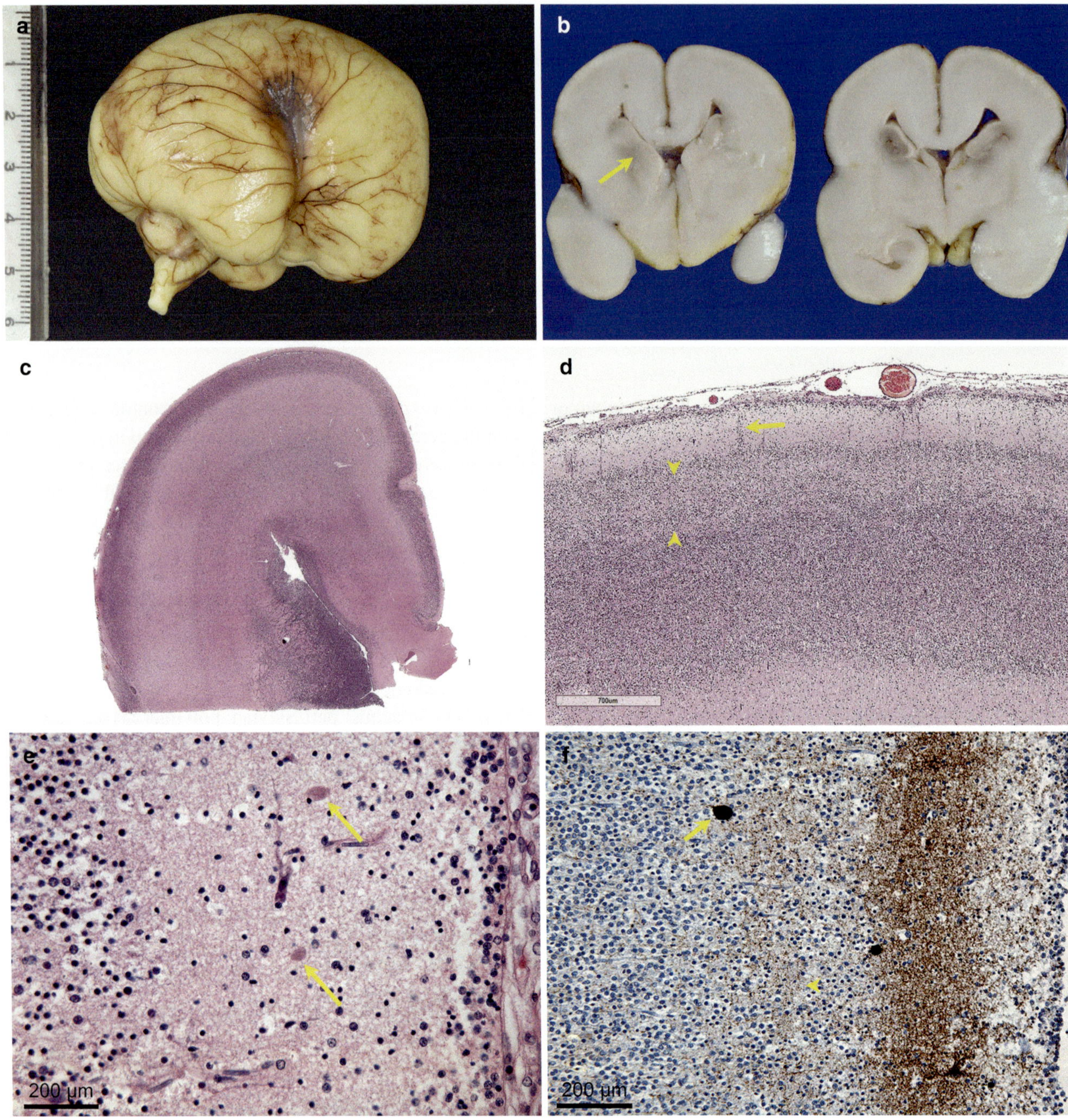

Fig. 5.1 (**a**) Megalencephaly at 22 weeks gestation with PIK3R2 activating germline mutation. The brain weight is over twice that expected for gestational age, with a massively and symmetrically expanded cerebrum with squared-off appearance of the frontal lobe and an almost vertical Sylvian fissure. (**b**) Coronal section of (**a**) demonstrating expanded cortical mantle and large germinal matrices. (**c**) Frontal cortex demonstrating premature and abnormal lamination with hypocellularity in future layer 3 (arrows). (**d**) Layer 1 of the illustrated cortex demonstrating numerous swollen processes. (**e**) Such swollen processes in this case stain for reelin, as do the Cajal–Retzius neurons (arrows). (**f**) Staining for synaptophysin (molecular layer to the right) demonstrates swollen processes and a premature band of staining (between arrows) corresponding to the layer between arrows in (**c**)

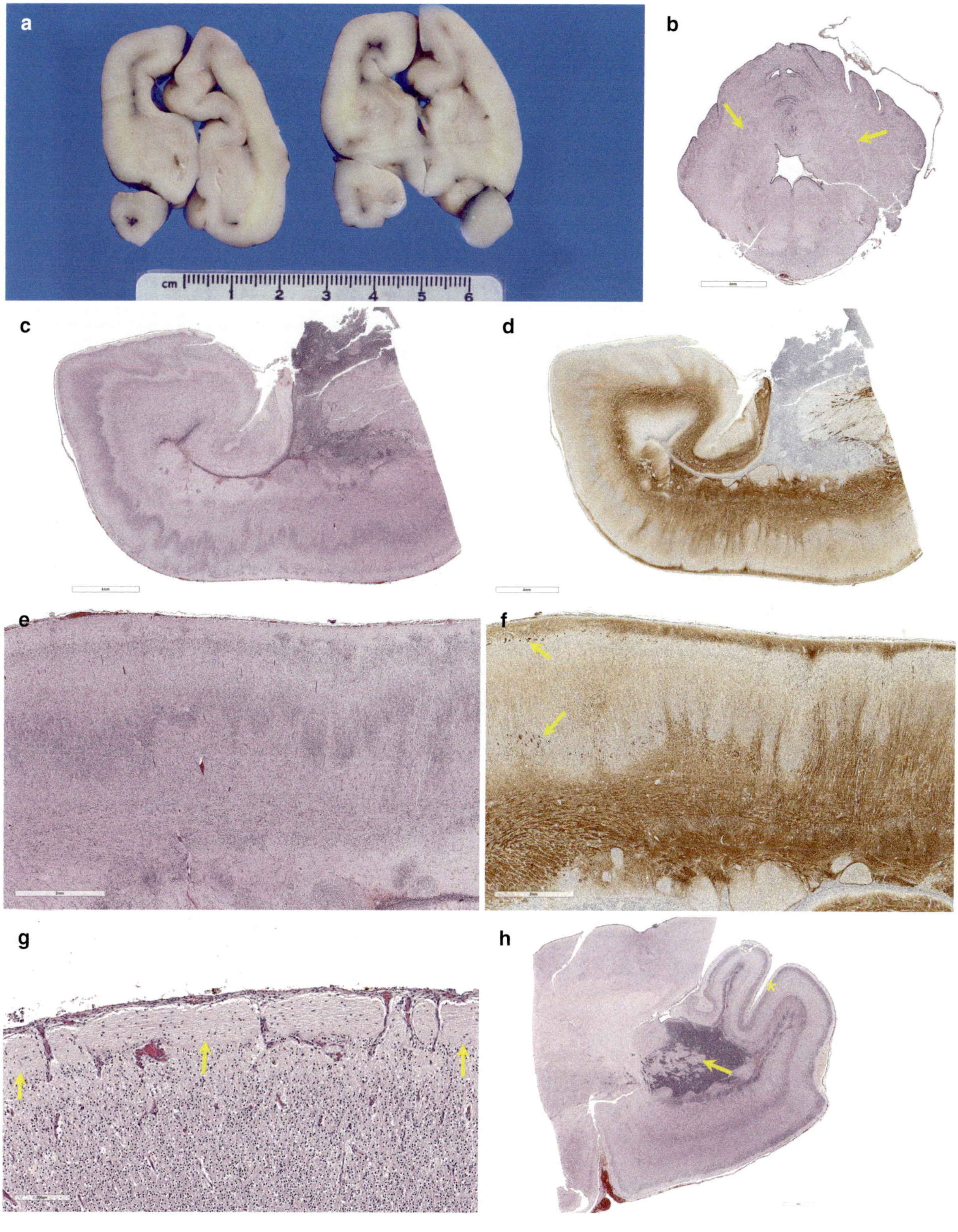

Fig. 5.2 (**a**) Megalencephaly at 18 weeks, with unknown genetic etiology. The supratentorial brain is irregularly expanded with ventriculomegaly, expanded germinal matrices, and agenesis of the corpus callosum. (**b**) The cerebellum demonstrates premature convolution and condensation of the dentate nuclei. (**c**) Hemispheric section (dorsal to the left, ventral to the right) demonstrating irregular cortical ribbon and expanded germinal matrix. (**d**) Immunohistochemistry for neurofilament light chain, demonstrating innumerable periventricular heterotopias and highlighting the irregular cortical ribbon. (**e**) Cortical mantle, demonstrating alternating cellular and acellular layers, suggesting possible band heterotopia morphology. (**f**) Immunohistochemistry for neurofilament light chain, demonstrating irregular numerous tangentially directed axonal tracts (arrows). (**g**) In multiple areas, there is a confluent superficial layer of axons sandwiched by a deep and superficial vascular network, suggesting leptomeningeal heterotopias. (**h**) Temporal lobe (medial is superior portion, and inferior is to right) demonstrating massive expansion of germinal matrix tissue with irregular nodular maturation (arrow) as well as premature deep sulcation (asterisk: compare to Fig. 5.6)

5.2 Hemimegalencephaly

In hemimegalencephaly, one cerebral hemisphere with or without the associated cerebellum is markedly enlarged compared to the contralateral hemisphere, and in dysplastic hemimegalencephaly, the enlargement is accompanied by cortical and subcortical abnormalities. Fetal cases are occasionally described, demonstrating periventricular nodular heterotopias, incipient polymicrogyria, double cortex-like heterotopias, and leptomeningeal glioneuronal heterotopias (Itoh et al. 2023). We have seen two cases of hemimegalencephaly—one at midgestation (Fig. 5.3a) with small predominantly frontal leptomeningeal heterotopias and an irregular arrangement of deep axonal tracts (Fig. 5.3b–d)—and the germinal matrix of the affected hemisphere was enlarged and demonstrated foci of necrosis. The neocortex demonstrated premature and irregular layering as well as poor distinction of the cortical plate from the subplate. Neuronal and glial cytological abnormalities were muted at midgestation. In one case in our experience, at term gestation, polymicrogyria with leptomeningeal overgrowth (Fig. 5.3e) and cortical disarray (Fig. 5.3f) with neuronal malorientation were also evident. In the other at midgestation the cerebellum was unaffected, but in the case at term, the cerebellum demonstrated extensive areas of dysplasia (Fig. 5.3g), although the dentate nucleus and inferior olivary nuclear complex were appropriate for age. The cortex in the enlarged cerebrum may be dysplastic, and contain dysmorphic neurons that may be tau immunoreactive (Winden et al. 2015).

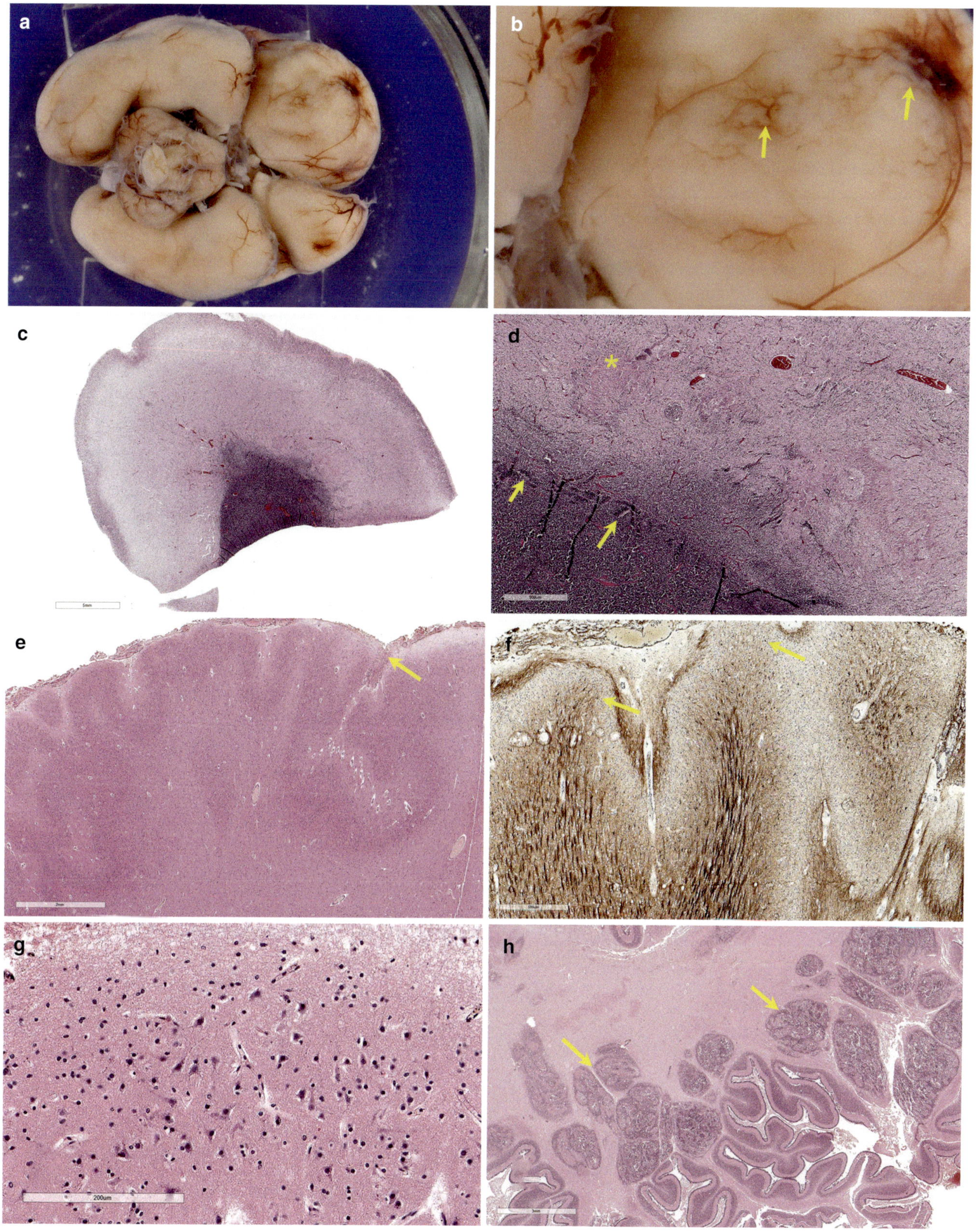

Fig. 5.3 (**a**) A 22-week-gestation fetus with hemimegalencephaly, demonstrating marked enlargement of the entire right hemisphere. (**b**) Numerous small leptomeningeal heterotopias (arrows) along the orbitofrontal cortex, with hypoplastic olfactory bulb and tract. (**c**) Affected frontal cortex with thickened cerebral mantle and markedly expanded germinal matrix. (**d**) Multiple foci of germinal matrix necrosis (arrows) and a chaotic arrangement of transitional zone axonal bundles are noted (asterisk). (**e**) Frontal neocortex from a 36-week-gestation fetus with megalencephaly, demonstrating polymicrogyria with fused gyri and thinned cortical ribbon, with areas of leptomeningeal overgrowth (arrows). (**f**) Neurofilament staining demonstrating radially directed axonal bundles extending from the cortex, many of which originate from enlarged superficial darkly staining neurons (arrows). (**g**) Superficial cortex demonstrates innumerable maloriented neurons in layer 2 (molecular layer at top of image). (**h**) Cerebellar cortex in the same case as (g), with large confluent islands of cerebellar dysplasia in the lateral neocerebellum

5.3 Tuberous Sclerosis

Tuberous sclerosis (TSC1 and TSC2, MIM #19110 61354) is a multisystem disease marked by proliferative benign lesions predominantly in the central nervous system, heart, skin, and lungs.

The histological hallmark of tuberous sclerosis in the central nervous system is the presence of a transmantle cerebral dysplasia characterized in the affected areas by aggregates of balloon cells (Fig. 5.4a). Balloon cells are possibly radial glia derivatives, although some have also hypothesized that at least a subpopulation of balloon cells represent abnormal progenitor cells (Yasin et al. 2010). Balloon cells show abundant glassy eosinophilic cytoplasm, tapering irregular cytoplasmic processes and one or more oval nuclei with nucleoli and oval nuclei. In our experience, these cells stain readily for nestin, alpha-beta crystallin, and vimentin and variably for GFAP (Fig. 5.4b). Balloon cells may form aggregates in ventricular zone (subependymal nodules and subependymal giant cell astrocytomas), in the transitional zone and subplate (neuroglial heterotopia), and in the cortical tubers, which give the disease its name (Park et al. 1997; Johnson et al. 2002; Magri et al. 2013).

The ventricular zone lesions in fetal specimens consist of variably sized aggregates of balloon cells that can adopt a variety of microscopic architectures; these can be partially calcified in the second trimester and presumably represent early subependymal nodules (Fig. 5.4c, d). However, they can also form substantial gross masses, which may relate to the subependymal giant cell astrocytomas encountered in pediatric patients. The subcortical heterotopias in fetal specimens generally consist of loose aggregates of balloon cells (Fig. 5.4e, f), which may show striking perivascular patterns, with aggregates of less differentiated precursors, and which may be in continuity with an overlying cortical tuber. Fetal cortical tubers correspond to infiltration of balloon cells into the cortex (Fig. 5.4g, h), accompanied by variable degrees of architectural distortion and a low-power impression of hypocellularity and loss of orderly lamination. Tubers can either be small and relatively subtle or massive enough to produce gross hemimegalencephaly (Fig. 5.5a, b) with extensive cortical involvement and transmantle extension (Fig. 5.5c, d). In fetal specimens, the neuronal abnormalities of tuberous sclerosis can be muted, but in close-to-term fetal brains, neuronal enlargement and abnormal cytology (Fig. 5.5e, f) become prominent. At the same time, the microvasculature becomes progressively more coarse, although excess reticulin is difficult to detect.

5.3.1 Genetics

Tuberous sclerosis is linked to constitutional loss of function mutations in TSC1 and TSC2, leading to overactivation of the mTOR complex. About 10–30% of familial cases and 10–15% of sporadic cases have mutations of TSC1 (Crino et al. 2006). Most cases, however, tend to be non-familial (Bundey and Evans 2007) with apparently de novo mutations. TSC2 mutations are found in 75–80% of sporadic cases (Curatolo et al. 2008), but in 15–20% of cases, no mutation is found, and these are probably somatic mutations. Somatic and germline mosaicism have been recorded. Both TSC1 and TSC2 appear to negatively regulate the PIK3–AKT–mTOR pathway, and it is thought that somatic inactivating mutations on the normal allele give rise to the various tumors and tumor-like lesions of tuberous sclerosis. Generally, more severe phenotypes are associated with TSC2 mutations (Au et al. 2007).

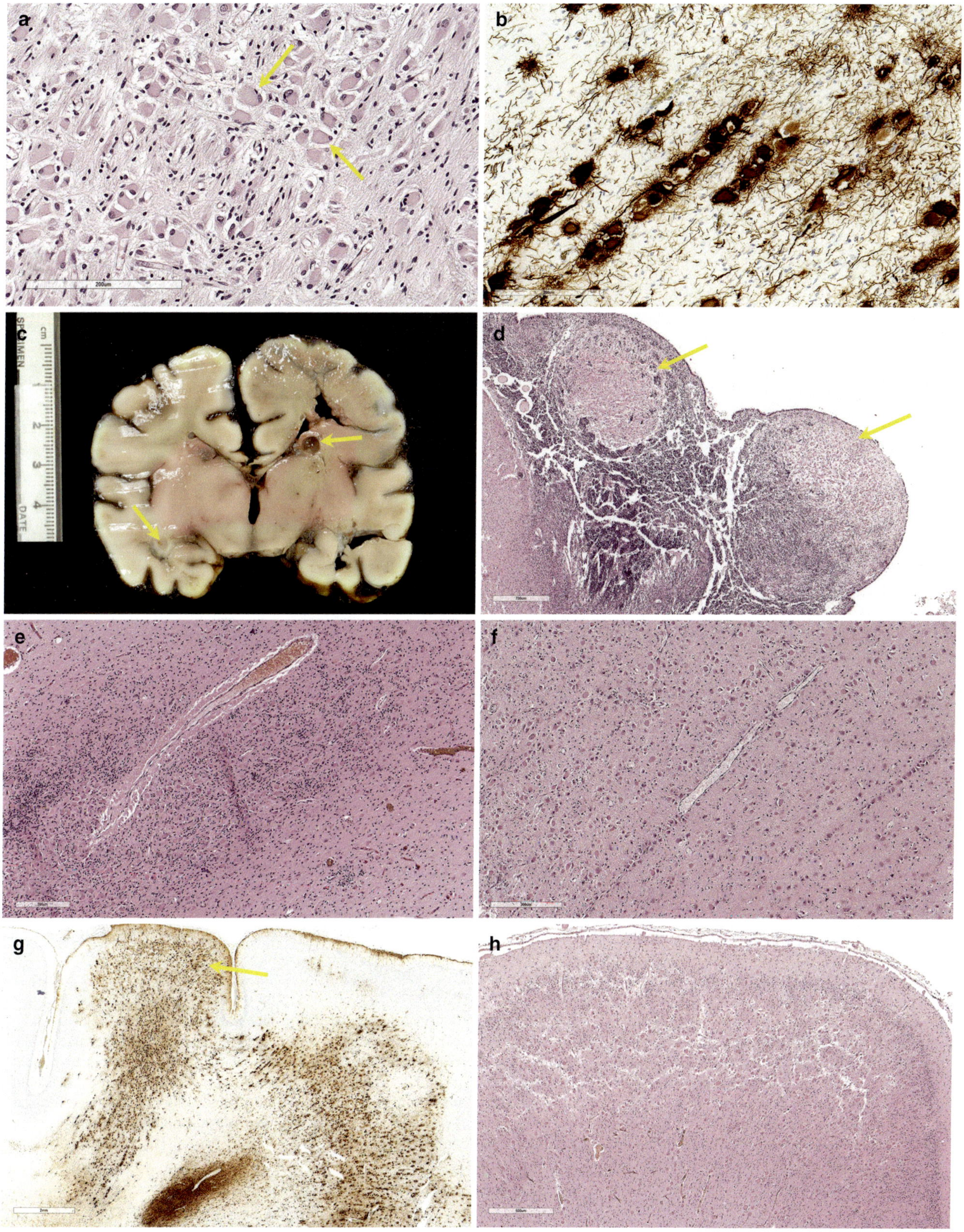

Fig. 5.4 (**a**) Tuberous sclerosis histology comprising of balloon cells with abundant glassy eosinophilic cytoplasm and peripherally placed, occasionally multiple nuclei. (**b**) Alpha-beta crystallin immunohistochemistry demonstrates a fine corona of irregular processes. (**c**) Brain of a 35-week gestation, with TSC2 deletion. Both cystic and solid large masses (arrows) distort the ventricle in the manner of subependymal giant cell astrocytomas. (**d**) Microscopy demonstrates innumerable subependymal nodules consisting of compact aggregates of balloon cells, sometimes with a spindled shape. (**e**) Transitional zone aggregates of balloon cells aligned roughly parallel to draining veins and admixed with spindled glia. (**f**) In the subplate, the radial orientation of the balloon cell aggregates along thin-walled vessels is apparent. (**g**) Balloon cells extending into the cortex of the medial orbital gyrus, in oblique continuity with subjacent heterotopia. (**h**) Cortical tuber with loss of lamination and hypocellularity and infiltration by balloon cells

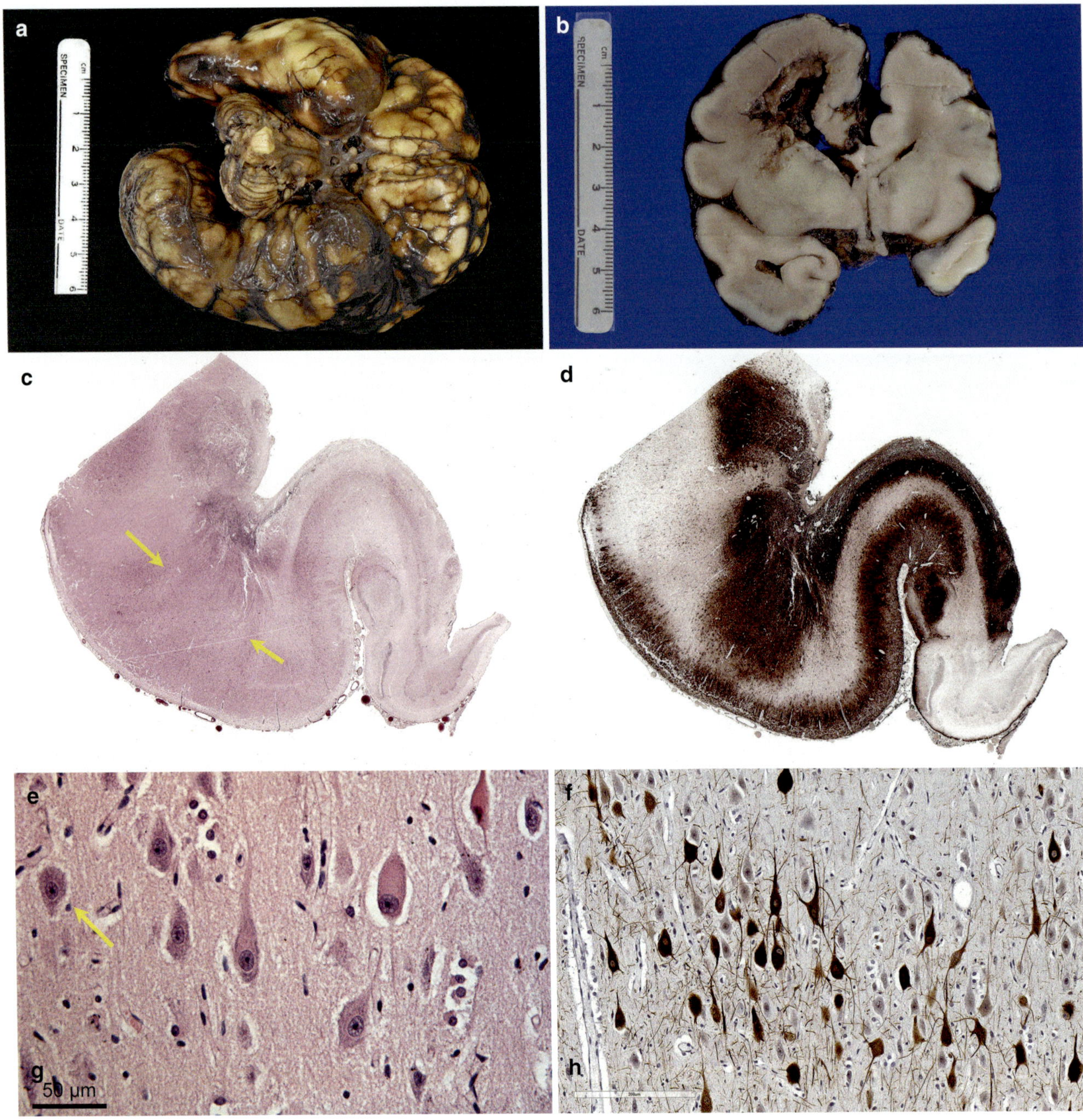

Fig. 5.5 (**a**) A 36-week gestation with TCS2. Massive right-sided hemispheric involvement by tuberous sclerosis, with effacement of cortical markings and mimicking hemimegalencephaly. (**b**) Coronal section demonstrating the expansion of cortical and subcortical brain. Cavitation on the left is postmortem artifact. Note the pale subependymal nodules (arrows). (**c**) Hippocampal formation with subependymal nodules (green arrow) and large area of transmantle abnormality (between arrows). (**d**) The same section as (**c**), stained with immunohistochemistry for alpha-beta crystallin, demonstrating massive periventricular and superficial populations of balloon cells and highlighting area of transmantle accumulation. (**e**) Cortical neurons in affected areas, with maloriented (arrow) enlarged and chromatolytic forms. (**f**) Alpha-beta crystallin staining demonstrating unusual neuronal morphologies

5.4 Temporal Lobe Overgrowth in Skeletal Dysplasias

Hyperplasia and cytoarchitectural dysplasia of the temporal lobe are characteristic, though not pathognomonic, of thanatophoric dysplasia and Apert syndrome.

Thanatophoric dysplasia (TD, types 1 and 2 (OMIM 187600, 187601)) is a short-rib brachymelic skeletal dysplasia characterized by striking epiphyseal cupping in the long bones and ribs as well as platyspondyly with a loss of the interpedical lumbar expansion. In our autopsy practices, it is the most commonly diagnosed severe skeletal dysplasia. Thanatophoric dysplasia consists of two forms, types 1 and 2, with type 2 distinguished clinically by the presence of a cloverleaf skull with craniosynostosis, less dramatic platyspondyly, and straight (as opposed to dramatically curved) femora. The central nervous system in both types is characterized by an enlarged brain with marked expansion of the temporal lobes and temporal germinal matrix, accompanied by distinctive radially oriented gyration on the surface of the inferior temporal lobes, which is well established by midgestation (Fig. 5.6a–c) (Hevner 2005). The hippocampal formations are dysplastic with widespread abnormal lamination and an absence of an orderly archicortex to neocortex progression (Fig. 5.6d, e). In general, TD type 2 demonstrates a larger and heavier brain than type 1, with a dramatic temporal lobe expansion such that the temporal pole extends anteriorly as far as the frontal pole, with abnormal, premature gyration extending to the paramedian parietal lobes (Fig. 5.6f, g). Other neuropathological findings of thanatophoric dysplasia include marked ventriculomegaly, leptomeningeal and periventricular nodular heterotopias, and more rarely agenesis of the corpus callosum, encephalocele, and holoprosencephaly. The spinal platyspondyly is accompanied by stenosis of the neural canal that may impinge on the spinal cord, especially at cervical levels (Faye-Petersen and Knisely 1991; see spinal cord and column malformations).

TD1 and TD2 are secondary to de novo mutations in FGFR3 (gene located on chromosome 4p16.3), which act in a dominant fashion and result in ligand-independent activation of fibroblast growth factor receptor 3 (FGFR3), a transmembrane tyrosine kinase. In the central nervous system, FGFR3 is expressed in the neuroepithelium of the dorsal and paramedian embryonic telencephalic vesicle, which subsequently expands into the temporal lobe. The activation of FGFR3 in neuroepithelium produces dimerization and serves as a proliferative signal in the affected brain (Thomson et al. 2009). The large majority of cases of TD1 result from missense mutations Y373C, R248C, and S249C, whereas TD2 demonstrates a K650E missense mutation (Wilcox et al. 1998).

In epiphyseal cartilage, abnormal stable dimerization and activation produced by the mutations of FGFR3 in TD1 prevent terminal chondrocyte differentiation and promote apoptosis (Legeai-Mallet et al. 1998; Delezoide et al. 1997), whereas the abnormal FGFR3 in TD2 is not dimerized but retained in the endoplasmic reticulum and activates STAT1, inhibits chondrocyte proliferation, and precipitates apoptosis (Lievens and Liboi 2003). Temporal lobe dysplasia can also be seen, although in a more subtle and muted form, in the allelic conditions of hypochondroplasia and achondroplasia (Kannu et al. 2005; Manikkam et al. 2018), which result from mutations giving ligand-dependent FGFR3 overactivation.

Apert syndrome is a skeletal dysplasia characterized by craniosynostosis with brachydactyly and oligosyndactyly in the hands and feet. In the brain, it is accompanied by temporal lobe pathology that in some cases is simply an expansion of the temporal lobe with a single radial groove anteriorly (Fig. 5.6h, i) but in other cases is grossly indistinguishable from TD type 1 (Fig. 5.6j, k) (Stark et al. 2015). Apert syndrome is characterized by activating mutations of FGFR2, but genotype—phenotype correlations are poor (Mantilla-Capacho et al. 2005). Temporal lobe expansion and dysplasia with radial grooves are not pathognomonic to TD and Apert syndrome; we have seen one case accompanied by numerous choroid plexus cysts in the context of fetal cleft palate and without other skeletal abnormalities and without genetic diagnosis (Fig. 5.6l).

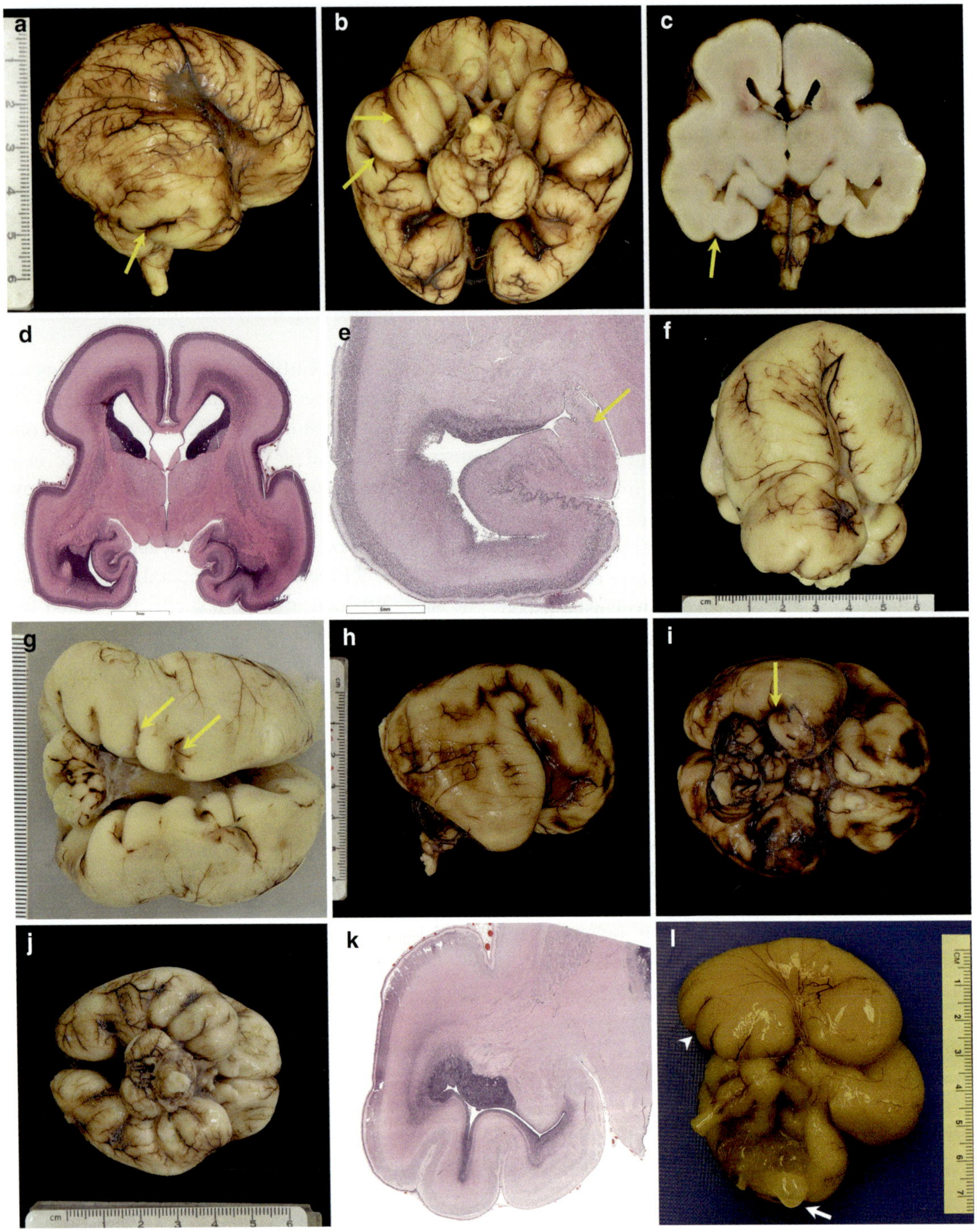

Fig. 5.6 (**a**) Thanatophoric dwarfism type 1 (TD1) at a 24-week gestation, with marked temporal lobe expansion and radial grooves along the inferior temporal lobe margin (arrow). (**b**) The premature irregular radial sulcation (arrows) is much more visible on the inferior aspects of the temporal lobes. (**c**) Coronal section, demonstrating dilation of temporal horns and indentation of the cortex along the premature sulcation. The discontinuity of the corpus callosum is artifact. (**d**) Whole mount of coronal section TD1 at a 20-week gestation, demonstrating enlarged temporal germinal matrices and asymmetric temporal sulcation. (**e**) Temporal lobe, 24-week gestation; there is a strip of small neurons resembling dentate granule cell neurons (arrow), but no normal hippocampal cytoarchitecture or orderly transition from the archicortex to neocortex is discernible. (**f**) Thanatophoric dysplasia type 2 (TD2) at a 25-week gestation, lateral view. Frontal pole is to the right; the temporal lobe is massively expanded inferiorly and anteriorly so that the temporal and frontal poles are nearly in the same coronal plane. (**g**) TD2, posterior aspect, cerebellum to the left. The radial grooves (arrows) proceed dorsally and anteriorly along the interhemispheric fissure. (**h**) Apert syndrome, a 24-week gestation, with expansion of the lateral aspect of temporal lobe. (**i**) Inferior surface of the same case, with single radially oriented temporal sulcus (arrow). (**j**) Apert syndrome, 24 weeks: this case is grossly indistinguishable from TD1 (compare with (b)). (**k**) Apert syndrome, 24 weeks; compare with (**d**) and (**e**). (**l**) Brain of a 22-week gestation fetus: this case lacked any skeletal dysplasia. Note the temporal lobe sulcation and overgrowth (arrowhead), as well as prominent choroid plexus cysts (arrow) in choroidal fissure. (Case courtesy of Dr. L Hamilton, Children's Hospital of Eastern Ontario, Ottawa)

References

Au KS, Williams AT, Roach ES, Batchelor L, Sparagana SP, Delgado MR, et al. Genotype/phenotype correlation in 325 individuals referred for a diagnosis of tuberous sclerosis complex in the United States. Genet Med. 2007;9:88–100.

Bundey S, Evans K. Tuberous sclerosis—a genetic study. J Neurol Neurosurg Psychiatry. 2007;32:591–603, 196.

Crino PB, Nathanson KL, Henske EP. The tuberous sclerosis complex. N Engl J Med. 2006;355:1345–56.

Curatolo P, Bombardieri R, Jozwiak S. Tuberous sclerosis. Lancet. 2008;372:657–68.

Delezoide A-L, Lasselin-Benoist C, Legeai-Mallet L, Brice P, Senee V, Yayon A, et al. Abnormal FGFR 3 expression in cartilage of thanatophoric dysplasia fetuses. Hum Molec Genet. 1997;6:1899–906.

Dobyns WB, Mirzaa GM. Megalencephaly syndromes associated with mutations of core components of the PI3K-AKT–MTOR pathway: PIK3CA, PIK3R2, AKT3, and MTOR. Am J Med Genet. 2019;Part C. 181C:582–90.

Faye-Petersen OM, Knisely AS. Neural arch stenosis and spinal cord injury in thanatophoric dysplasia. Am J Dis Child. 1991;145(1):87–9. https://doi.org/10.1001/archpedi.1991.02160010093023. PMID: 1985437

Hevner RF. The cerebral cortex malformation in thanatophoric dysplasia: neuropathology and pathogenesis. Acta Neuropathol. 2005;110(3):208–21.

Itoh K, Pooh R, Shimokawa O, Fushiki S. Somatic mosaicism of the PI3K-AKT-MTOR pathway is associated with hemimegalencephaly in fetal brains. Neuropathology. 2023;43:190–6.

Johnson MW, Miyata H, Vinters HV. Ezrin and moesin expression within the developing human cerebrum and tuberous sclerosis-associated cortical tubers. Acta Neuropathol. 2002;104(2):188–96.

Kannu P, Hayes IM, Mandelstam S, Donnan L, Savarirayan R. Medial temporal lobe dysgenesis in hypochondroplasia. Am J Med Genet A. 2005;138(4):389–91.

Legeai-Mallet L, Benoist-Lasselin C, Delezoide AL, Munnich A, Bonaventure J. Fibroblast growth factor receptor 3 mutations promote apoptosis but do not alter chondrocyte proliferation in thanatophoric dysplasia. J Biol Chem. 1998;273(21):13007–14. https://doi.org/10.1074/jbc.273.21.13007. Erratum in: J Biol Chem 1998 Jul 24;273(30).

Lievens PM, Liboi E. The thanatophoric dysplasia type II mutation hampers complete maturation of fibroblast growth factor receptor 3 (FGFR3), which activates signal transducer and activator of transcription 1 (STAT1) from the endoplasmic reticulum. J Biol Chem. 2003;278(19):17344–9.

Magri L, Cominelli M, Cambiaghi M, Cursi M, Leocani L, Minicucci F, et al. Timing of mTOR activation affects tuberous sclerosis complex neuropathology in mouse models. Dis Model Mech. 2013;6(5):1185–97.

Manikkam SA, Chetcuti K, Howell KB, Savarirayan R, Fink AM, Mandelstam SA. Temporal lobe malformations in achondroplasia: expanding the brain imaging phenotype associated with FGFR3-related skeletal dysplasias. AJNR Am J Neuroradiol. 2018;39(2):380–4.

Mantilla-Capacho JM, Arnaud L, Diaz-Rodriguez M, Barros-Nunez P. 2005 Apert syndrome with preaxial polydactyly showing the typical mutation Ser252Trp in the FGFR2 gene. Genet Counsel. 2005;16:403–6.

Mirzaa GM, Conti V, Timms AE, Smyser CD, Ahmed S, Carter M, et al. Characterisation of mutations of the phosphoinositide-3-kinase regulatory subunit, PIK3R2, in perisylvian polymicrogyria: a next-generation sequencing study. Lancet Neurol. 2015;14(12):1182–95.

Mirzaa GM, Conway RL, Gripp KW, Lerman-Sagie T, Siegel DH, deVries LS, et al. Megalencephaly-capillary malformation (MCAP) and megalencephaly-polydactyly-polymicrogyria-hydrocephalus (MPPH) syndromes: two closely related disorders of brain overgrowth and abnormal brain and body morphogenesis. Am J Med Genet. 2012;158A:269–91.

Park SH, Pepkowitz SH, Kerfoot C, De Rosa MJ, Poukens V, Wienecke R, et al. Tuberous sclerosis in a 20-week gestation fetus: immunohistochemical study. Acta Neuropathol. 1997;94(2):180–6.

Sarnat HB, Flores-Sarnat L, Trevenen CL. Synaptophysin immunoreactivity in the human hippocampus and neocortex from 6 to 41 weeks of gestation. J Neuropathol Exp Neurol. 2010;69(3):234–45.

Stark Z, McGillivray G, Sampson A, Palma-Dias R, Edwards A, Said JM, et al. Apert syndrome: temporal lobe abnormalities on fetal brain imaging. Prenat Diagn. 2015;35(2):179–82.

Thomson RE, Kind PC, Graham NA, Etherson ML, Kennedy J, Fernandes AC, et al. FGF receptor 3 activation promotes selective growth and expansion of occipitotemporal cortex. Neural Dev. 2009;4:4. https://doi.org/10.1186/1749-8104-4-4. PMID: 19192266; PMCID: PMC2661882.

Wang X, Zhang Z, Peng P, Peng J. The phenotypic and genetic spectrum of AKT3-related neurodevelopmental condition. Sci Rep. 2025;15(1):7484.

Wilcox WR, Tavormina PL, Krakow D, Kitoh H, Lachman RS, Wasmuth JJ, et al. Molecular, radiologic, and histopathologic correlations in thanatophoric dysplasia. Am J Med Genet. 1998;78(3):274–81.

Winden KD, Yuskaitis CJ, Poduri A. Megalencephaly and macrocephaly. Semin Neurol. 2015;35(3):277–87.

Yasin SA, Latak K, Becherini F, et al. Balloon cells in human cortical dysplasia and tuberous sclerosis: isolation of a pathological progenitor-like cell. Acta Neuropathol. 2010;120(1):85–96.

6 Prosencephalic Malformations

At embryonic stage 10, roughly 4 weeks post conception, the rostral neural folds begin to fuse, and the major components of the forebrain (the prosencephalon) are first discerned. At this point, the notochord extends rostrally to the oropharyngeal membrane, ventral to neuromeres D2 and D1. The primary prosencephalon divides into the caudal diencephalon and the rostral secondary prosencephalon. The prechordal portion of the neural tube develops into the rostral diencephalon or hypothalamus, the optic vesicles, the preoptic region, and the future telencephalon. The most rostral portion of the brain forms the telencephalon (the order from caudal to rostral being D2, D1, and telencephalon). Neuromere D2 gives rise to the future thalamus, epithalamus, hypothalamus, globus pallidus, and amygdaloid body and D1 to the optic primordia connected basally by the chiasmatic plate. The telencephalon will consist of the olfactory bulbs and tracts, basal forebrain, striatum, and cerebral cortex (du Plessis and Volpe 2018). The development of the prosencephalon can be thought of as consisting of three sequential events: formation, cleavage, and midline development (Volpe 2000). Horizontal cleavage gives rise to olfactory bulbs and tracts and optic vesicles, while transverse cleavage also gives rise to the telencephalon and diencephalon. Midline development is thought to occur from sixth to seventh week of gestation onward and is comprised of formation of commissural, chiasmatic, and hypothalamic plates, which, respectively, give rise to the corpus callosum and septum pellucidum, optic nerve and chiasm, and hypothalamus (du Plessis and Volpe 2018).

Abnormalities in prosencephalic formation can be categorised by the agenesis or dysgenesis of the major structures comprising the prosencephalon.

6.1 Aprosencephaly

In aprosencephaly, prosencephalic (i.e., both diencephalic and telencephalic) structures rostral to the midbrain are absent or dysplastic and rudimentary (Lurie et al. 1979), while with atelencephaly, diencephalic structures are present but telencephalic are absent. In reports of aprosencephaly, the rostral neural mass may demonstrate glioependymal cysts, rudimentary eyes, and disorganized neural masses to which it may be challenging to assign normal anatomical homologues. As in atelencephaly (see below), foci of calcification and gliosis may be encountered (Fallet-Bainco 2018; Kim et al. 1990; Garcia and Duncan 1977; Harris et al. 1994; Iivanainen et al. 1997; Siebert et al. 1986), leading some to speculate that the malformation is secondary to an embryonic-phase vascular event. However, dystrophic calcifications are generally not infrequent in holoprosencephaly (HPE) (see below) and in the absence of other corroborative findings should be interpreted with caution. In some cases, the presence of dysplastic prosencephalic elements militates against a true failure of formation of a prosencephalic anlage, and such cases might represent extreme forms of HPE (Sergi and Schmitt 2000). Certainly, in our experience with some cases of aprosencephaly, the examination of the fetal rudimentary forebrain demonstrates that both dorsal and ventral aspects of the brain are formed of choroid plexus (Fig. 6.1a–c), suggesting that a lack of patterning in the rostral neural tube, rather than a strict agenesis or a destruction of prosencephalic primordia, leads to the observed pathology.

P. Shannon et al., *Atlas of Neurodevelopmental Pathology*, https://doi.org/10.1007/978-3-032-14148-4_6

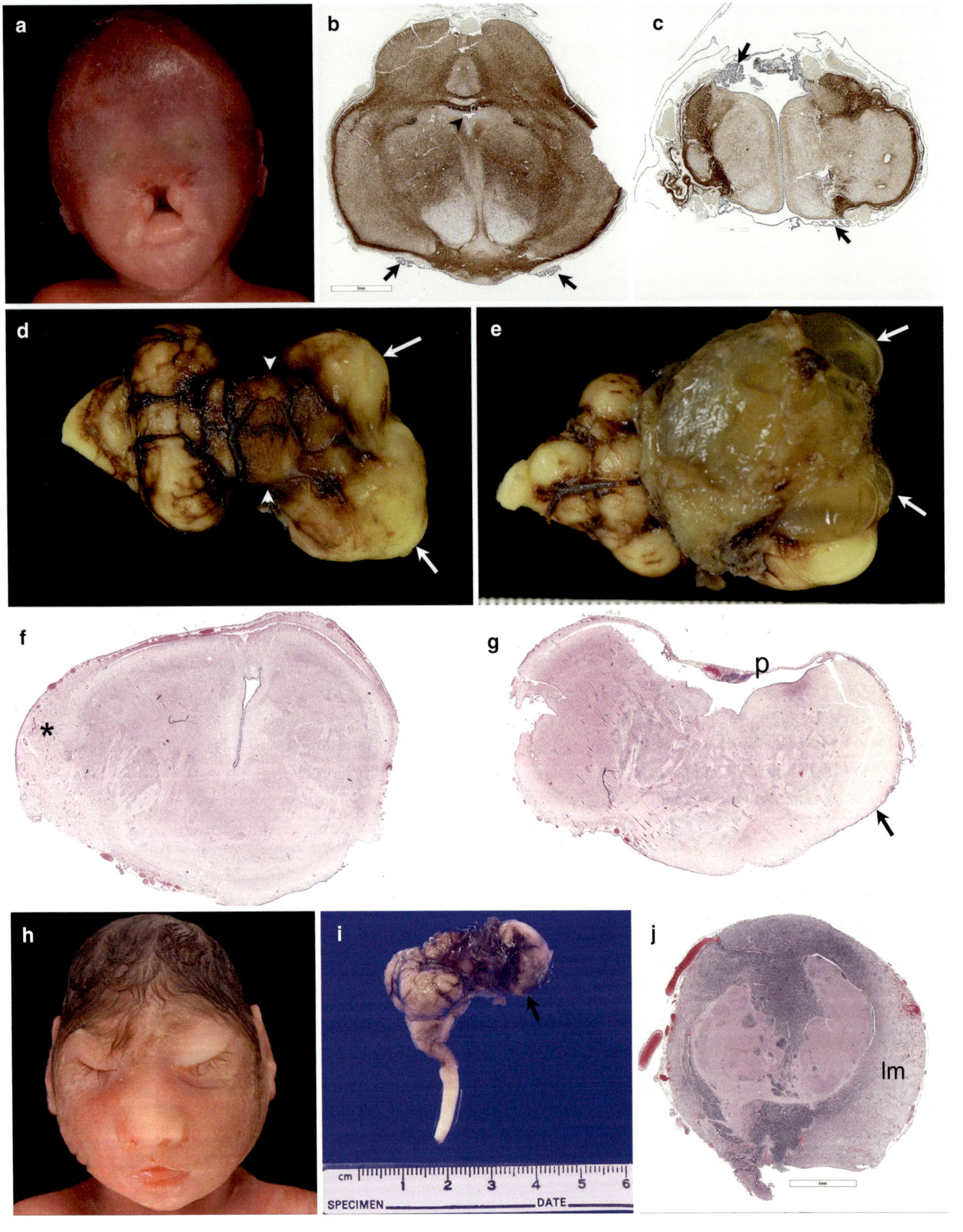

Fig. 6.1 (**a**) An anopthalmic fetus with rostral brain in coronal sections. (**b**) Coronal sections demonstrating rudimentary midbrain development with a suggestion of dorsal collicular and posterior commissure development (arrowhead) and ventral choroid plexus attachment. (**c**) The most rostral brain demonstrates dorsal and ventral choroid plexus with a midline slit-like ventricle. (**d**) Atelencephaly with tubular midbrain-like structure (arrowheads) and irregularly lobed rostral enlargement (arrows). (**e**) Ventral surface of (**d**) demonstrating rostral and ventral choroid plexus cysts (arrows). (**f**) Cross section through (**d**) demonstrating slit-like ventricle, irregular deep masses (asterisk), and extensive leptomeningeal heterotopias. (**g**) Section through bilobed rostral aspect, demonstrating pineal gland (p) and irregular neuronal masses covered ventrally by tightly applied choroid plexus (arrow). (**h**) Atelencephaly with asymmetric microphthalmia. (**i**) The rostral brain of (**h**) is an irregular globoid neural mass (arrow). (**j**) The rostral mass consists of irregular deep neural masses surrounded by leptomeninges (lm) infiltrated by heterotopic neurons and glia and apparent precursors

6.2 Atelencephaly

Atelencephaly demonstrates morphological overlap with aprosencephaly in that in both conditions, the rostral neural mass is hypoplastic and demonstrates disorganized elements, but in atelencephaly, one has organized deep structures that resemble thalami rostral to the midbrain (Fig. 6.1d–f); organized cerebral cortex and olfactory bulbs and tracts are absent, as are corticofugal tracts. The eyes are variably affected (Fig. 6.1g–i), while the brainstem and cerebellum are generally preserved. We have seen one midgestation case in which a complete absence of the telencephalon was accompanied by a rostral open neural tube defect, with herniation of choroid plexus and scant neural elements (Fig. 6.2a–e). The open rostral neuropore might presumably lead to both poor local patterning with herniation and destruction of the brain, and differentiating the relative contribution of each would seem speculative.

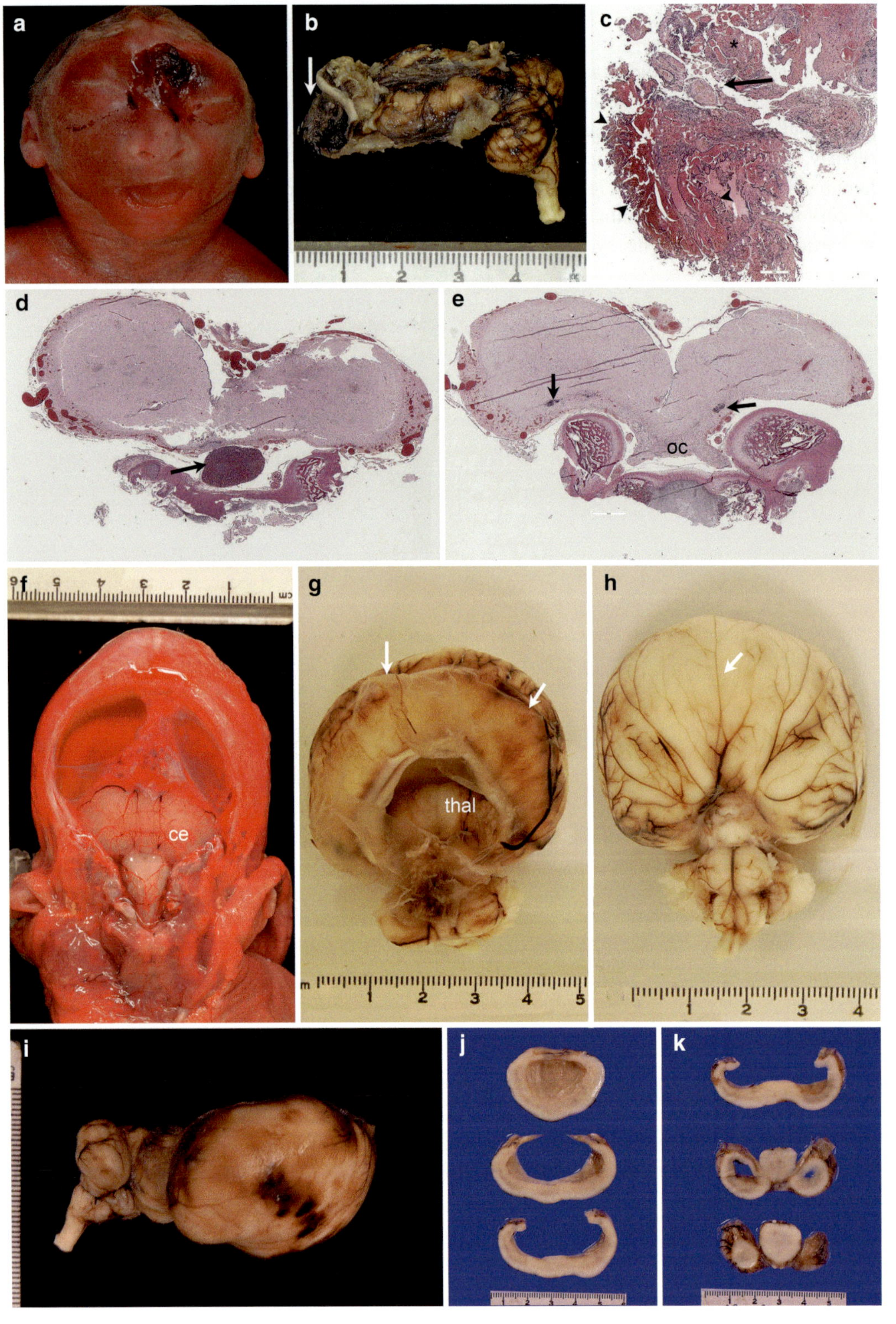

Fig. 6.2 (**a**) Fetus with marked microcephaly and a midline hemorrhagic forehead mass. (**b**) Explanted brain demonstrating absent cerebral hemispheres. The rostral mass (arrow) is in continuity with the brain through a defect in the skin. (**c**) Sagittal sections through the rostral mass demonstrate congested choroid plexus (arrowheads), small nodules of neural tissue (asterisk), and embedded vernix with reaction (arrow). (**d**) The coronal section through the sella demonstrates an intact pituitary (arrow) and a bilobed neural mass with a midline ventricle as well as basal and lateral leptomeningeal heterotopias. (**e**) Somewhat caudally, the optic chiasm is intact (OC), and basal calcifications are present (arrows). (**f**) Alobar HPE: midgestation fetus case with the occipital bone removed demonstrating relatively normal cerebellum (CE) and a very large dorsal cyst filled with clear cerebrospinal fluid occupying the intracranial vertex. (**g**) Same case as (**f**), with dorsal surface demonstrating redundant cyst wall (arrows), here opened with a small fused thalamus (thal) visible underneath, and a large horseshoe-shaped posterior opening into the holoventricle. (**h**) Ventral view of (**g**) with single anterior cerebral artery (arrow) and absent anterior communicating artery. (**i**) Lateral aspect of alobar HPE: the holosphere is often elongated with a concave rounded ventral surface. (**j**) Coronal sections of the anterior holosphere, anterior to posterior (top to bottom). (**k**) The same case as (**j**), with coronal sections of the posterior holosphere and thalamus, anterior to posterior (top to bottom), demonstrating the small fused thalami and slender attachment of the holosphere to the remainder of the brain

6.3 Holoprosencephaly

In HPE, there is a failure of cleavage of the prosencephalon into two distinct hemispheres, with no septal leaflets, and the forniceal leaves and columns are indistinct. Consequently, the lateral ventricles are fused frontally to form a holoventricle. In the usual forms, the olfactory bulbs and tracts are always absent or at the least hypoplastic. The usual classification follows the degree of separation of the forebrain into distinct hemispheres, with complete fusion of the hemispheres (alobar HPE), posterior separation with hypoplastic falx cerebri (semilobar HPE), and complete dorsal separation (lobar HPE). In general, the derangement of facial, ophthalmic, and subcortical architecture follows the severity of derangement of cortical separation, but this is only a rule of thumb, so these categories should be thought of as general descriptions and not discrete diagnostic categories, nor can one expect every case to fall neatly into one or the other category.

6.3.1 Alobar HPE

In alobar HPE, the brain is usually small, and the cerebrum is reduced to a single mushroom-cap-shaped anterior mass without median or Sylvian fissure and with markedly reduced or irregular sulcation. This holosphere opens posteriorly and dorsally into a membranous cyst lined with ependymal or choroid plexus-type epithelium that may occupy most of the intracranial space (Fig. 6.2f–h). This cyst can be very large relative to the holosphere and can occupy the majority of a relatively normally sized or even expanded intracranial space, giving rise to an ultrasonographic impression of hydranencephaly. Within the holosphere, the single ventricle is U-shaped, without a septum and with anteriorly fused or absent striatum; the palladium is usually absent, and the hypothalamus is often dysplastic. The holosphere is perched ventrally and rostrally and attached to the rest of the brain by a narrow ventral peduncle. The telencephalic flexure is usually lost (Fig. 6.2f-k). Basal and perimesencephalic leptomeningeal heterotopias are common and may be dramatic. Both ventral (hypothalamic) and dorsal (thalamic) heterotopic neuronal masses are common (Fig. 6.3). Particularly when ophthalmic abnormalities are marked, the optic nerves may be fused, and ventral masses with neuroepithelial and even retinal differentiation may form. The thalami are generally reduced and are often at least partially fused. The holosphere is bounded posteriorly and dorsally by an arched posterior opening from which the cyst wall originates; the rim of the arch often demonstrates a superficial fiber system, and if sectioned perpendicularly to its surface, the underlying brain may demonstrate a hippocampal architecture (Fig. 6.4a–c). Dystrophic calcifications may be prominent (Fig. 6.4d).

The telencephalic commissural and projecting fiber systems are reduced or absent. The cortical cytoarchitecture is variable from case to case (Fig. 6.4e, f); it may demonstrate an apparently ordered six-layered structure with an orderly transition to archicortex, or there may be widespread abnormalities with microcolumnar and nodular architectures, heterotopic or maloriented magnocellular neurons, or a paucity of calretinin (+) neurons and synaptic maturation may be accelerated (Sarnat et al. 2014). Polymicrogyria may develop. The germinal matrix is often small and may disappear prematurely, and the external granular cell layer may be absent even at midgestation, suggesting an absent ventral stream. The peduncle connecting the holosphere to the rest of the brain often appears to be a chaotic mass of axonal tracts. The thalamus is often fused and may be coated with leptomeningeal heterotopia. Aqueductal pathology may be severe, with atresia or forking (see Chap. 7), and if there is aqueductal pathology, there is frequently mesencephalosynapsis (Fisher et al. 2024; Sarnat and Flores-Sarnat 2001). The brainstem and cerebellum are often relatively well preserved, but dentato-olivary dysplasia, cerebellar hypoplasia, and Dandy–Walker-like malformations may be encountered. The corticospinal tracts are generally absent or hypoplastic (Fallet-Bainco 2018, pers. Obs.). The venous anatomy is distorted following the cerebral abnormality; in common with semilobar HPE, there are not well-formed internal cerebral veins, the deep venous network being irregular, and a vein of Galen is also absent. In common with semilobar and some lobar HPE, the circle of Willis is incomplete anteriorly, and frequently, only one anterior cerebral artery fans out to supply all or most of the orbitofrontal cortex.

6.3.2 Semilobar HPE

In semilobar HPE, the interhemispheric fissure is present posteriorly together with a short falx, although the inferior sagittal sinus is absent. The frontal lobe, the underlying frontal recesses of the lateral ventricles, and the striatum are usually fused. The olfactory bulbs and tracts are usually absent or hypoplastic, and the septum is absent, such that a holosphere is obvious. Temporal lobes may be developed, and there may be rudimentary occipital lobes. There is generally a posterior opening to the holosphere as in alobar HPE, but the posterior cyst is not usually as dramatic, particularly if the third ventricle and aqueduct are preserved. The thalamus may be small and fused. Ventriculomegaly may still be so dramatic as to cause macrocephaly (Varma et al. 2022). Posteriorly, a corpus callosum-like commissure may be present. In general, the brainstem and cerebellum are preserved, although absent or hypoplastic corticospinal tracts are still common. The inferior sagittal sinus is usually not present, nor are there well-formed internal cerebral veins, and vein of Galen is also absent. In common with alobar HPE, the circle of Willis is incomplete anteriorly, and frequently, only one anterior cerebral artery fans out to supply all or most of the orbitofrontal cortex.

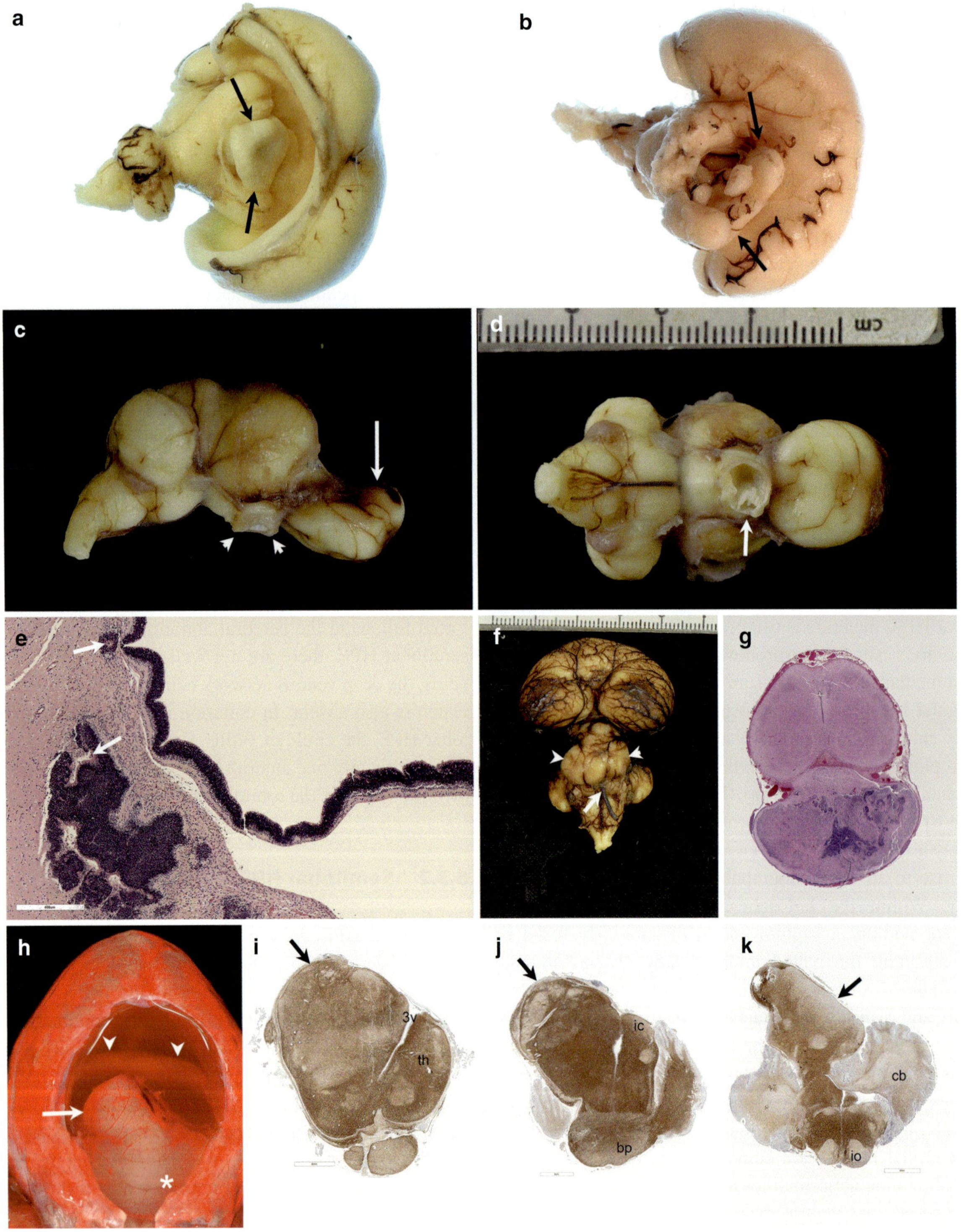

Fig. 6.3 (**a**) Alobar HPE: dorsal surface with dorsal cyst wall removed; note the heterotopic neuronal mass in the dorsal thalamus (arrows). (**b**) The same case as (**a**) with irregular ventral neuronal mass. (**c**) Alobar HPE with minute telencephalon (arrow) and broad ventral cystic mass (small arrows). (**d**) Ventral irregular cystic mass in the same case as (**c**). (**e**) Microscopy of cyst wall, demonstrating rosette and neuroepithelial differentiation (arrows). (**f**) Alobar HPE: 23 weeks' gestation with irregular ventral mass covering and engulfing basilar artery (arrow). (**g**) Section at level marked by arrowheads in (**f**), demonstrating hamartomatous mass anterior to the preserved midbrain architecture. (**h**) Alobar HPE: a 22-week-gestation fetus with the occipital bone removed (compare with (**f**)). Arrowheads mark the dorsal lip of the posterior holosphere opening, visible through cyst fluid. The arrow marks a large mass dorsal and rostral to the cerebellum (asterisks). (**i**) Section of the caudal thalamus (immunohistochemistry for calretinin) with left mass (arrow) separated from contralateral thalamus (th) by a narrow third ventricle (3v). (**j**) Section of pons at the level of the inferior colliculus (ic) and basis points (bp), showing mass on the left (arrow) (immunohistochemistry for calretinin). (**k**) Section of the medulla and cerebellum, showing mass on the left (arrow) in continuity with thalamic mass (immunohistochemistry for calretinin)

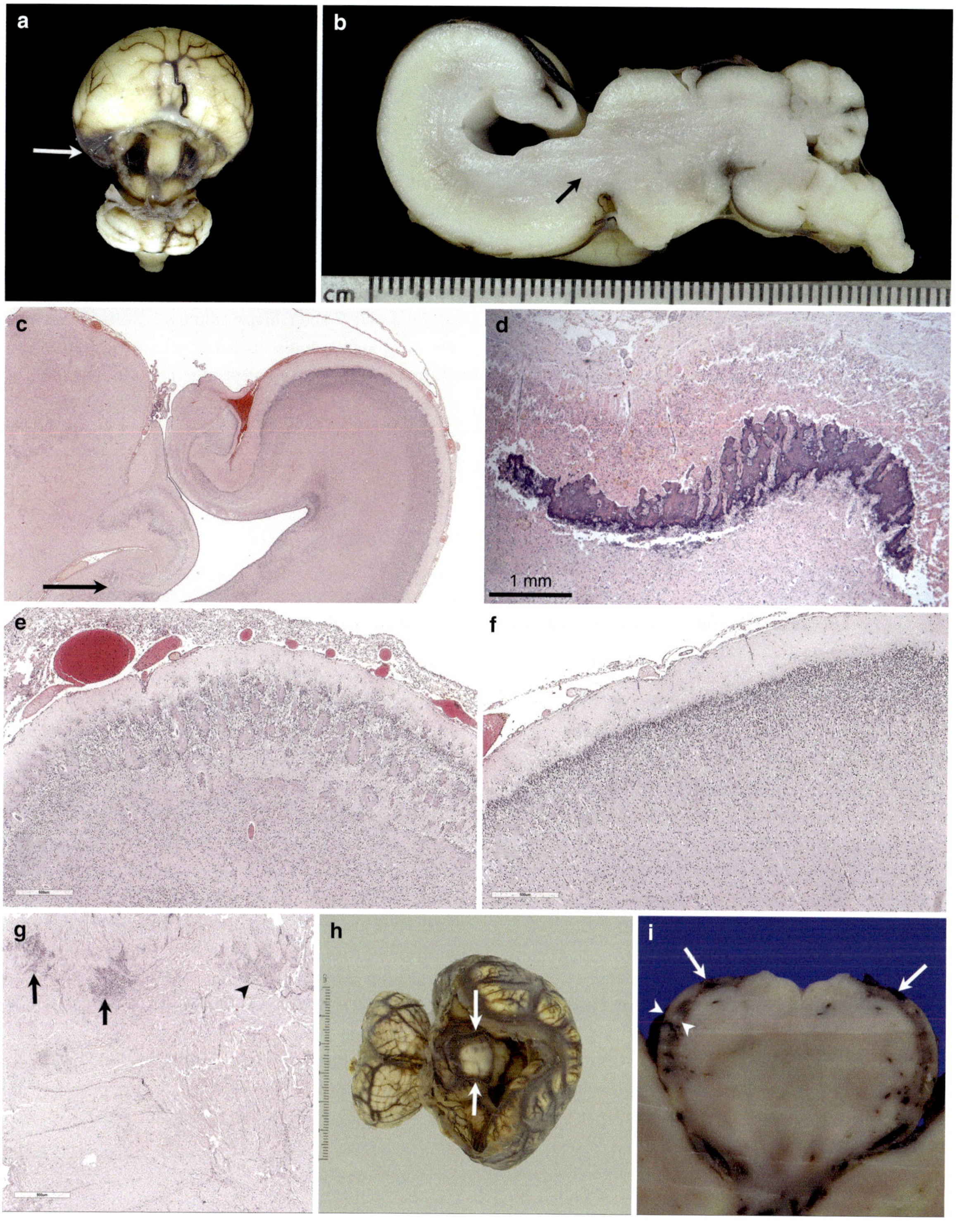

Fig. 6.4 (**a**) Alobar HPE, 24 weeks of gestation, dorsal view. (**b**) Sagittal section of (**a**), demonstrating rostral holosphere attached by a narrow peduncle (arrow) to the thalamus. (**c**) Transverse section of the specimen in (**a**), demonstrating hippocampal architecture and lateral thalamic attachment of the holosphere by medial cerebrum, demonstrating architecture resembling the hippocampus (arrow). (**d**) Massive cortical calcification in alobar HPE in a 26-week-gestation fetus with digynic triploidy. (**e**) Holoprosencephaly, 23 weeks, trisomy 13, posteroinferior and lateral cortex with irregular columnar architecture. (**f**) The same case as (**e**): dorsomedial cortex, with thinning and poor delimitation from the underlying fiber tracts. Note that the external granular cell layer is absent in both (**e**) and (**f**). (**g**) The same case as (**b**): section through ventral peduncle indicated in (**b**), demonstrating patchy areas of calcification (arrows) as well as a cluster of neurons (arrowhead) apparently unconnected to any larger adjacent structure on deeper sections. (**h**) A 38-week gestation with trisomy 13: the brain is small and the thalamus fused; arrows indicate deep cerebral veins on either side of a pale area, which represents the roof of the fused third ventricle. (**i**) The same case as (**h**); arrows indicate deep cerebral veins; laterally, the brain is obscured by leptomeningeal heterotopias (arrowheads), and medially, the pale area is the roof of the fused thalamus bounded by the attachments of the choroid plexus

6.3.3 Lobar HPE

In lobar HPE (Fig. 6.5), the external division of the hemispheres is complete on external examination, although the septum pellucidum is absent and the olfactory bulbs and tracts are hypoplastic or absent. There may be cortical continuity across the corpus callosum anteriorly (cingulosynapsis).

6.3.4 Middle Hemispheric HPE

In middle hemispheric HPE (also called syntelencephaly), the base of the forebrain separates, and there are usually olfactory bulbs and tracts, but the posterior frontal and parietal regions do not separate, leading to a hypoplastic falx anteriorly, cortical continuity across the posterior frontal and parietal lobes, and the replacement or effacement of the corpus callosum in these areas with a well-defined splenium and genu. The Sylvian fissures may be connected dorsally across the midline, and the neocortex lining the interhemispheric fissure may be thickened. Internally, the basal ganglia and thalami may be fused. Chiari type 1 or 2 malformations and cerebellar vermis hypoplasia have been reported (Barcovich and Quint 1993; Simon et al. 2002).

6.3.5 Septo-preoptic Holoprosencephaly

In this variant, the nonseparation of cerebral hemispheres is limited to septal, subcallosal, and/or preoptic regions. The rostrum and genu of the corpus callosum are hypoplastic with a normal body and splenium, or the body may be abnormally thickened. The thalami may be fused (Koob et al. 2012; Hahn et al. 2010).

6.3.6 TBC1D32-Related Disease and Thalamic Fusion

The HPE reported with accompanying homozygous mutations of TBC1D132 (c.2650C>T p.(Arg884Trp)) has externally complete separation of the cerebral hemispheres along with absent olfactory bulbs and tracts, small dysplastic temporal lobes, membranous corpus callosum, massive ventriculomegaly, a small fused thalamus, dysplastic hypothalamus with absent pituitary and microphthalmia with a fused optic nerve containing ciliated neuroepithelial tubules and rosettes (Harris et al. 2023) (Fig. 6.6a–c) as well as aqueduct stenosis with mesencephalosynapsis (Fisher et al. 2025), and a poorly demarcated cerebellar vermis. Note that the fusion of the thalami is frequent in HPE and generally is accompanied by micrencephaly and basal heterotopias. However, it is not specific to HPE and can accompany severe Chiari malformations (Fig. 6.6e), and sometimes seems to supervene on thalami that are roughly appropriate in size and shape (Fig. 6.6f) but in which the third ventricle, having formed, is subsequently filled by heterotopic neural tissue instead of its walls becoming fused.

6.3.7 Pathogenesis

Holoprosencephaly is thought to be related to the failure of midline induction by the prechordal plate, leading to abnormal cleavage of the prosencephalon. It is associated with common aneuploidies, such as trisomy 13 and 16, and has been associated with cytogenetic deletions and/or duplications on almost every chromosome. Genes reported in association with classical forms of HPE include SHH, ZIC2, SIX3, FGF8, CDON, CNOT1, DISP1, DLL1, FGFR1, KMT2D, PPP1R12A, RAD21, SMC1A, SMC3, STAG2, STIL, and TGIF1 (Daly et al. 2020; Barratt et al. 2022; Harris et al. 2022). The middle interhemispheric variant is associated particularly with mutations in ZIC2 gene (Brown et al. 1998). ZIC2 acts in dorsal midline to promote differentiation of roof plate (Simon et al. 2002) and is involved in neural tube roof plate closure, which may explain the association of MIH with cephaloceles, myelomeningocele, and/or Chiari type 2 malformation. TBC1D32 is a ciliary protein known to be expressed in the hypothalamus and thalamus at least at Carnegie stage 23 and probably interacts with SHH signaling (Hietamaki et al. 2020).

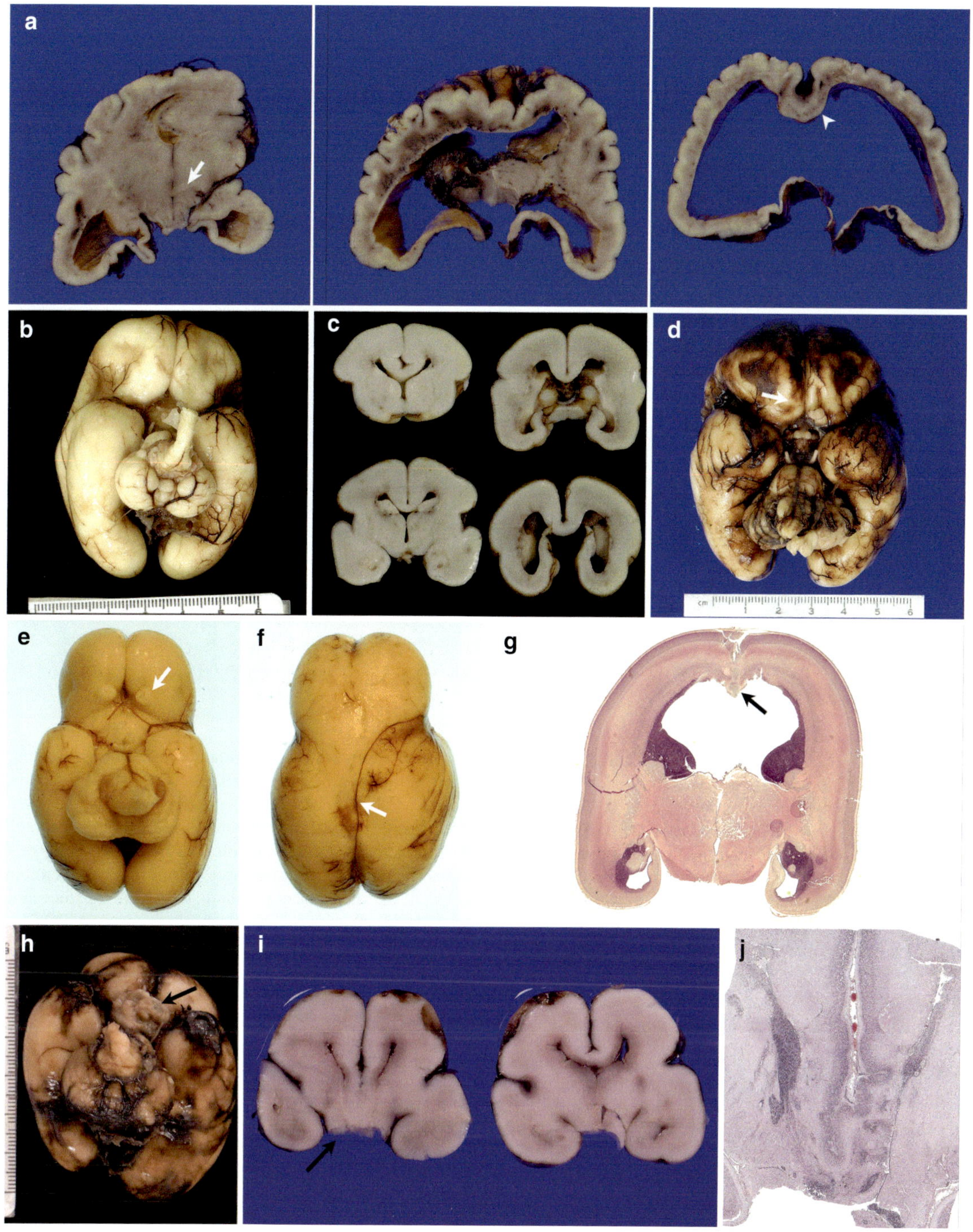

Fig. 6.5 (**a**) Lobar HPE, 39 weeks gestation, anterior to posterior in the coronal section. Rudimentary temporal lobes are present as is an anterior commissure (arrow), while posteriorly, there is a rudimentary corpus callosum (arrowhead). The thalamus is fused and the holoventricle ballooned posteriorly. (**b**) Lobar HPE, 22 weeks' gestation: ventrally, the rostral and caudal interhemispheric fissure is well marked, and the external morphology is roughly normal, although no olfactory bulbs or tracts are present. (**c**) Coronal sections of (**b**), demonstrating mild ventriculomegaly with septal agenesis and without fornices. (**d**) A 26-week gestation, with a unilateral absence of the olfactory bulb and tract (arrow). Note the ipsilateral absent gyrus rectus. (**e**) A 20-week gestation, with syntelencephaly; note the olfactory bulbs are present (arrow) as is the anterior communicating cerebral artery with well-marked anterior and posterior interhemispheric fissure. (**f**) Dorsal view of (**e**) with poorly marked midportion of interhemispheric fissure. Note the branch of the middle cerebral artery (arrow) crossing to the contralateral hemisphere. (**g**) Whole-mount coronal section of (**e**) at the mid-thalamus, demonstrating absent septum, ventriculomegaly, and dysplastic fusion of hemispheres at midline with heterotopic neuronal mass (arrow). (**h**) Septo-preoptic HPE, with interhemispheric fissure well marked ventrally and large artifactually disrupted anterior ventral mass and absent olfactory bulbs and tracts. (**i**) Coronal sections of (**h**): the arrow indicates disrupted basal preoptic mass with septal agenesis and cortical continuity across the corpus callosum. (**j**) Whole mount of basal frontal lobes, demonstrating irregular cortical and ventral fusion with disorganization and heterotopic germinal elements

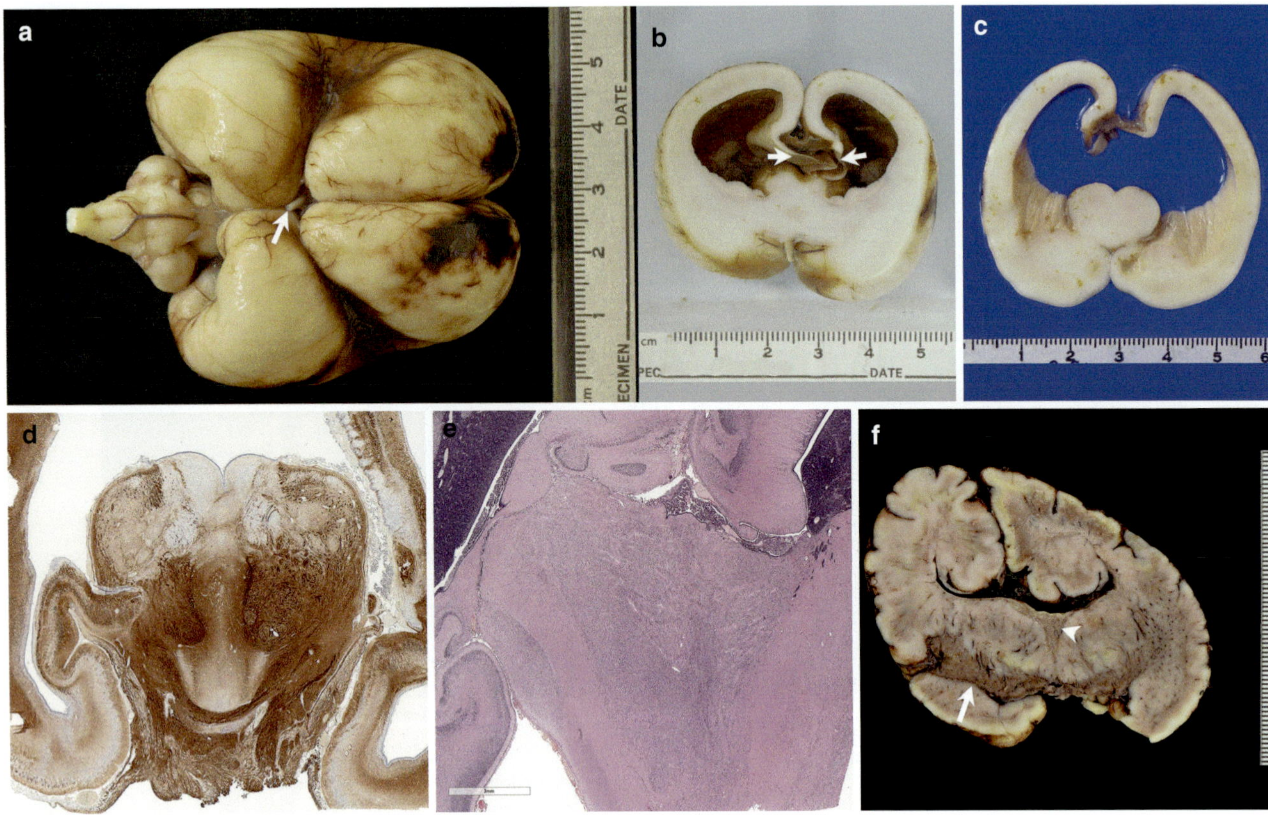

Fig. 6.6 (**a**) TBC1D32-related malformation, 22 weeks' gestation, with interhemispheric fissure well marked anteriorly and posteriorly, and with short temporal lobes touching in the midline; the arrow indicates fused single optic nerve. (**b**) The same case as in (**a**), with the coronal section demonstrating membranous midline structures continuous caudally with hippocampal formations as in fornices but lined by leptomeninges dorsally. (**c**) The same case as in (**b**) looking anteriorly, demonstrating fused thalamus and massive holosphere. (**d**) A 23-week gestation, trisomy 13, with immunohistochemical staining for neurofilament light chain, demonstrating a symmetrical fused thalamus, with extensive basal and ventral leptomeningeal heterotopias. (**e**) Fused thalamus in Chiari malformation at the level of the suprapineal recess. (**f**) Term infant with ACC and olfactory bulb agenesis (not shown) with massive, almost tumefactive basal leptomeningeal heterotopias (arrows) as well as disorganized neural tissue filling the third ventricle (arrowhead)

6.4 Arrhinencephaly

The agenesis of the olfactory bulbs and tracts (arhinencephaly), when it occurs in concert with other CNS malformations, usually accompanies HPE but may be present in septo-optic dysplasia (SOD) or other forebrain malformations, such as hypothalamic hamartomas (HH). It is usually bilateral but can be unilateral and may accompany CHARGE syndrome (CHD7), Waardenburg syndrome (SOX10), Kallmann syndrome (PROKR2), Acrocallosal syndrome, or Greig cephalopolysyndactyly syndrome (GLI2, allelic with Pallister–Hall) (Fallet-Bainco 2018).

6.5 Corpus Callosum and Septum Pellucidum Development

The development of the corpus callosum begins with a posterior thickening of the lamina terminalis (the thin rostral wall of the telencephalon), resulting in the formation of the lamina reuniens. Infolding at the superior aspect of the lamina reuniens creates the sulcus medianus telencephali medii (SMTM). The SMTM is filled with cell masses and the superior banks fuse to form the massa commissuralis, also known as the commissural plate. The commissural plate becomes the bed for ingrowing fibers of the developing cerebral hemispheres.

At 11–12 weeks of gestation, the pioneer callosal fibers begin to enter the commissural plate. By 12–13 weeks, a definite corpus callosum is formed in the region of the commissural plate, which will become the genu of the corpus callosum and is present just anterior to the foramen of Monro. Growth continues over the next 5–7 weeks in a caudal direction, reflecting the rapid rate of caudal growth of the cerebral hemispheres. Growth of the corpus callosum is primarily from anterior to posterior with the genu forming first and then the anterior body, posterior body, and splenium. The exception to this rule involves the rostrum, which is the last to develop by 18–20 weeks of gestation by belated thickening of the ventral component of the most rostral part of the plate (Barcovich and Norman 1988; Rakic and Yakovlev 1968).

As the cortical plates of the cerebral hemispheres get larger, axons extend as association fibers, the majority of which cross to the contralateral hemisphere through the corpus callosum, resulting in the thickening and enlargement of the corpus callosum.

The cavum septum pellucidum (CSP) is bordered laterally by the anterior horns of the lateral ventricles, superiorly by the corpus callosum, and inferiorly by the fornix. The CSP is visible in normal fetal brain at 6 months of gestation but begins to close posteriorly such that the cavum vergae is obliterated at term. The CSP is usually present at birth but continues to shrink and is present in about 20% of adults (Loeser and Alvord 1968).

6.6 Agenesis of the Corpus Callosum

The agenesis of the corpus callosum (ACC) may be complete (Fig. 6.7a–d) or partial. Agenesis can be an isolated finding or can be observed in association with a large number of other CNS malformations, including HPE, interhemispheric cysts, neuroaxonal dystrophies and lissencephaly, and Dandy–Walker malformations. Generally, in partial agenesis, the splenium is absent or short.

6.6.1 Neuropathology

Early in gestation, the angles of the lateral ventricles point apically, the occipital horn and atrium may be dilated (colpocephaly), and the pericallosal artery has a characteristically vertical course. Either immediately near the medial surfaces of the hemispheres or sometimes partially slightly buried within the subcortical white matter, there are parallel longitudinally directed bundles of axons (Probst bundles). These are usually evident by midgestation and can even be present when a destructive process has apparently prevented the formation of the corpus callosum (Fig. 6.7e–g). By term, there is a radially directed gyral pattern on the medial surface of the cerebral hemispheres, and a well-formed continuous cingulate gyrus is absent. ACC may accompany other disorders of tract formation, and other commissural tracts (anterior, hippocampal) may also be absent (Loeser and Alvord 1968). The dorsal dilation of the third ventricle is invariably present (Loeser and Alvord 1968). In a short or dysplastic corpus callosum, Probst-like bundles may be present, although they are much more subtle (Fig. 6.8a, b).

6.6.2 Pathogenesis

Abnormalities in the guidance and growth of axonal fibers, mass, mechanical or local signaling effects by lipomas or hamartomatous lesions (Fig. 6.7c, d), and potentially any insult to the SMTM can result in ACC. Because of the

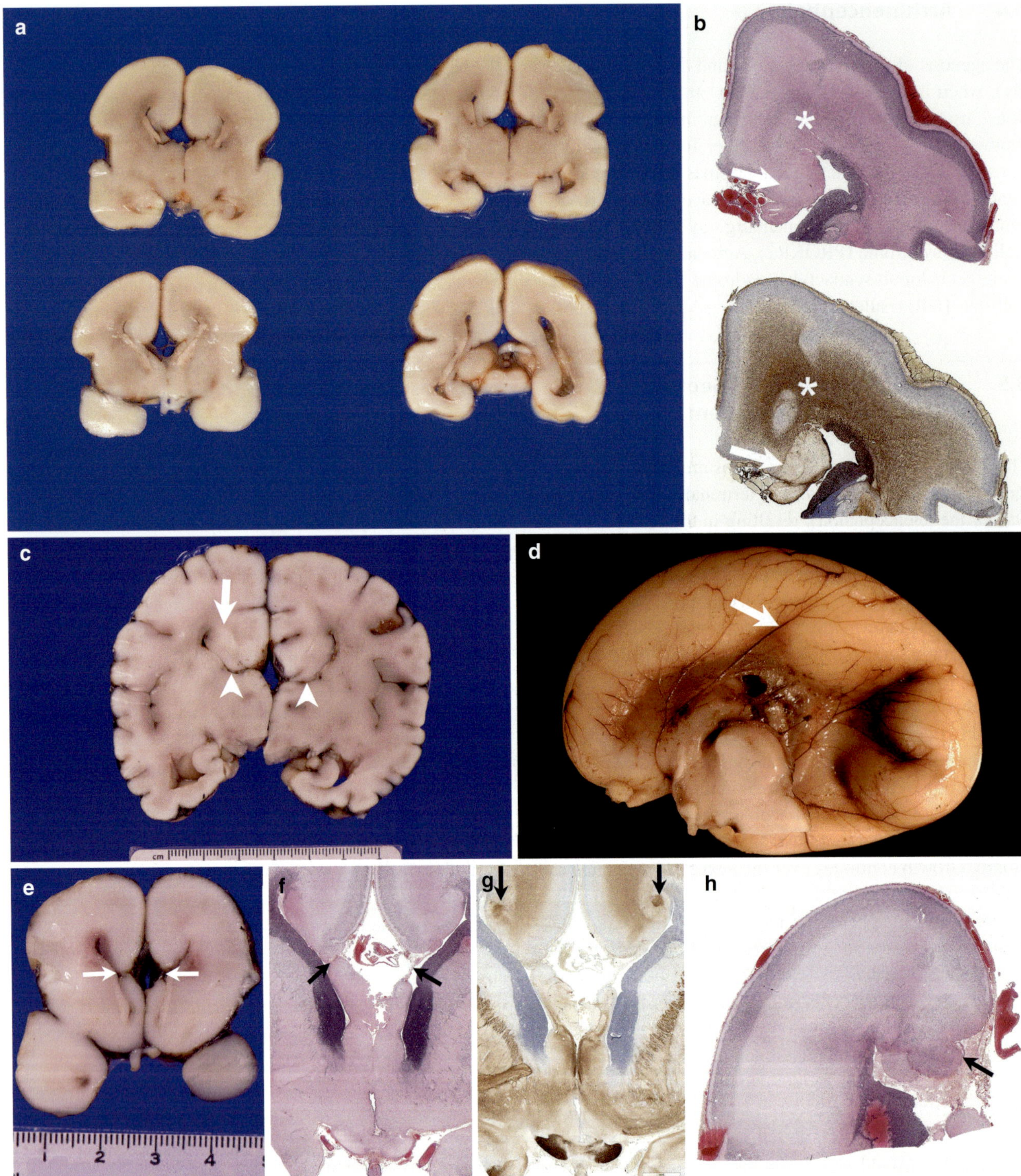

Fig. 6.7 (**a**) Agenesis of the corpus callosum, 23 weeks' gestation; the frontal horns of the lateral ventricles point medially at their dorsal extent. (**b**) Coronal section of (**a**), demonstrating anteroposteriorly directed subcingulate axonal bundle (arrow) on H + E (top) and outlined by glial and vascular immunohistochemical staining for vimentin (lower). Note the fornix attached medially and inferiorly by a broad-based, horizontally oriented, and short septum. In this case (asterisk), there is a subcortical neuronal heterotopia. (**c**) Agenesis of the corpus callosum, 37 weeks' gestation; the subcingulate Probst bundles are more readily visible as masses indenting the medial aspect of the lateral ventricles (arrows), and the fornices are oriented mediolaterally (arrowheads). Note the temporal horns are large. (**d**) Agenesis of the corpus callosum, 22 weeks' gestation; midsagittal cut demonstrating the characteristic vertical course of the pericallosal artery (arrow). We do not usually encourage this mode of sectioning of the cerebral hemispheres, as it can disrupt the fragile rostral brainstem and basal midline anatomy and interfere with the assessment of the aqueduct. (**e**) Absent corpus callosum, 24 weeks' gestation; ultrasonographic examination prior to chorionic villus sampling at 13 weeks was normal, but repeat examination at 19 weeks demonstrated absent corpus callosum. The medial ventricular wall is present frontally but focally thinned (arrows). (**f**) Whole mount of (**e**) demonstrates bilateral pori (arrows). (**g**) Immunohistochemical staining for neurofilament light chain demonstrates small Probst bundles bilaterally. (**h**) The same case as (**e**) more posteriorly demonstrating incipient polymicrogyria (arrow) adjacent to the medial porus. The interpretation is an early post-embryonic insult interrupted the formation of the corpus callosum and yielded bilateral porencephaly

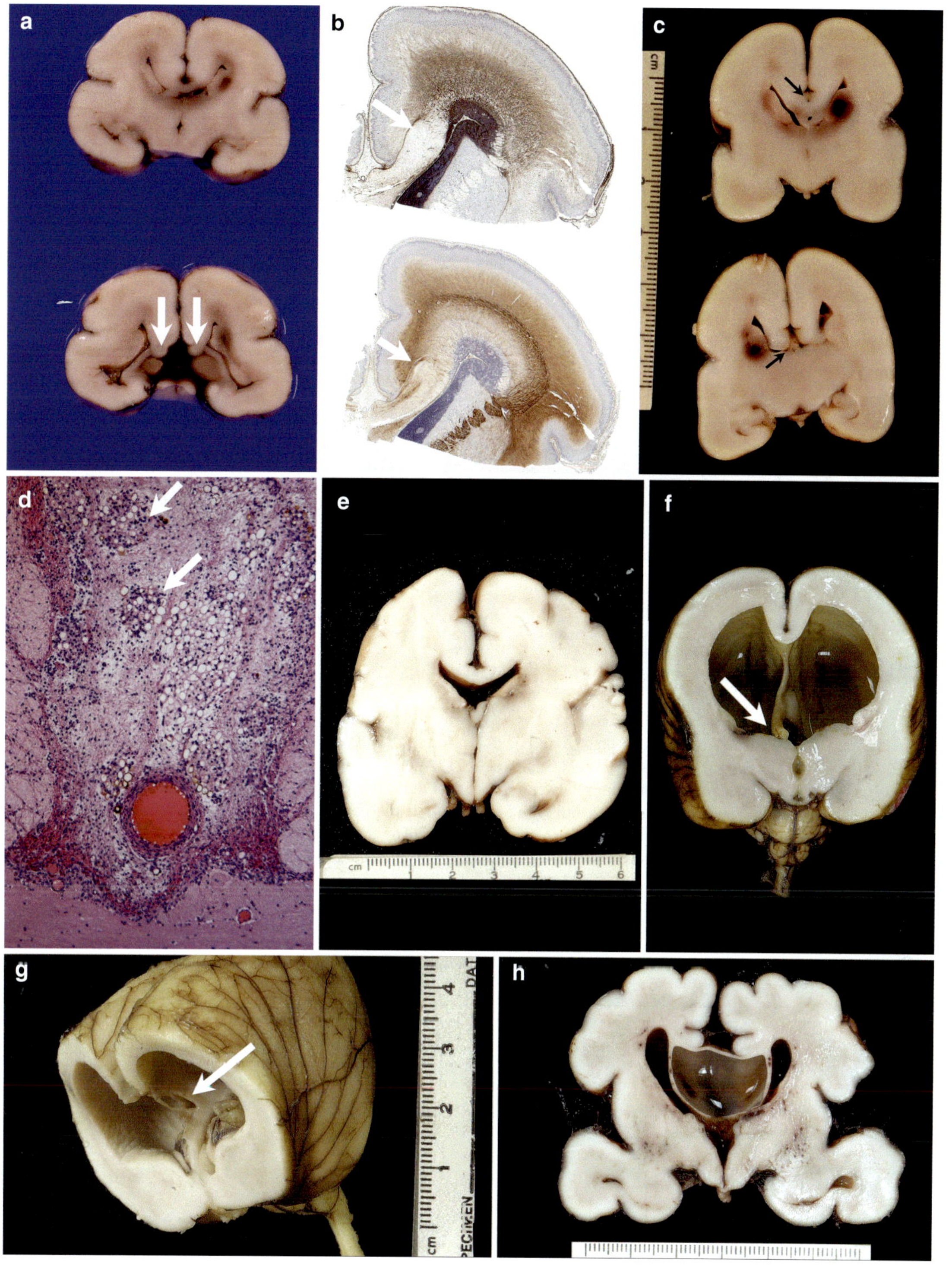

Fig. 6.8 (**a**) Dysplastic corpus callosum, 24 weeks' gestation; the corpus callosum is irregular in thickness anteriorly, and posteriorly, the splenium does not extend as far as the caudal pulvinar and pineal but ends as bundles (arrows). (**b**) The same case as (**a**); immunohistochemistry for vimentin (top) demonstrates abnormal delimitation of frontal corpus callosal fibers (arrow) from subcingulate white matter by glial/vascular condensation; staining for neurofilament light chain (bottom) demonstrates displacement of normal fiber architecture by longitudinally oriented fibers (arrow). (**c**) Callosal lipoma, 22 weeks' gestation; the arrow demonstrates minute callosal mass (arrow) with short anteroposterior corpus callosum and mass in continuity with the roof of the third ventricle. The germinal matrix hematomas are acute. (**d**) Same cases as (**c**), demonstrating lobules of lipoblasts (arrows) in fibromyxoid stroma, attached to the dorsal surface of the corpus callosum. The pigment is formalin pigment. (**e**) Absent septum pellucidum, 26 weeks' gestation; the corpus callosum and fornices are normal, and there is little other pathology in the brain. (**f**) Incomplete (perforated) septum in aqueduct stenosis. There is massive lateral and third ventricular dilation, the fornices (arrow) are fused and descended, and the septum is incomplete. (**g**) Fenestrated septum (arrow) in X-linked aqueduct stenosis. The septum has multiple irregular fenestrae (arrow). (**h**) Massive CSP, here with a thin corpus callosum, in a case of pachygyria of unclear origin

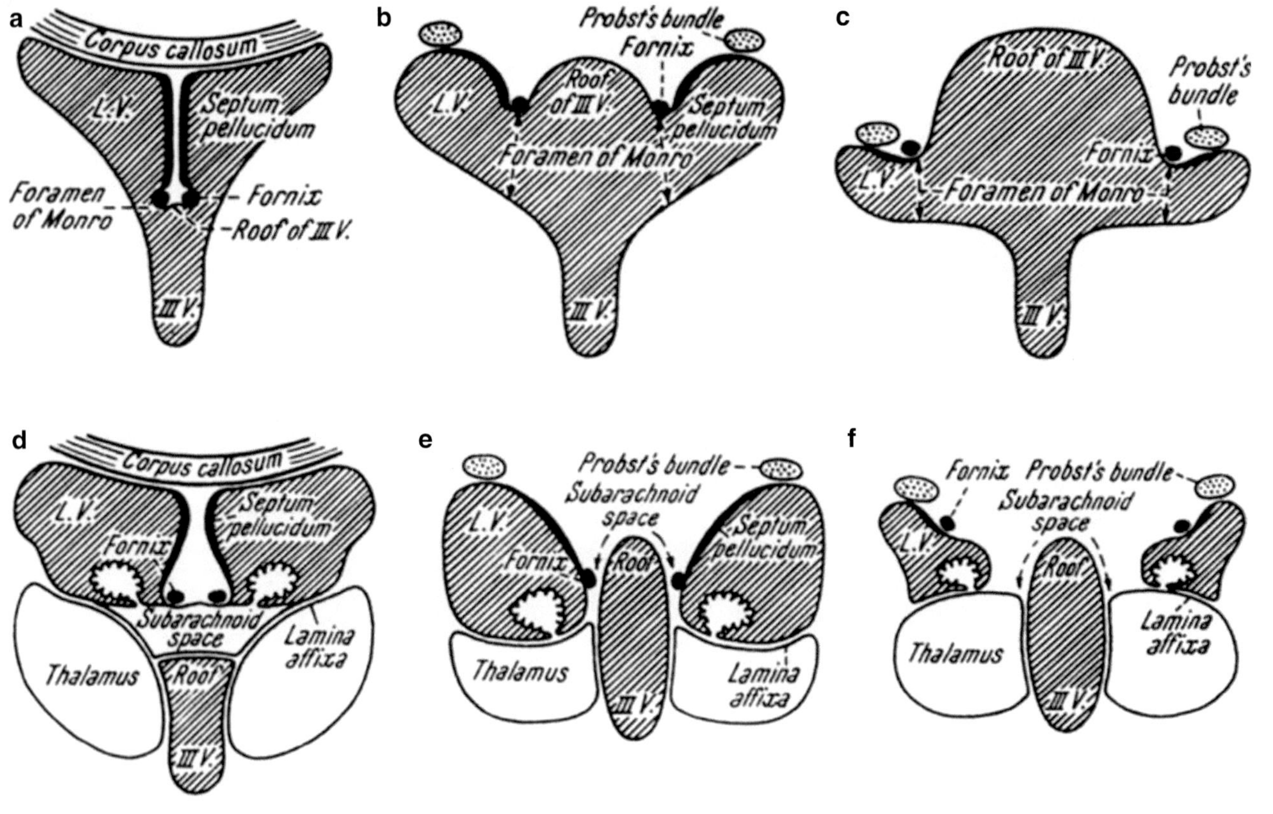

Fig. 6.9 Schematic drawings of coronal sections of normal and acallosal brains. (**a–c**) At the level of the foramen of Monro. (**a**) Normal. (**b**) Agenesis of the corpus callosum with septum pellucidum between fornices and Probst bundles. (**c**) Agenesis of the corpus callosum with fornices apposed to Probst bundles and no septum pellucidum. Note the change in orientation of the septum pellucidum and the preservation of anatomical relationships. (**d–f**) Posterior to the foramen of Monro. (**d**) Normal. (**e**) Agenesis of the corpus callosum with septum pellucidum. (**f**) Agenesis of the corpus callosum without septum pellucidum. Note that the subarachnoid space overlies the roof of the third ventricle even though the cavum velum interpositum is not present in an acallosal brain. The bare area of the thalamus is also greatly reduced in the acallosal brain (From Loeser and Alvord (1968); with permission)

predominantly posterior growth of the corpus callosum, partial agenesis almost always involves the splenium. Genetic syndromes include the Aicardi, Andermann, acrocallosal, and Meckel syndromes.

The acallosal brain does have septi pellucidi, but their course is directed sharply laterally (Fig. 6.7b). It appears as if the callosal fibers maintain a midline orientation for the septum, and the failure to decussate permits lateral placement of the remaining callosal fibers (Probst bundle) with the attached septum pellucidum. The absence of the splenium is responsible for the marked mesial dilatation of the lateral ventricle trigone.

6.7 Agenesis of the Septum Pellucidum

Antenatal observation of septum pellucidum agenesis is often used asa clue to the presence of other associated anomalies (e.g., HPE, ACC, SOD)(Sundarakumar et al. 2015), but itcan be an isolated anomaly (Fig. 6.10e) or may accompany obstructive hydrocephalus, either of post-encephaloclastic origin, post-obstructive hydrocephalus with multiple anomalies, or apparently isolated aqueductal stenosis (personal observation) (Fig. 6.8f, g). Occasionally, one encounters a very capacious cavum (Fig. 6.8h), but the significance of such a finding is unclear.

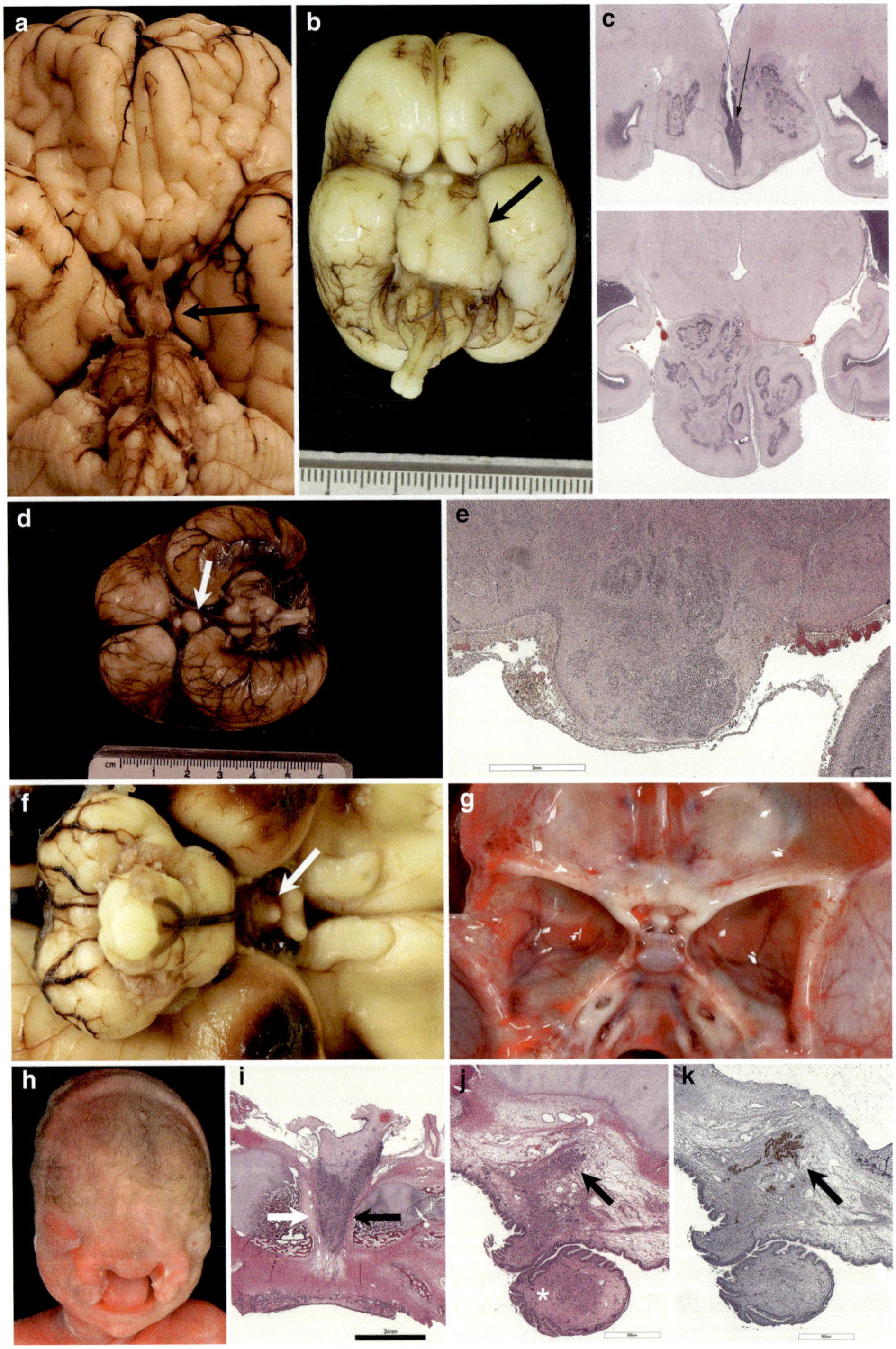

Fig. 6.10 (**a**) Small pedunculated HH (arrow); a term infant with otherwise isolated agenesis of the olfactory bulbs and tracts. (**b**) Massive HH (arrow), 18 weeks' gestation, in GLI3-related Pallister–Hall syndrome. (**c**) Whole mounts of the anterior (top) and posterior (bottom) aspect of the hypothalamus, with heterotopic germinal matrix tissue in the third ventricle and with disorganized neural masses in the lateral hypothalamus and in the hamartoma, with areas of cerebral cortical differentiation. (**d**) Anterior HH in TBC1D32-related disease. (**e**) Histology of hamartoma replacing the neurohypophysis and accompanying agenesis of the pituitary. (**f**) Blunt-ended neurohypophysis in pituitary agenesis. (**g**) Sella of the case in (**f**), demonstrating bony floor of the sella with no pituitary tissue. (**h**) Split-face malformation with central wide cleft lip and palate, agenesis of the nasal septum and striking hypertelorism. (**i**) Coronal section through the sella demonstrating hypothalamus and adenohypophysis (arrows) between sphenoid ossification centers extending to the submucosa of the nasopharynx below. (**j**) Roof of the nasopharynx displaying fibroepithelial and smooth muscle nodular mass (asterisk) with heterotopic pituitary in the submucosal tissue immediately below the cartilage of the anterior sphenoid. (**k**) The same section as (**j**), stained immunohistochemically with synaptophysin antibody, demonstrating a nest of heterotopic pituitary gland (arrow)

6.8 Septo-optic Dysplasia (Also Known as de Morsier Syndrome)

Septo-optic dysplasia comprises a triad, which is complete clinically in only a minority of cases (Morishima and Aranoff 1986) consisting of optic hypoplasia, pituitary dysfunction, and absent septum pellucidum. Midline forebrain anomalies include hypothalamic gliosis, hypoplasia or nuclear dysplasia, hypoplasia/absence of the neurohypophysis or hypoplasia of the adenohypophysis, third ventricular fusion, absent olfactory bulbs and/or tracts, thin corpus callosum, and hippocampal hypoplasia or dysplasia. These abnormalities may be accompanied by retinal dysplasia or hypoplasia, hypoplastic optic chiasm or nerves, lateral geniculate hypoplasia, cerebral heterotopias, reduced white matter volume, shallow cerebral fissuring or gyration, HPE, porencephaly, schizencephaly, polymicrogyria, cerebral cortical dyslamination, basal ganglia gliosis or calcification, ependymal denudation, and subependymal gliosis. Brainstem abnormalities recorded may include the full triad, which is seen in 30% of patients. The triad may be associated with small medullary pyramids, disorganized corticospinal tracts, dentato-olivary dysplasia, cerebellar hypoplasia and dysplasia, small brainstem, and tonsillar grooving (Blackburn et al. 2021; Roessmann et al. 1987). Clearly, the literature as a whole may not be describing a unitary developmental entity.

6.8.1 Pathogenesis/Embryology

Septo-optic dysplasia is sometimes thought to occur after failure in forebrain development from 4 to 6 weeks of gestation, when the anterior plate undergoes morphogenesis (Webb and Dattani 2010). Genetic, acquired (e.g., fetal viral infections), and environmental factors (e.g., antenatal drug and alcohol) (Barcovich and Lindan 1994; Lippe et al. 1979; Riedl et al. 2008) may play a role. Early vascular disruption, particularly of the anterior circulation, has been suggested as a unifying hypothesis (Chiaramonte et al. 2013; Lubinsky 1997; Stevens and Dobyns 2004; Lubinsky and Encha-Razavi 2022) in carefully delineated cases (Lubinsky and Encha-Razavi 2022).

6.8.2 Genetics

Septo-optic dysplasia has been associated with abnormalities in HESX1, SOX2, SOX3, and OTX2 (Kelberman and Dattani 2007; Webb and Dattani 2010) and TAX1BP3 (dilated cardiomyopathy with SOD (Reinstein et al. 2015)). Caveats as to etiopathogenesis (above) apply.

6.9 Hypothalamic Hamartoma

These are variably sized masses of poorly organized neural tissue, typically attached near the posterior hypothalamus (Fig. 6.9a), but can incorporate or even efface the infundibulum (Fig. 6.9b–e). Non-syndromic hamartomas are generally smaller and associated with gelastic seizures and precocious puberty than those accompanying familial conditions.

6.9.1 Neuropathology

These masses generally are attached by a narrow or broad stalk to the posterior hypothalamus in the area of the mammillary bodies. The neuropathology varies with the size of the lesion. Some describe a circumferential layer of myelinated fibers in the peripheral region of the tissue mass, with clusters of small neurons intermixed with glia and a spongy neuropil and relatively sparse large neurons (Kerrigan et al. 2017; Coons et al. 2007). Cystic change and prominent masses of fibrous tissue or other mesenchymal elements can sometimes be seen (Prasad et al. 2000). The arrangement of neurons can vary from small nodules of a few neurons tightly grouped in a grape-like manner to large arrays; in Pallister–Hall syndrome, the masses of neurons can be very large, and cerebral cortical differentiation with areas of neuroepithelium and germinal matrix tissue can be seen in early fetal cases (Dunham et al. 2018, personal observation).

6.9.2 Genetics

Hypothalamic hamartomas are most commonly sporadic. Where they are seen with other malformations, we have seen them most commonly with HPE (see above), ACC, and Joubert-type pathology in the cerebellum and brainstem. Approximately 5% of cases of HH are associated with Pallister–Hall syndrome, with mutation in the *GLI3* gene (Kang et al. 1997).

6.9.3 Other Hypothalamic Abnormalities

The congenital absence of the pituitary can be related to the anterior HH (Fig. 6.9d, e) in TBC1D32-related disease or with a simple blunt-ended neurohypophysis (Fig. 6.9f, g). In wide middle facial defects, the hypothalamus may be tightly tethered to the base of the skull by a midline cleft sphenoid containing neurohypophysis and heterotopic pituitary in the roof of the nasopharynx (Fig. 6.9h–k).

References

Barcovich AJ, Norman D. Anomalies of the corpus callosum: correlation with further anomalies of the brain. AJR Am J Roentgenol. 1988;151(1):171–9.

Barcovich AJ, Quint DJ. Middle interhemispheric fusion: an unusual variant of holoprosencephaly. AJNR Am J Neuroradiol. 1993;14(2):431–40.

Barkovich AJ, Lindan CE. Congenital cytomegalovirus infection of the brain: imaging analysis and embryologic considerations. AJNR Am J Neuroradiol. 1994;15(4):703–15.

Barratt K, Drover KA, Thomas ZM, Arkell RM. Patterning of anteroventral mammalian brain: lessons from holoprosencephaly comparative biology in man and mouse. WIREs Mech Dis. 2022:e1552. https://doi.org/10.1002/wsbm.1552.

Blackburn J, Thomas DL, Hughes A, Pierson CR. Neuropathology of Septo-optic dysplasia: a report of 4 autopsy cases. J Child Neurol. 2021;36(2):105–15.

Brown SA, Warburton D, Brown LY, Yu CY, Roeder ER, Stengel-Rutkowski S, Hennekam RC, Muenke M. Holoprosencephaly due to mutations in ZIC2, a homologue of drosophila odd-paired. Nat Genet. 1998;20(2):180–3.

Chiaramonte I, Cappello G, Uccello A, et al. Vascular cerebral anomalies associated with septo-optic dysplasia. A case report. Neuroradiol J. 2013;26(1):66–70.

Coons SW, Rekate HL, Prenger EC, Wang N, Drees C, Ng YT, Chung SS, Kerrigan JF. The histopathology of hypothalamic hamartomas: study of 57 cases. J Neuropathol Exp Neurol. 2007;66(2):131–41.

Daly T, Roberts A, Yang E, Mochida GH, Bodamer O. Holoprosencephaly in Kabuki syndrome. Am J Med Genet A. 2020;182(3):441–5.

du Plessis AJ, Volpe JJ. Prosencephalic development. In: Volpe's neurology of newborn. 6th ed. Elsevier Inc.; 2018.

Dunham C, McFadden D, Dahlgren L, Butler B, Hamilton S, McKinnon M. Congenital hypothalamic "hamartoblastoma" versus "hamartoma": suggestions for neuropathologic terminology emanating from a mid-gestational autopsy case of Pallister-Hall syndrome. Pediatr Dev Pathol. 2018;21(3):324–31.

Fallet-Bainco C. Neuropathology of Holoprosencephaly. Am J Med Genet C Semin Med Genet. 2018;178(2):214–28.

Fisher Y, Shannon P, Greenberg O, Chitayat D, Chong K, Blaser S, Shinar S. Mesencephalosynapsis and aqueductal stenosis. J Neuropathol Exp Neurol. 2024; Online ahead of print.

Fisher Y, Shannon P, Greenberg O, Chitayat D, Chong K, Blaser S, Shinar S. Mesencephalosynapsis and aqueductal stenosis. J Neuropathol Exp Neurol. 2025;84(3):195–209.

Garcia CA, Duncan C. Atelencephalic microcephaly. Dev Med Child Neurol. 1977;19(2):227–32.

Hahn JS, Barnes PD, Clegg NJ, Stashinko EE. Septopreoptic holoprosencephaly: a mild subtype associated with midline craniofacial anomalies. AJNR Am J Neuroradiol. 2010;31(9):1596–601.

Harris CP, Townsend JJ, Norman MG, White VA, Viskochil DH, Pysher TJ, Klatt EC. Atelencephalic aprosencephaly. J Child Neurol. 1994;9(4):412–6.

Harris E, Richardson R, Annavarapu S, Tellez J, Butteriss D, Hannon T, Splitt M. Mosaicism in Hartsfield syndrome. Eur J Med Genet. 2022;65(5):104491. https://doi.org/10.1016/j.ejmg.2022.104491.

Harris SC, Chong K, Chitayat D, Gilmore KL, Jorge AAL, Freire BL, Lerario A, Shannon P, Cope H, Gallentine WB, Le Guyader G, Bilan F, Létard P, Davis EE, Vora NL. Diagnosis of TBC1D32-associated conditions: expanding the phenotypic spectrum of a complex ciliopathy. Am J Med Genet A. 2023;191(5):1282–92.

Hietamäki J, Gregory LC, Ayoub S, Iivonen AP, Vaaralahti K, Liu X, Brandstack N, Buckton AJ, Laine T, Känsäkoski J, Hero M, Miettinen PJ, Varjosalo M, Wakeling E, Dattani MT, Raivio T. Loss-of-function variants in TBC1D32 underlie syndromic hypopituitarism. J Clin Endocrinol Metab. 2020;105(6):1748–58.

Iivanainen M, Haltia M, Lydecken K. Atelencephaly. Dev Med Child Neurol. 1997;19(5):663–8.

Kang S, Allen J, Graham JM Jr, et al. Linkage mapping and phenotypic analysis of autosomal dominant Pallister-Hall syndrome. J Med Genet. 1997;34(6):441–6.

Kelberman D, Dattani MT. Genetics of septo-optic dysplasia. Pituitary. 2007;10(4):393–407.

Kerrigan JF, Parsons A, Tsang C, et al. Hypothalamic hamartoma: neuropathology and epileptogenesis. Epilepsia. 2017;58(Suppl 2):22–31.

Kim TS, Cho S, Dickson DW. Aprosencephaly: review of the literature and report of a case with cerebellar hypoplasia, pigmented epithelial cyst and Rathke's cleft cyst. Acta Neuropathol. 1990;79(4):424–31.

Koob M, Weingertner AS, Gasser B, Oubel E, Dietemann JL. Thick corpus callosum: a clue to the diagnosis of fetal septopreoptic holoprosencephaly? Pediatr Radiol. 2012;42(7):886–90.

Lippe B, Kaplan SA, LaFranchi S. Septo-optic dysplasia and maternal age. Lancet. 1979;2(8133):92–3.

Loeser JD, Alvord EC Jr. Agenesis of the corpus callosum. Brain. 1968;91(93):553–70.

Lubinsky MS. Hypothesis: septo-optic dysplasia is a vascular disruption sequence. Am J Med Genet. 1997;69(3):235–6.

Lubinsky M, Encha-Razavi F. Delineating septo-optic dysplasia. Birth Defects Res. 2022;114(20):1343–53.

Lurie W, Nedzved MK, Lazjuk GI, Kirillova IA, Cherstvoy ED. Aprosencephaly-atelencephaly and the aprosencephaly (XK) syndrome. Am J Med Genet. 1979;3(3):217–316.

Morishima A, Aranoff GS. Syndrome of septo-optic-pituitary dysplasia: the clinical spectrum. Brain Dev. 1986;8(3):233–9.

Prasad S, Shah J, Patkar D, et al. Giant hypothalamic hamartoma with cystic change: report of two cases and review of the literature. Neuroradiology. 2000;42(9):48–50.

Rakic P, Yakovlev P. Development of the corpus callosum and cavum septi in man. J Comp Neurol. 1968;132(1):45–72.

Reinstein E, Orvin K, Tayeb-Fligelman E. Mutations in TAX1BP3 cause dilated cardiomyopathy with septo-optic dysplasia. Hum Mutat. 2015;36(4):439–42.

Riedl S, Vosahlo J, Battelino T, et al. Refining clinical phenotypes in septo-optic dysplasia based on MRI findings. Eur J Pediatr. 2008;167(11):1269–76.

Roessmann U, Velasco ME, Small EJ, Hori A. Neuropathology of "septo-optic dysplasia" (de Morsier syndrome) with immunohistochemical studies of the hypothalamus and pituitary gland. J Neuropathol Exp Neurol. 1987;46(5):597–608.

Sarnat HB, Flores-Sarnat L. Neuropathologic research strategies in holoprosencephaly. J Child Neurol. 2001;16(12):918–31.

Sarnet HB, Resch L, Flores-Sarnat LF, Yu W. Precocious synapses in 13.5-week fetal holoprosencephalic cortex and cyclopean retina. Brain Development. 2014;36(6):463–71.

Sergi C, Schmitt HP. The vesicular forebrain (pseudo-aprosencephaly): a missing link in the teratogenetic spectrum of the defective brain anlage and its discrimination from aprosencephaly. Acta Neuropathol. 2000;99(3):277–84.

Siebert JR, Warkany J, Lemire RJ. Atelencephalic microcephaly in a 21-week human fetus. Teratology. 1986;34(1):9–19.

Simon EM, Hevner RF, Pinter JD, Clegg NJ, Delgado M, Kinsman SL, Hahn JS, Barkovich AJ. The middle interhemispheric variant of holoprosencephaly. AJNR Am J Neuroradiol. 2002;23(1):151–6.

Stevens CA, Dobyns WB. Septo-optic dysplasia and amniotic bands: further evidence for a vascular pathogenesis. Am J Med Genet A. 2004;125A(1):12–6.

Sundarakumar DK, Farley SA, Smith CM, et al. Absent cavum septum pellucidum: a review with emphasis on associated commissural abnormalities. Pediatr Radiol. 2015;45:95–964.

Varma A, Mishra GV, Dhande R, Lakhkar BB. Varied presentation of lobar holoprosencephaly as a cause of macrocephaly in a neonate. BMJ Case Rep. 2022;15(1):e248024. https://doi.org/10.1136/bcr-2021-248024.

Volpe JJ. Overview: normal and abnormal human brain development. Ment Retard Dev Disabil Res Rev. 2000;6:1–5.

Webb EA, Dattani MT. Septo-optic dysplasia. Eur J Hum Genet. 2010;18(4):393–7.

Midbrain and Hindbrain Malformations

7

The development of the midbrain and hindbrain occurs between the fifth and tenth weeks of gestation as part of ventral induction. As the neural tube closes, three primary cephalic vesicles develop—prosencephalon, mesencephalon, and rhombencephalon (Cotes et al. 2015). The mesencephalon and rhombencephalon are separated rostrally from the prosencephalon by the cephalic flexure and separated caudally from the spinal cord by the cervical flexure.

The mesencephalon differentiates into midbrain structures. The aqueduct of Sylvius develops by the narrowing of the central canal. Migrating neuroblasts from the alar plate form the superior and inferior colliculi as well as the red nucleus and substantia nigra. The tegmentum develops from the basal plate (Fotos et al. 2011).

The rhombencephalon further develops into hindbrain structures. Its rhomboid shape is formed by the separation of the lateral walls. The pontine flexure forms and divides the rhombencephalon between the rostral metencephalon and caudal myelencephalon. The thickening of the floor and lateral walls of the metencephalon and myelencephalon gives rise to the pons and medulla oblongata, respectively (Shekdar 2011).

The thinning and widening of the rhombencephalic roof plate form the fourth ventricle. At 10 weeks of gestation, the tissue that will subsequently develop into the choroid plexus creates the plica choroidalis, an indentation in the thinned roof plate that divides it into the anterior and posterior membranous areas. The anterior membranous area subsequently merges into the choroid plexus, while the posterior membranous area forms Blake's pouch. The accumulation of the cerebrospinal fluid in this area results in the cisterna magna that will later regress to form the foramen of Magendie. The Luschka foramina develop from the lateral angles of the rhomboid fossa (Cotes et al. 2015).

7.1 Aqueductal Stenosis and Mesencephalosynapsis

Stenosis of the aqueduct of Sylvius is a common finding in obstructive hydrocephalus. Mesencephalosynapsis refers to the absence of the dorsal median glial septum of the midbrain, resulting in a failure of cleavage of the superior and/or inferior colliculi. All reported cases of mesencephalosynapsis to date are accompanied by aqueductal stenosis and are commonly associated with other brain malformations (Fisher et al. 2025).

Aqueductal stenosis is considered a spectrum, ranging between complete atresia of the aqueduct to slit-like elongated aqueducts, and aqueducts that are indefinite for stenosis but appear abnormal to the experienced eye (Fig. 7.1a–g). The incidence of mesencephalosynapsis increases with the severity of stenosis. Atresia of the aqueduct, with or without rudimentary ependymal rosettes, often accompanies pervasive brain malformations such as holoprosencephaly or rhombencephalosynapsis but has also been reported in cases of severe ischemic injury with gliosis of the tegmentum (Fisher et al. 2025). Careful consideration and clinical correlation should be applied when diagnosing aqueductal stenosis in the presence of maceration, as this might be artifactual.

Forking refers to the separation of the aqueduct into two or more channels. A dorsoventral split to two channels in the caudal midbrain is a result of the normal anatomy of the aqueduct and should not be considered an abnormality (Fig. 7.1h) (Friede 1961; Fisher et al. 2025). True forking or atresia–forking refers to the splitting of the aqueduct into small channels and/or ependymal nests without the associated gliosis (Fig. 7.1i–k). Gliosis or webbing of the aqueduct with glial septa is usually associated with infectious disease but is occasionally seen with other malformations, such as

P. Shannon et al., *Atlas of Neurodevelopmental Pathology*, https://doi.org/10.1007/978-3-032-14148-4_7

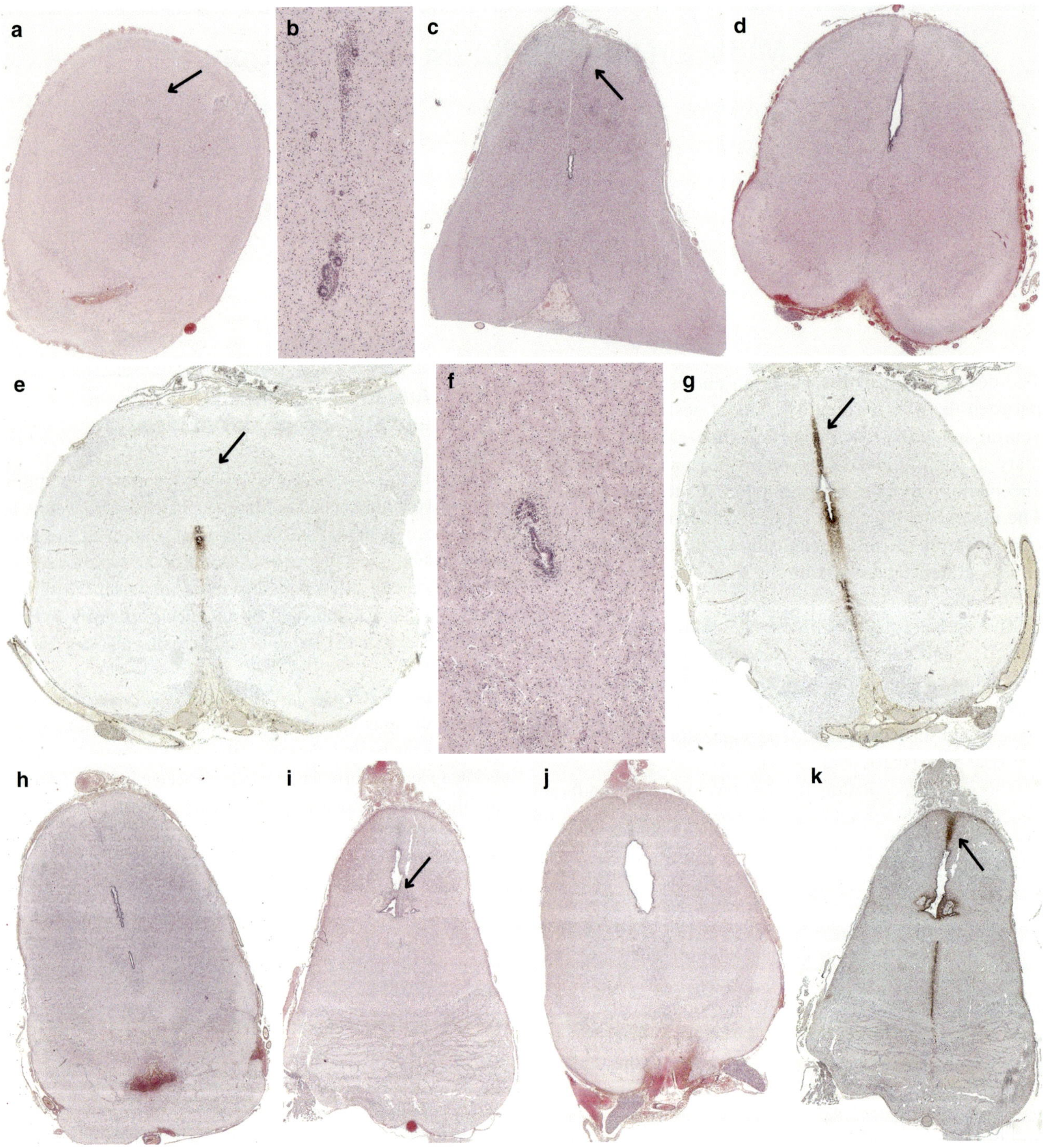

Fig. 7.1 Aqueductal stenosis. (**a**, **b**) Atresia and forking of the aqueduct of a 22-week-gestation fetus with amniotic rupture sequence. The median dorsal glial raphe is absent (arrow), and the tectum is dome-shaped. (**c**) Mild aqueductal stenosis of a 20-week-gestation fetus with an occipital meningocele and hydrocephalus. The glial raphe is present (arrow). (**d**) Simplified and distorted aqueduct of a 19-week-gestation fetus with multiple congenital anomalies and ventriculomegaly. (**e–g**) Severe aqueductal stenosis in a 22-week-gestation fetus with trisomy 18. There is mesencephalosynapsis at the level of the superior colliculi (**e**); however, the median glial raphe is present at the level of the inferior colliculi (**g**) (arrows) (vimentin). (**h**) Trivial forking of the aqueduct. (**i**) Glial web in the aqueduct of a 22-week-gestation fetus, with hydrocephalus. (**j**) The rostral aqueduct is dilated and simplified. (**k**) The median glial raphe is intact (arrow, nestin)

rhombencephalosynapsis and Chiari type 2 malformation (Russell 1949; Ellison et al. 2013; Fisher et al. 2025).

Although aqueductal stenosis is described in a number of genetic diseases (e.g., X-linked hydrocephalus due to *L1CAM* mutation), in most cases, a recurrent genetic aberration is not found (Adle-Biassette et al. 2013). Mesencephalosynapsis is considered a result of abnormal dorsoventral patterning, explaining its association with holoprosencephaly and rhombencephalosynapsis (Sarnat and Flores-Sarnat 2008).

7.2 Chiari Malformations

Chiari malformations, initially described by Hans Chiari in 1891, are a group of malformations that have in common the herniation of the cerebellar tonsils below the foramen magnum (Chiari 1891). Chiari type 1 involves slight displacement of the tonsils below the foramen magnum. It is usually asymptomatic in infancy and rarely encountered in the fetal autopsy service (Sarnat 2008; Cesmebasi et al. 2015).

Chiari type 2 is the most common type observed in fetal autopsy and is usually associated with an open neural tube defect, often in the lumbosacral spine (see Chap. 3). Chiari type 3 is rare and represents the most severe form, usually associated with occipital encephalocele or cervical myelomeningocele. Chiari type 4 was added by Chiari to his original description in 1895; it represents cerebellar hypoplasia without caudal displacement, unlike the other types (Chiari 1895).

On macroscopic examination (Fig. 7.2), when viewing the exposed posterior fossa, the cerebellar vermis and obex appear caudally displaced through the foramen magnum. The brainstem structures are elongated, and the aqueduct of Sylvius varies between mildly stenotic, slit-like, and patent. Rarely, there may be a point obstruction of the aqueduct due to a glial web; however, mesencephalosynapsis is not observed (Fisher et al. 2025). The pons is flat, and the cranial nerve roots are ascending. Often, there is a kink in the caudal medulla. The cerebellum assumes a conical structure, occasionally wrapping around the brainstem. The posterior fossa itself is small. Chiari malformations are commonly associated with hydrocephalus, often with periventricular nodular heterotopia or nodular excrescences along the ventricular wall. The thalami often appear fused with an enlarged massa intermedia (Cesmebasi et al. 2015).

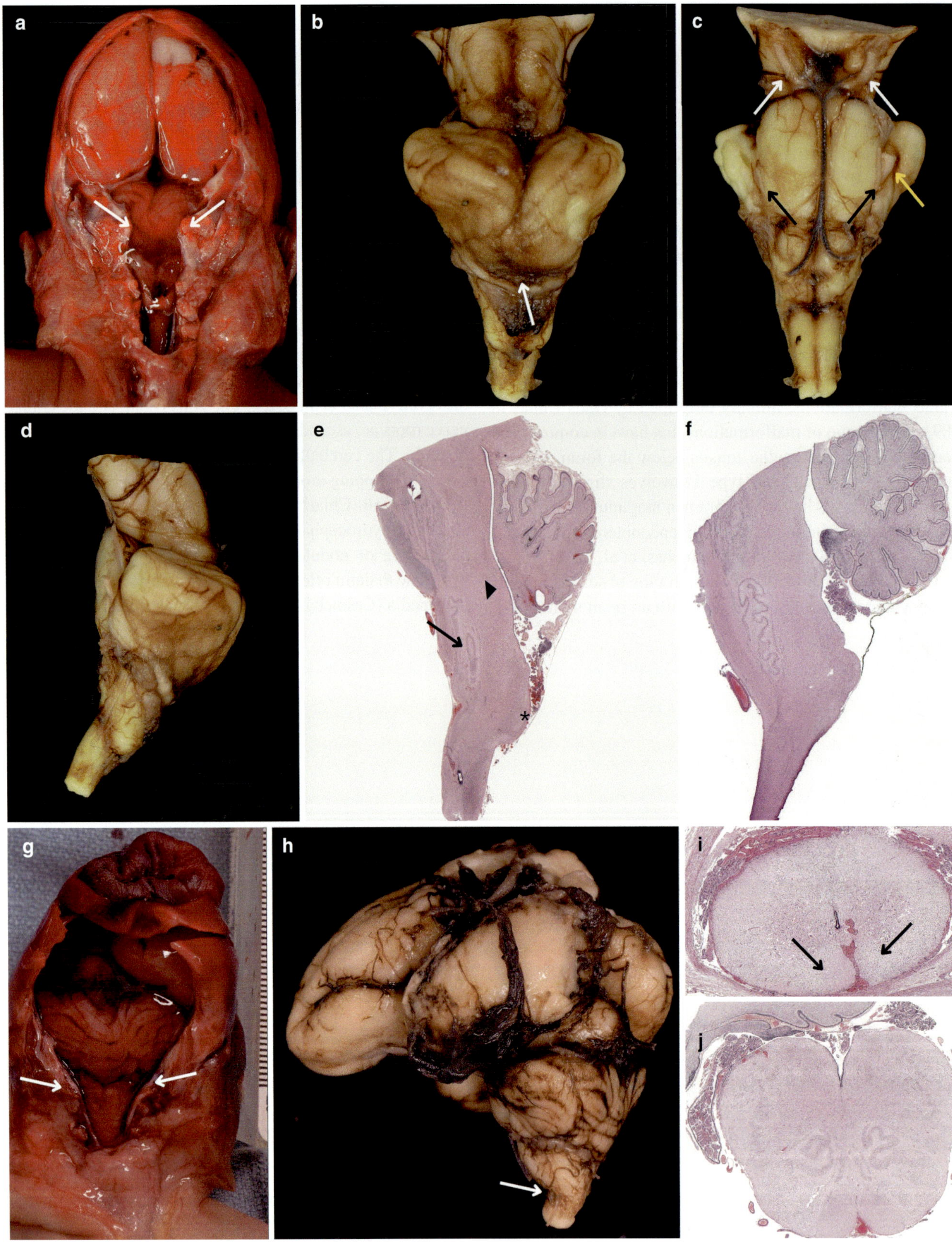

Fig. 7.2 Chiari malformations. (**a**) Chiari type 2 malformation in a 22-week-gestation fetus. The cerebellar vermis and obex are herniated through the foramen magnum (arrows). (**b**) The cerebellum is conical with a caudally displaced vermis (arrow). (**c**) The cranial nerves III (white arrows), V (yellow arrow), and VII or VIII (black arrows) are oriented in an ascending trajectory. (**d**) The midbrain is elongated and "towering," the pons is flattened, and the cerebellar hemispheres are wrapped around the brainstem. (**e**) The medulla is elongated, and the inferior olives are caudally displaced compared to an age-matched normal control (**f**). The fastigial angle of the cerebellum is flattened (arrowhead). (**g**) Chiari type 3 malformation in a 22-week-gestation fetus with an occipital encephalocele. The vermis is caudally displaced to the verge of the foramen magnum (arrows). (**h**) The cerebellum is conical and the medulla is kinked (arrow). (**i**) The anterior columns of the spinal cord are asymmetric due to non-decussation of the corticospinal tracts (arrows), (**j**) despite symmetrical pyramids

7.3 Brainstem Dysplasia

Brainstem dysplasia is a broad term that encompasses various morphologic patterns, involving the different structures of the brainstem: the brainstem nuclei including cranial nerve nuclei and the various tracts of the brainstem. Brainstem dysplasia is often associated with cerebellar and cerebral malformations but may also be an isolated finding. Some genetic syndromes are associated with specific patterns of brainstem dysplasia. The following sections describe these patterns and their associations.

7.3.1 Tract Abnormalities

The most prominent tracts in the ventral brainstem are the corticospinal (or pyramidal) tracts (Fig. 7.3a–c). The absence or hypoplasia of these tracts (Fig. 7.3d–f) may occur as part of genetic syndromes—such as X-linked hydrocephalus with *L1CAM* mutations—or result from pervasive brain anomalies, i.e., aprosencephaly, holoprosencephaly, or severe cortical malformations (Chatron et al. 2019; Pirot et al. 2016; Florell et al. 1996; Adle-Biassette et al. 2013). Occasionally, tract loss may be unilateral, or the tracts may be present but appear dysplastic (Fig. 7.3g, h).

Other tracts running through the brainstem tegmentum may be absent or exhibit an anomalous course (Fig. 7.3i–k). These are more difficult to identify on H&E stains, and the use of immunohistochemical stains, such as for neurofilament light chain, is helpful.

7.3.2 Nuclear Abnormalities

Dysplasia of brainstem neuronal groups may be part of many brain malformations. These abnormalities are difficult to identify in fetal cases and require meticulous comparison with age-matched and level-matched normal controls. Abnormalities of the inferior olivary nuclear complexes are more prominent and are described separately below. Other nuclear abnormalities are usually associated with additional brainstem abnormalities and will be demonstrated in the following sections.

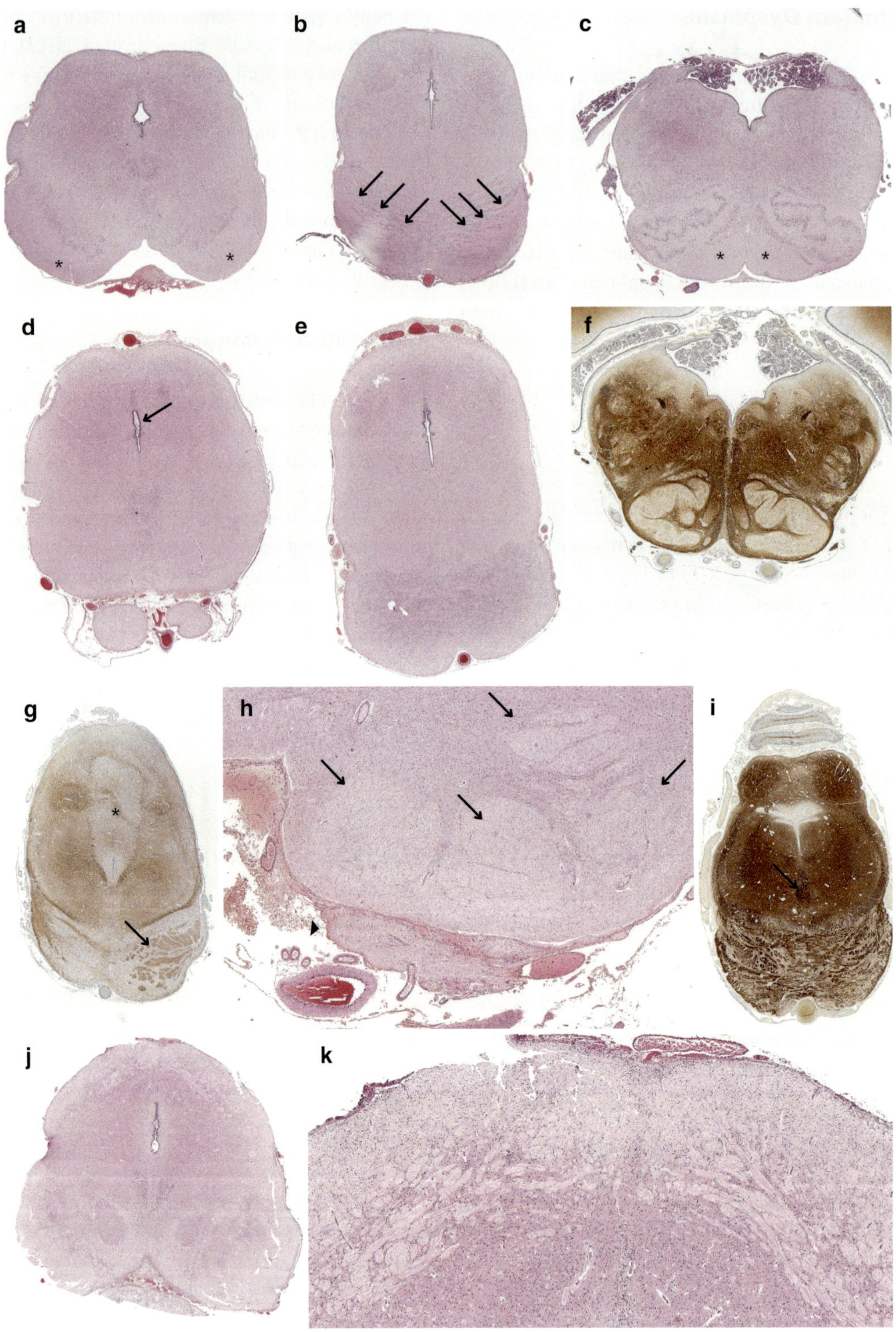

Fig. 7.3 Tract abnormalities. (**a–c**) Normal anatomy of the corticospinal tracts. (**a**) Midbrain: the corticospinal tracts are located in the cerebral peduncles, ventral to the substantia nigra (asterisks). (**b**) Pons: the corticospinal tracts course between the neurons of the nucleus basis pontis (arrows). (**c**) Medulla: the corticospinal tracts are bundled in the pyramids, ventromedial to the inferior olives (asterisks). (**d–f**) Absent corticospinal tracts in a male fetus with X-linked hydrocephalus. (**d**) The ventral midbrain is flattened due to the absence of the cerebral peduncles, and the aqueduct is slit-like (arrow). (**e**) In the pons, the neurons of the nucleus basis pontis are densely packed due to the absence of the dissecting corticospinal tracts. (**f**) In the medulla, the pyramids are absent (neurofilament light chain). (**g**) Asymmetric corticospinal tracts present in one side of the basis pontis (arrow) in a fetus with amniotic rupture sequence. The periaqueductal gray is disorganized (asterisk) (neurofilament light chain). (**h**) Fragmented cerebral peduncles (arrows) in a fetus with polymicrogyria, aqueductal stenosis, and perimesencephalic brainstem heterotopia (arrowhead). The pyramidal tracts were absent in the medulla. (**i**) An abnormal tract in the central pontine tegmentum (arrow), possibly an abnormal medial longitudinal fasciculus. (**j, k**) In this midbrain, an aberrant tract appears to decussate in the tectum, dorsal to the superior colliculi

7.4 Brainstem Heterotopia and Hamartoma

As in other parts of the CNS, leptomeningeal heterotopia can be seen around the brainstem, most often ventral to the midbrain (Fig. 7.4a). This is a relatively common finding in holoprosencephaly, as well as in genetic syndromes, including mutations in tubulin and alpha-dystroglycan genes (Mizuguchi et al. 1994; Fallet-Bianco et al. 2014; Devisme et al. 2012).

Within the brainstem parenchyma, the most common forms of heterotopia are nodular heterotopia adjacent to the aqueduct of Sylvius (Fig. 7.4b, c) and olivary heterotopia (see below). Nodular heterotopia in the aqueduct may occur in various conditions, including type 2 lissencephaly and porencephaly, or as an isolated finding. It often obstructs the aqueduct, resulting in hydrocephalus (Fisher et al. 2025). Apart from these, heterotopia in the brainstem is a rare finding (Fig. 7.4d).

Occasionally, hamartomas may also be observed in the brainstem. The most common location is the caudal tectum; this may be an isolated finding but often accompanies holoprosencephaly (Akman et al. 2002; Ramelli et al. 2011). Histologically, brainstem hamartomas are masses comprised of lipomatous tissue and may contain other components, such as fibrous tissue, striated muscle, cartilage, and osseous tissue (Fig. 7.4e–g) (Budka 1974; Kim et al. 1996; Schuhmann et al. 1997; Fix et al. 1989). The mass may compress the aqueduct or rostral fourth ventricle and cause hydrocephalus (Ternier et al. 2006). Hamartomas may also arise in other locations around the brainstem, such as a medullary hamartoma in a case of Klippel–Feil anomaly (described in Chap. 10).

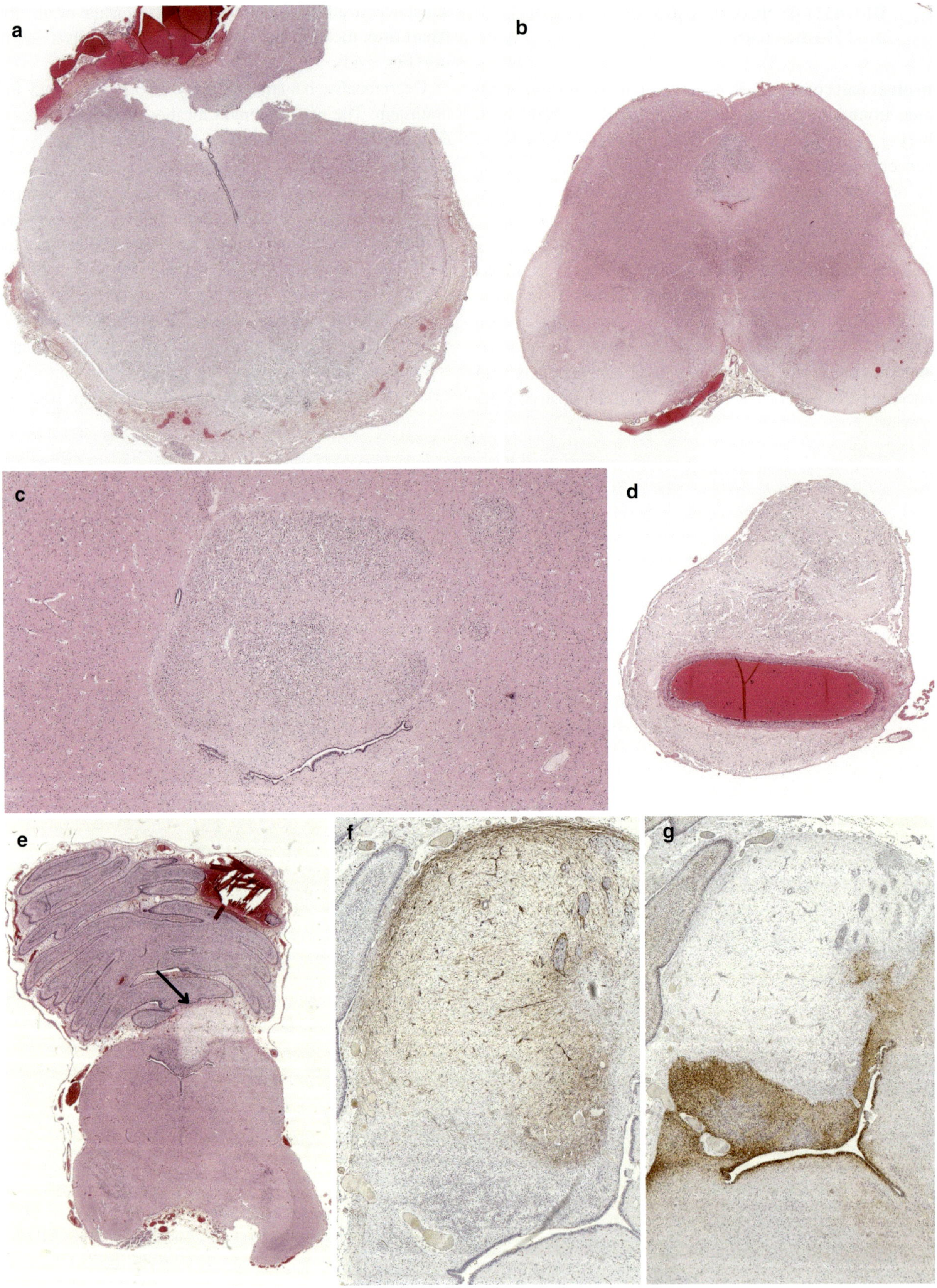

Fig. 7.4 Brainstem heterotopia and hamartoma. (**a**) Perimesencephalic leptomeningeal heterotopia in a fetus with holoprosencephaly. (**b**, **c**) Nodular heterotopia obstructing and fragmenting the aqueduct in a fetus with obstructive hydrocephalus. (**d**) This was accompanied by a nodular heterotopia encasing an artery near the cervicomedullary junction. There were no other systemic or CNS malformations. (**e**) Lipomatous hamartoma in the caudal tectum (arrow) obstructing the rostral fourth ventricle, resulting in hydrocephalus. (**f**) The cells are positive for CD34 and (**g**) negative for GFAP

7.5 Olivary Dysplasia and Heterotopia

Dysplasia of the inferior olivary nuclei is often associated with dysplastic dentate nuclei (see Chap. 7) but may also occur independently. This is often a subtle finding, and its identification in fetal autopsy requires familiarity with the developmental process and comparison with age-matched controls. Dysplasia may appear in the form of excessive undulation or simplification of the architecture, with the most severe forms assuming a "hook-like" shape (Fig. 7.5; see also Fig. 7.11 in cerebellar malformations) (Friede 1989). In most cases, the neurons of the inferior olives appear cytologically normal; however, rare descriptions have shown binucleation (Fig. 7.5e) (Tateishi et al. 1979).

Olivary heterotopia is a form of olivary dysplasia in which nodules of neurons morphologically resembling the structure and cytoarchitecture of the inferior olivary nuclei are seen in abnormal locations. These are usually located along the path of migration between the lateral floor of the fourth ventricle and the location of the inferior olivary nuclear complex (Fig. 7.5e, f) (Friede 1989).

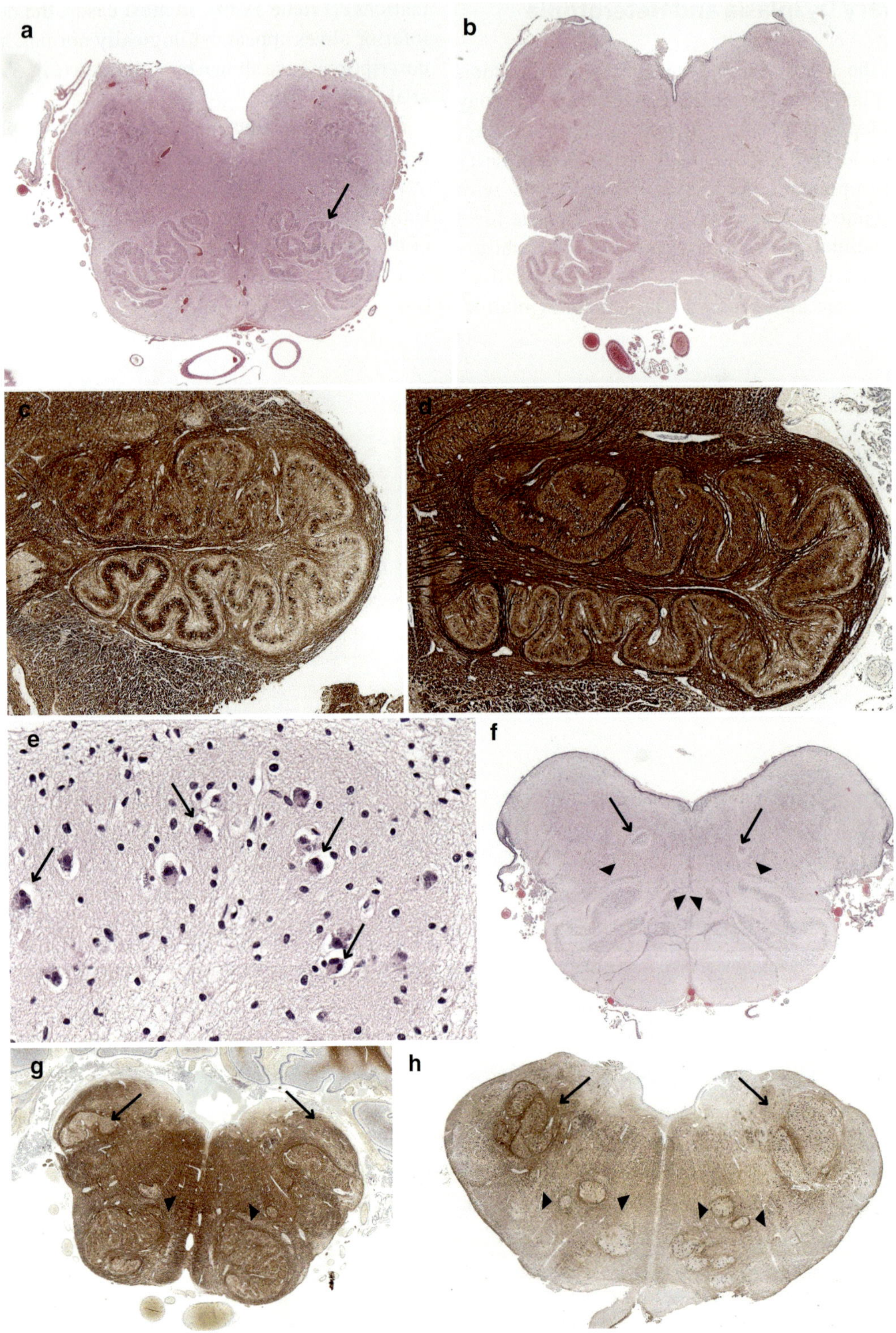

Fig. 7.5 Olivary dysplasia and heterotopia. (**a**) Olivary dysplasia in a 32-week-gestation fetus. The inferior olives are hyperconvoluted, irregular, and focally duplicated (arrow). The dysplasia is better appreciated when compared to (**b**), an age-matched control. (**c**) Mildly dysplastic inferior olive of a 28-week-gestation fetus. The ribbon-like structure is thin and slightly hypoconvoluted compared to (**d**) an age-matched control (neurofilament light chain). (**e**) High magnification of the inferior olives from case (**c**) reveals abnormal binucleate neurons (arrows). (**f**) Olivary dysplasia in a 21-week-gestation fetus with trisomy 13. The inferior olivary nuclei are simplified; the dorsal and medial accessory olives are present (arrowheads). There is an olivary heterotopia in the tegmentum (arrows). (**g**) Dysplastic olives with a thick posterior limb in a fetus with loss of heterozygosity in a segment of chromosome 11 associated with uniparental disomy. Olivary heterotopias are present in the dorsolateral (arrows) and central (arrowheads) tegmentum. (**h**) Large olivary heterotopia in the dorsolateral medullary tegmentum (arrows) and smaller olivary heterotopic nodules in the central tegmentum (arrowheads) in a case of Miller–Dieker lissencephaly syndrome due to a microdeletion in chromosome 17p13.3. There are small rudimentary olivary structures in the usual location of the inferior olivary nuclear complexes (neurofilament light chain)

7.6 Joubert Malformation

Marie Joubert et al. (1969) described four siblings in a family of French–Canadian descent with agenesis of the cerebellar vermis (Joubert et al. 1969). To date, aberrations in more than 40 genes have been associated with Joubert syndrome, all sharing in common dysfunction of the motile cilium (Glass et al. 2025; Van De Weghe et al. 2022). Subsequent descriptions of Joubert syndrome in the literature discuss its clinical and radiological features, with only limited reports on the neuropathological features. Joubert syndrome can be pure with only brainstem manifestations, or it can be associated with other malformations involving the eyes (posterior colobomata and retinal degeneration), kidneys (cystic dysplasia and nephronophthisis), liver (congenital hepatic fibrosis or ductal plate malformation), polydactyly, and orofacial clefts (Hevner et al. 2018; Poretti et al. 2017; Lopez et al. 2014). Other genetic syndromes have overlapping characteristics with Joubert, sometimes noted as Joubert-related disorders. One of these is Meckel syndrome, characterized by a combination of occipital encephalocele, cystic dysplasia of the kidneys, ductal plate malformation of the liver, and polydactyly (Van De Weghe et al. 2022). This is a genetically diverse group of syndromes, and some subtypes are associated with Joubert malformation. Since the characteristic brainstem Joubert-type malformation is similar in Joubert and Joubert-related disorders, for the purpose of our morphologic review, we will discuss the morphology of Joubert malformation (Fig. 7.6).

The diagnostic hallmark of Joubert malformation is the neuroimaging "molar tooth sign" comprised of an enlarged fourth ventricle, thick and vertically oriented superior cerebellar peduncles, and a hypoplastic cerebellar vermis (Fig. 7.6h) (Maria et al. 1999; Juric-Sekhar et al. 2012). At autopsy, the hallmarks of Joubert are best demonstrated in axial sections of the brainstem and cerebellum, including non-decussation of the superior cerebellar peduncles (Fig. 7.6g), vermian dysplasia and hypoplasia (Fig. 7.6i, k, l), and an abnormally shaped, enlarged fourth ventricle described as "bat-wing" or "inverted umbrella" (Fig. 7.6k, l) (Hevner et al. 2018). Other consistent findings include a deep interpeduncular fossa due to the separation between the corticospinal tracts and dysplasia of the nuclei gracilis and cuneatus in the dorsal caudal medulla (Fig. 7.6m) (Hevner et al. 2018; Yachnis et al. 1999). The latter corresponds to the posterior medullary protuberance seen in MRI.

These are associated with many additional findings in the cerebellum, brainstem, and supratentorial brain. The cerebellar hemispheres range from atrophic to enlarged and display dysplasia, neuronal heterotopia, atrophic cortex, and fragmented dentate nuclei (Hevner et al. 2018; Poretti et al. 2017). The brainstem nuclei are also affected, with hypoplasia or dysplasia in the pontine nuclei, inferior olivary complexes, and solitary nuclei, as well as fragmentation of the spinal trigeminal nuclei (Hevner et al. 2018). The corticospinal tracts do not decussate at the cervicomedullary junctions, resulting in bulky anterior columns in the spinal cord (Juric-Sekhar et al. 2012). Supratentorial anomalies are less common and may include ventriculomegaly, agenesis or dysgenesis of the corpus callosum, hippocampal malrotation, polymicrogyria, periventricular nodular heterotopia, and hypothalamic hamartoma (Fig. 7.6j, o) (Hevner et al. 2018; Cauley et al. 2019; Lopez et al. 2014; Poretti et al. 2017).

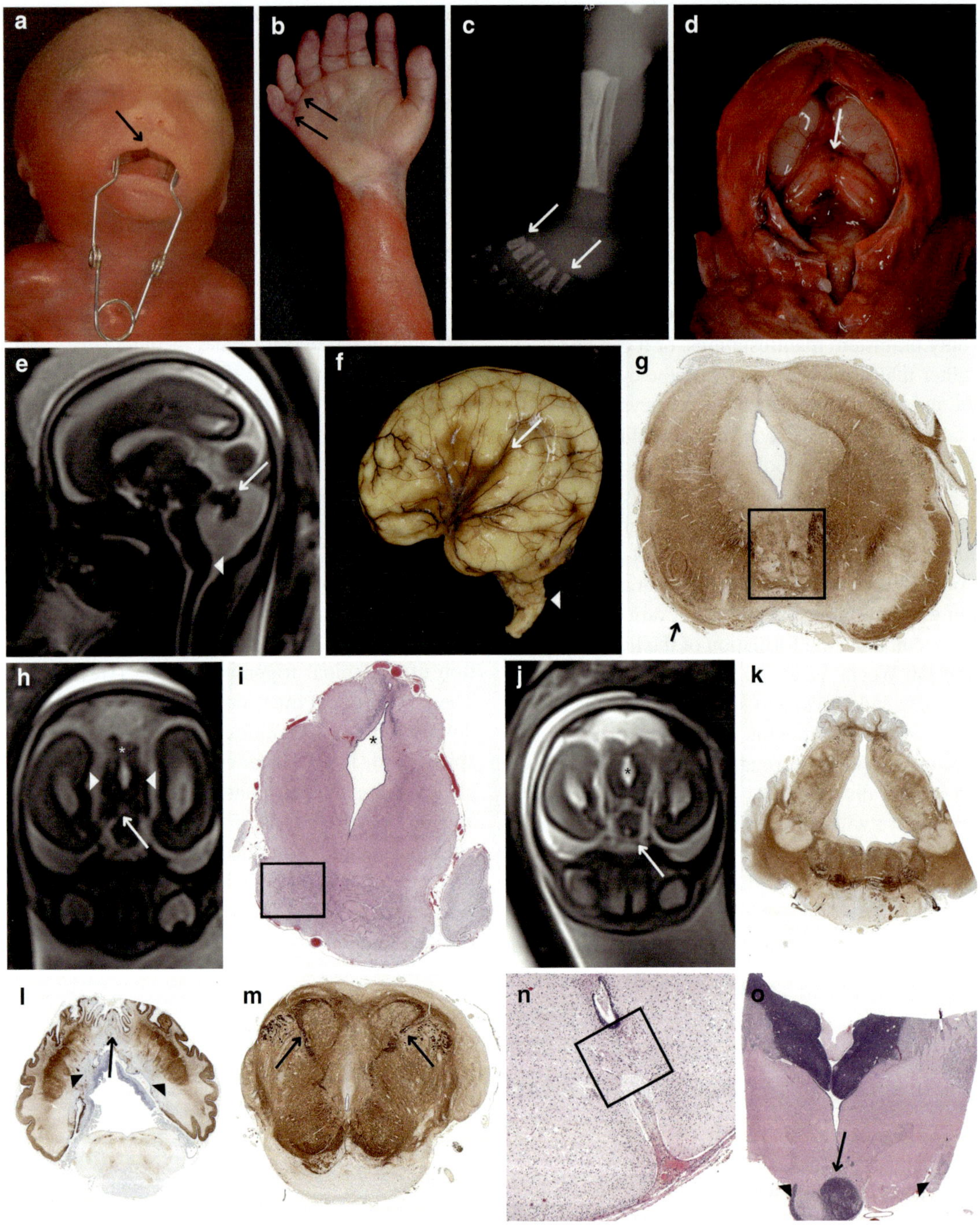

Fig. 7.6 Joubert syndrome. (**a**) Male fetus of 24 weeks' gestation with a compound heterozygous mutation in *C5orf42*, corresponding to oral–facial–digital type 6 syndrome, a Joubert syndrome-related disorder (Lopez et al. 2014). There is a partial cleft in the lip and a central cleft palate (arrow). (**b**, **c**) There is preaxial and postaxial polydactyly in the hands and feet (arrows). (**d**) The opening of the fourth ventricle is enlarged and triangular, and the vermis is small (arrow). (**e**) MRI shows an enlarged posterior fossa with a hypoplastic vermis (arrow). There is a protuberance in the dorsal medulla (arrowhead). (**f**) The cerebral hemispheres display an irregular sulcation pattern; the Sylvian fissure is dysplastic (arrow), and the dorsal medulla is prominent (arrowhead). (**g**) In the midbrain, the decussation of the superior cerebellar peduncles is absent, and the cranial nerve III nuclei are fragmented (rectangle). One cerebral peduncle is aplastic (arrow) (neurofilament light chain). (**h**) Axial MRI section shows the "molar tooth sign" with a deep interpeduncular fossa (arrow), thick and vertically oriented superior cerebellar peduncles (arrowheads), and a hypoplastic vermis (asterisk). (**i**) The basis pontis is asymmetric due to unilateral hypoplasia of the corticospinal tracts (rectangle), and the rostral fourth ventricle is enlarged dorsally (asterisk). (**j**) A slightly more caudal MRI section demonstrates the enlarged fourth ventricle (asterisk) and shows a hypothalamic hamartoma anterior to the brainstem (arrow). (**k**) The distorted fourth ventricle assumes a triangular configuration (asterisk), and the superior cerebellar peduncles are vertically oriented (neurofilament light chain). (**l**) Calbindin staining shows an irregular distribution in the vermian cortex (arrow) and fragmentation of the dentate nuclei (arrowheads). (**m**) The dorsal column nuclei are dysplastic (arrows), and the inferior olivary nuclear complexes are absent (neurofilament light chain). (**n**) The decussation of the corticospinal tracts is absent at the cervicomedullary junction (rectangle). (**o**) In the supratentorium, there is a hypothalamic hamartoma (arrow) and asymmetry of the cerebral peduncles (arrowheads). MRI images are courtesy of Drs. C. Rutten and E. Miller, Department of Radiology, The Hospital for Sick Children, Toronto, Ontario, Canada

7.7 Brainstem Dysplasia in Other Ciliopathies

Other ciliopathies are associated with brainstem dysplasia in patterns distinct from Joubert malformation. They all share in common abnormal tract organization, simplification of the tegmentum, and hypoplasia or dysplasia of the nuclei. Another recurring feature seems to be simplification of the aqueduct, which ranges from stenotic to dilated.

Mutations in *TBC1D32*, a primary ciliary protein, are associated with holoprosencephaly (see also Chap. 5) and a distinct form of brainstem dysplasia. This includes aqueductal atresia, chaotic organization of the brainstem, and vermian dysplasia (Fig. 7.7a–f) (Harris et al. 2023). Another group of ciliopathy-associated syndromes is short-rib thoracic dysplasia. Although this is primarily a skeletal ciliopathy, some cases are associated with brain anomalies (Cideciyan et al. 1993; Córdova-Fletes et al. 2018; Simonini et al. 2022). Reports of neuropathological studies of these cases are sparse. We provide an example of a case of short-rib thoracic dysplasia without polydactyly, with neuronal migration anomalies, cerebellar dysplasia, and hypoplasia of brainstem nuclei, including the inferior olives, dentate nuclei, and nucleus basis pontis (Fig. 7.7g–j).

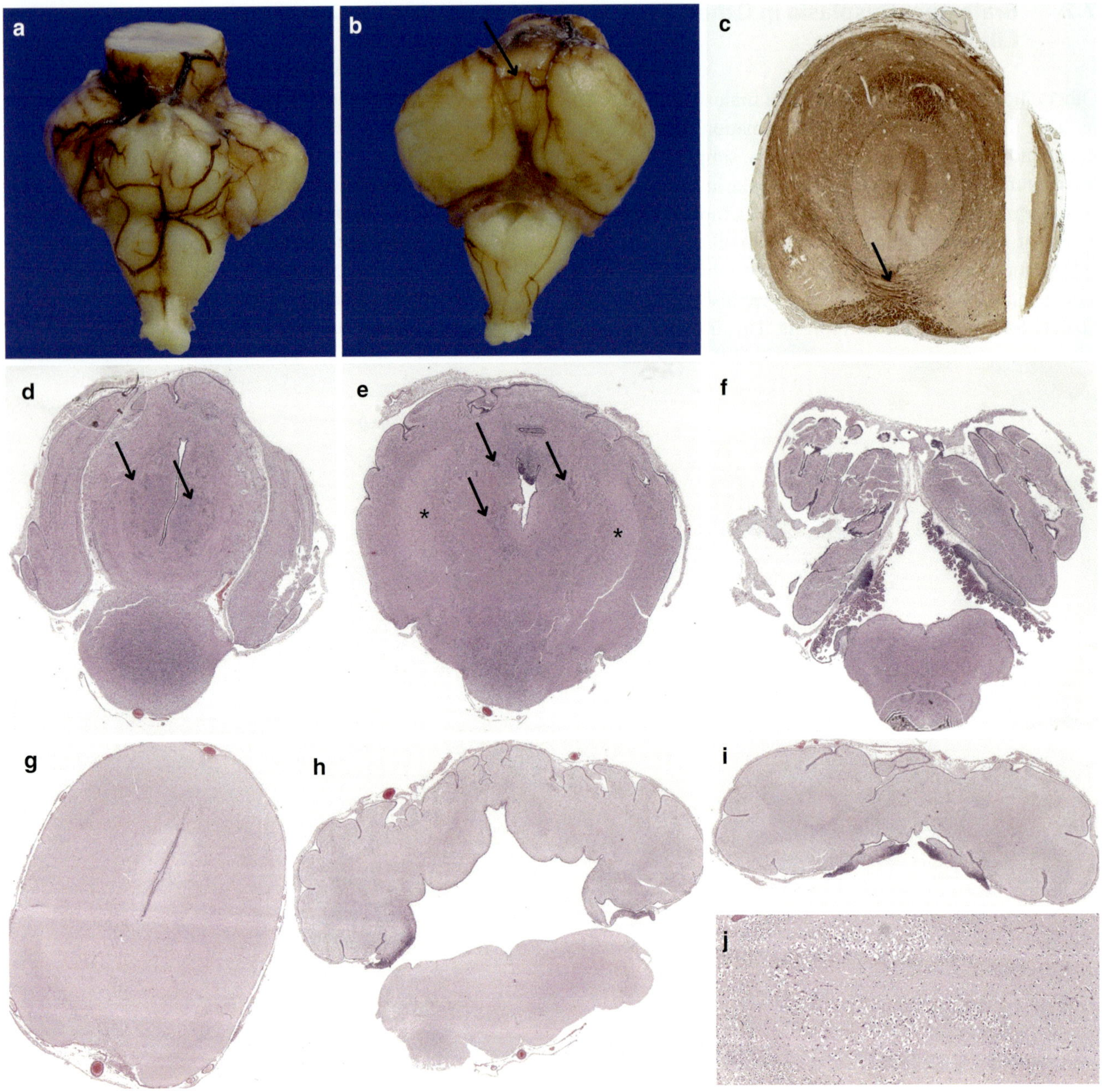

Fig. 7.7 Brainstem dysplasia in other ciliopathies. (**a**–**f**) TBC1D32 ciliopathy. (**a**) The midbrain has a round contour, and the pons is globose. (**b**) The vermis is hypoplastic (arrows). (**c**) The cerebral peduncles are absent, and there is a decussation of tracts in the ventral tegmentum, possibly of the superior cerebellar peduncles (arrow). There is aqueductal atresia and mesencephalosynapsis (neurofilament light chain). (**d**) The cerebellar hemispheres are wrapped around the pons. The nucleus basis pontis is compact due to a lack of descending tracts and appears as a rounded mass. The tegmentum is disorganized with dysplastic neuronal groups (arrows) on either side of the distorted, slit-like fourth ventricle. (**e**) The border between the cerebellum and the tegmentum is poorly demarcated, and the vermis is narrow. The dentate nuclei are simplified (asterisks), and dysplastic neuronal structures are observed in the chaotic tegmentum (arrows). (**f**) The posterior vermis is absent, and the cerebellar hemispheres are splayed. (**g**–**j**) Short-rib thoracic dysplasia. (**g**) In the midbrain, the cerebral peduncles are hypoplastic, and the aqueduct is slit-like and simplified. The tegmentum is simplified. (**h**) The nucleus basis pontis is hypoplastic. The cerebellar vermis is small and dysplastic, and the fourth ventricle is enlarged. (**i**) The dentate nuclei are simplified, and (**j**) the inferior olives are hypoplastic

7.8 Brainstem Cap Dysplasia

Several different malformations of the brainstem share the neuroradiological characteristic of a cap protruding either anteriorly in anterior mesencephalic cap dysplasia (AMCD) or posteriorly in pontine tegmental cap dysplasia (PTCD) and medullary tegmental cap dysplasia (MTCD) (Arrigoni et al. 2017; Barth et al. 2007; Gafner et al. 2023). Diffusion tensor imaging studies on AMCD and PTCD demonstrate aberrant axonal tracts with a horizontal transverse orientation, suggesting the pathogenesis involves defective axonal guidance (Figs. 7.8 and 7.9) (Barth et al. 2007; Jissendi-Tchofo et al. 2009; Arrigoni et al. 2017; Chan et al. 2019; Raghuveer et al. 2023). To date, only a handful of fetal autopsy cases have been published, including cases of PTCD and MTCD. Abnormal axonal tracts were confirmed in PTCD; however, the MTCD cases seemed more diverse and included both hamartomas and axonal abnormalities, suggesting different etiologies in this subgroup (Harding et al. 2016; Gafner et al. 2023). Both AMCD and MTCD were linked to Joubert syndrome (Arrigoni et al. 2017; Gafner et al. 2023). In one case of PTCD, a microdeletion of 2q13 was identified. This involved the *NPHP1* gene, also associated with Joubert syndrome (Picker-Minh et al. 2017). Another case carried a deletion of 16p13.1 including the *STUB1* and *WDR24* genes that affect hindbrain development (Macferran et al. 2010). No genetic findings were reported for other cases.

The morphologic description of PTCD is best delineated (Fig. 7.8). Pontine tegmental cap dysplasia is characterized by a flat ventral pons with a dysplastic "vaulted" tegmentum (Barth et al. 2007). The structures of the tegmentum are displaced by a mass of immature neurons, which project into the fourth ventricle, forming the cap seen in a median sagittal view, and a flattened appearance of the floor of the fourth ventricle on the axial section (Fig. 7.8b, h, i). The superior cerebellar peduncles are hypoplastic and may give rise to a neuroradiological "molar tooth" appearance (Barth et al. 2007; Jissendi-Tchofo et al. 2009; Harding et al. 2016). The middle cerebellar peduncles are absent, and the inferior cerebellar peduncles are hypoplastic (Fig. 7.8c, i) (Barth et al. 2007; Jissendi-Tchofo et al. 2009; Harding et al. 2016). The transverse pontine fibers are absent, and irregular horizontal bands of axon form in aberrant locations (Fig. 7.8c, g–i) (Harding et al. 2016). The cerebellum is often small, the vermis is hypoplastic, and there is dentato-olivary dysplasia (Barth et al. 2007; Jissendi-Tchofo et al. 2009; Harding et al. 2016). In severe cap dysplasia, the fourth ventricle can be occluded by the "cap," and the cerebellar vermis may be virtually absent, resulting in rhombencephalosynapsis (Fig. 7.9d–h).

In AMCD, there are abnormal transverse fibers forming a cap ventral to the midbrain or pons. These can be demonstrated in both sagittal and axial sections, and the use of neurofilament light chain immunohistochemistry helps highlight them (Fig. 7.9a–c).

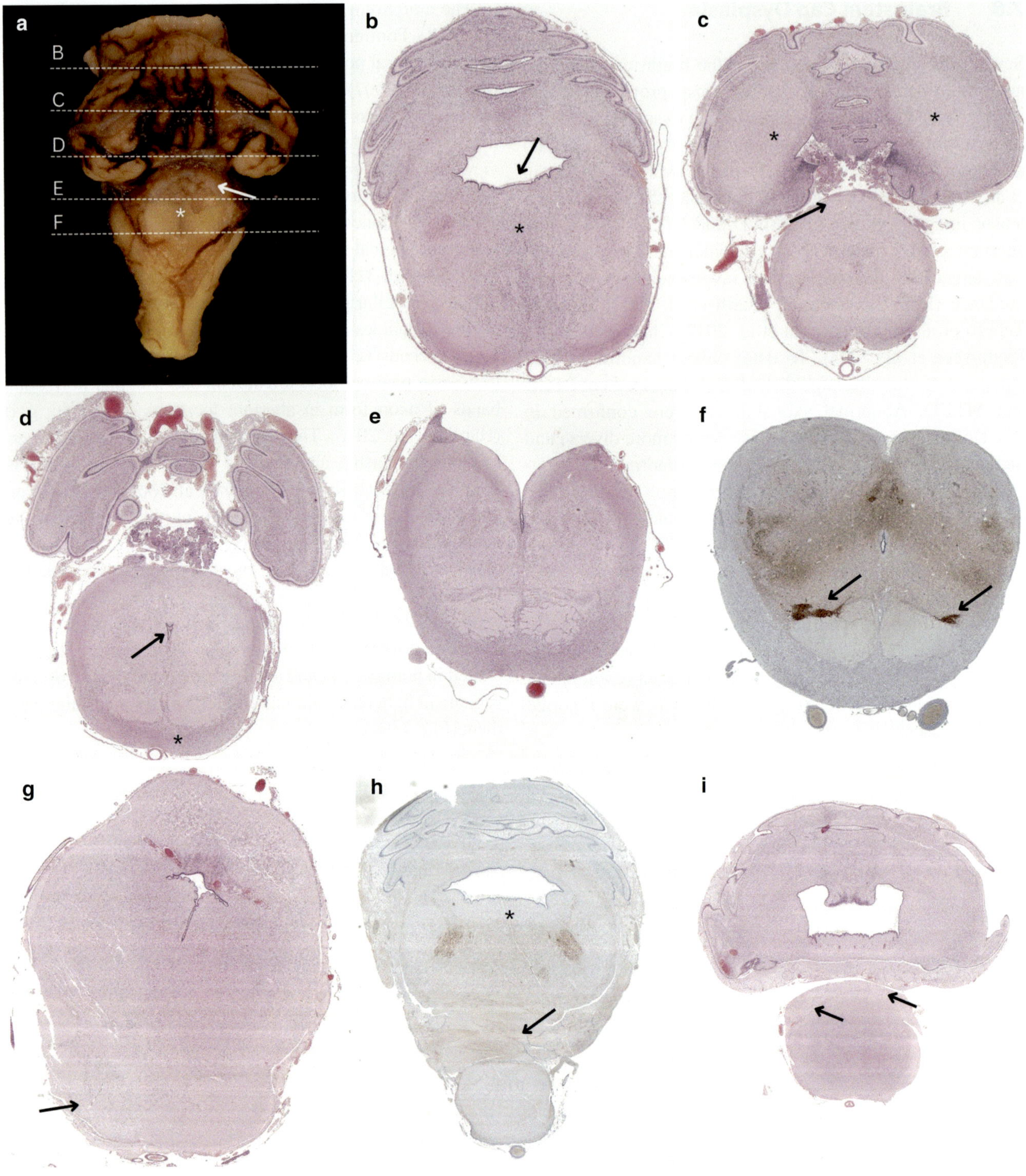

Fig. 7.8 Pontine tegmental cap dysplasia. (**a**) The brainstem of a 22-week-gestation female fetus. The opening of the fourth ventricle is wide, and the choroid plexus is dangling outside of it (asterisk). There is excess tissue on the dorsal pons that forms a "cap" and separates between the pontine and cerebellar portions of the fourth ventricle (arrow). The plane of section of the following images is shown. (**b**) The rostral pontine tegmentum is occupied by disorganized immature neurons (asterisk) that project into the floor of the fourth ventricle and flatten it (arrow). The nucleus basis pontis is absent at this level. (**c**) The middle cerebellar peduncles are absent, and the caudal pons appears detached from the cerebellum. There are tracts of unmyelinated axons in the dorsal pons running perpendicular to the fourth ventricle, corresponding to the "cap" seen in the macroscopic figure (arrow). The cerebellum is small, and the dentate nuclei are simplified (asterisks). (**d**) The neurons of the nucleus basis pontis begin to appear at the mid-caudal pons (asterisk). In the center of the pons, there is a rudimentary pontine fourth ventricle (arrow), separated from the larger cerebellar portion by the tegmental "cap." (**e**) At the pontomedullary junction, the corticospinal tracts are bundled (arrows) dorsal to the nucleus basis pontis, which is caudally displaced, and the inferior olives are not seen. (**f**) In the rostral closed medulla, the inferior olives are severely hypoplastic (arrows) (calbindin). (**g**) In another case of a 23-week-gestation fetus with multiple congenital anomalies, the rostral pons is distorted, and there is an aberrant axonal tract ventral to the pons. (**h**) Lower in the pons, the dysplastic axonal tract is expanded (arrow) and seems to divide the pons into a ventral nucleus basis pontis and a dorsal tegmentum. The floor of the fourth ventricle at this level is obscured (asterisk) (neurofilament light chain). (**i**) The caudal pons is separated from the cerebellum by horizontal axonal tracts in the leptomeninges (arrows). The middle cerebellar peduncles are absent

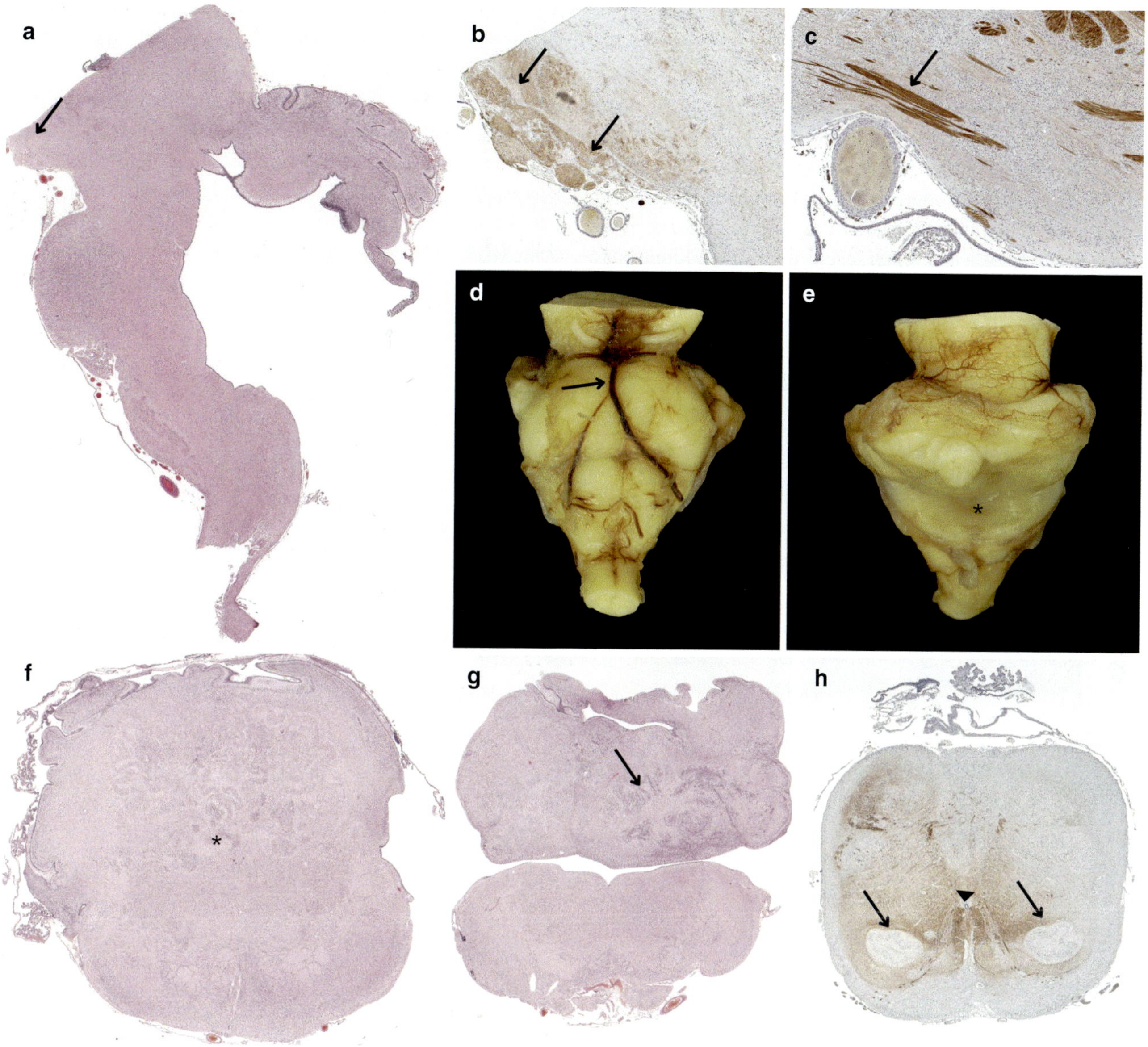

Fig. 7.9 Brainstem cap dysplasia. (**a**) Median section of a Joubert malformation. The midbrain is protruding ventrally (arrow), and the vermis is severely dysplastic. (**b**) Section of the ventral midbrain stained for neurofilament light chain shows abnormal transverse fibers consistent with an AMCD. (**c**) Transverse fibers in an axial section of the rostral pons of another fetus with Joubert malformation. (**d**–**h**) The brainstem of a 23-week-gestation fetus with a complex CNS malformation, which shares features of pontine cap dysplasia. (**d**) The pons appears irregular, and the basilar artery is short (arrow). (**e**) The cerebellum is irregular with the absence of the posterior cerebellum and exposed fourth ventricle (asterisk). The foliation is poor, and the vermis is not well defined. (**f**) The dorsal pons is fused with the cerebellum, completely occluding the fourth ventricle (asterisk). The vermis is not seen, and the cerebellar hemispheres are fused. (**g**) The middle cerebellar peduncles are absent, and the caudal pons is detached from the cerebellum. The deep cerebellar nuclei are dysplastic (arrow). (**h**) The neurons of the nucleus basis pontis are caudally displaced to the medulla (asterisk), and the inferior olives are hypoplastic (arrows). The medial lemniscus is present (arrowhead), but the pyramids and medial longitudinal fasciculus are absent. The medulla appears encased in an excess tissue, creating a square contour (neurofilament light chain)

7.9 Tubulinopathies

Mutations in the tubulin genes are associated with microlissencephaly with cerebellar hypoplasia (see also Chaps. 4 and 7). Fallet-Bianco et al. (2014) described the phenotypic differences according to the mutated gene (Fallet-Bianco et al. 2014). Herein, we summarize the common features. The brainstem in tubulinopathies often exhibits significant hypoplasia and dysplasia and, when severe, may appear kinked into a Z shape macroscopically (Fig. 7.10a). Both ascending and descending tracts are hypoplastic, disorganized, or completely absent (Fig. 7.10b–i) (Fallet-Bianco et al. 2008, 2014; Laquerriere et al. 2016). Various neuronal groups within the brainstem are hypoplastic and dysplastic, including the pontine nuclei, olivary nuclei, and cranial nerve nuclei. Olivary heterotopias are frequently observed (Fig. 7.10b–i) (Fallet-Bianco et al. 2008, 2014). Occasionally, neuronal overgrowth into the leptomeninges surrounding the brainstem is observed (Fig. 7.10i) (Fallet-Bianco et al. 2014). The structures of the tectum are relatively preserved (Fallet-Bianco et al. 2008).

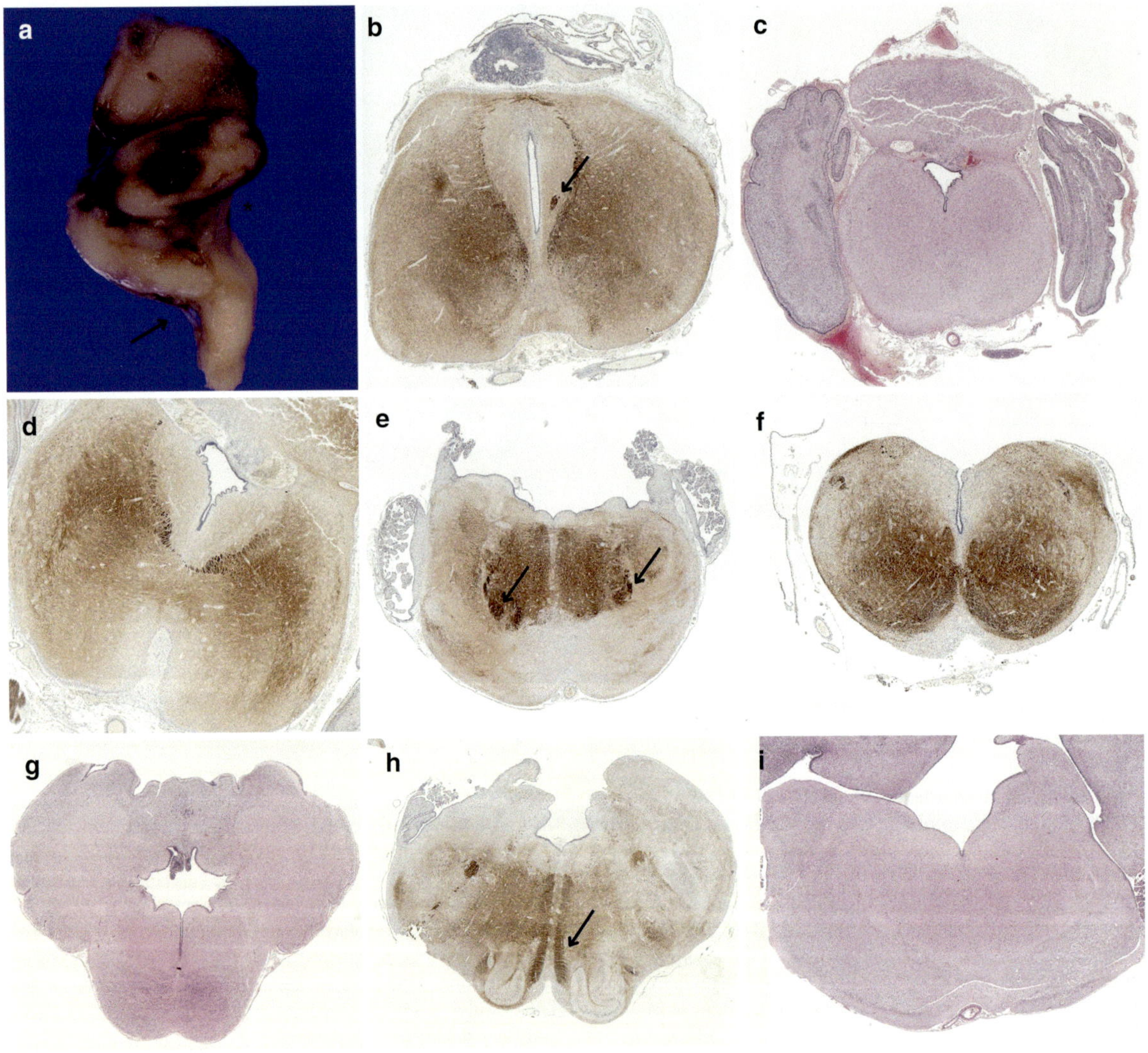

Fig. 7.10 Tubulinopathies. (**a**) Lateral view of a kinked (arrow) Z-shaped brainstem of a 23-week-gestation fetus. The pons is irregular, and the medulla is hypoplastic. The cerebellum is small and discoid, and the opening of the fourth ventricle is enlarged (asterisk). (**b**) In the midbrain, the red nuclei and substantia nigra are absent. The aqueduct is simplified, and the periaqueductal gray is well defined but contains a unilateral aberrant tract (arrow). The corticospinal tracts and major brainstem tracts are absent (neurofilament light chain). (**c**) The rostral pons is flat due to the absence of the corticospinal tracts and hypoplasia of the nucleus basis pontis. The tegmentum is simplified, and the major neuronal groups are not discernible. (**d**) The tracts of the tegmentum, including the central tegmental tract, medial longitudinal fasciculus, and medial and lateral lemniscus tracts, are absent (neurofilament light chain). (**e**) The nucleus basis pontis is present in the caudal pons, and hypoplastic tracts are present in the tegmentum (arrows), although their exact nature is unclear. (**f**) In the medulla, the pyramids and the inferior olivary nuclei are absent. The dorsal tegmental structures are poorly defined (neurofilament light chain). (**g**) In another fetus (22 weeks) with a tubulinopathy, the nucleus basis pontis is present, but the corticospinal tracts are severely hypoplastic, and the tegmentum is small and simplified, as are the cerebellum and dentate nuclei. (**h**) In the medulla, the inferior olives are simplified, and the pyramids are absent. The arcuate nucleus and medial lemniscus are present (arrows). The dorsal tegmental structures are poorly defined. (**i**) Neuronal overgrowth into the leptomeninges in another fetus (also 22 weeks) with a tubulinopathy. The basis pontis and corticospinal tracts are hypoplastic, and the tegmentum is simplified

7.10 Other Brainstem Dysplasias

Brainstem dysplasia may be part of many CNS malformations and genetic syndromes. Some of these may resemble the patterns described above, and others may involve only part of the brainstem. In this section, we present various cases of brainstem dysplasia that did not fit any of the previously described patterns.

Structural anomalies, including anencephaly, and caudal regression syndrome may be associated with abnormal brainstems (Fig. 7.11a–c). The brainstem may also appear dysplastic in cases of neuroaxonal dystrophy. In these cases, the tracts and neuronal groups appear hypoplastic similar to brainstem dysplasia; however, dystrophic axons can be identified when using higher magnification (Fig. 7.11d–f).

Pontocerebellar hypoplasia is a group of diseases defined radiologically by a reduced volume of the pons and cerebellum. Genetically defined pontocerebellar hypoplasia syndromes include at least 28 entries in the OMIM; however, the correlation with the radiologic diagnosis is poor (Zakaria et al. 2024). Fetal autopsy cases are rarely reported in the medical literature, and we did not identify any genetically confirmed cases in our archives.

Brain malformations of different etiologies may be associated with hypoplasia of the pons and cerebellum, with or without micrencephaly. These include chromosomal aberrations, single-gene diseases, and acquired conditions (Zakaria et al. 2024). Examples include the Seckel and Neu–Laxova syndromes, which may feature hindbrain abnormalities that include pontocerebellar hypoplasia, along with micrencephaly and other findings (Fitzgerald et al. 2012; Ostrovskaya et al. 1988).

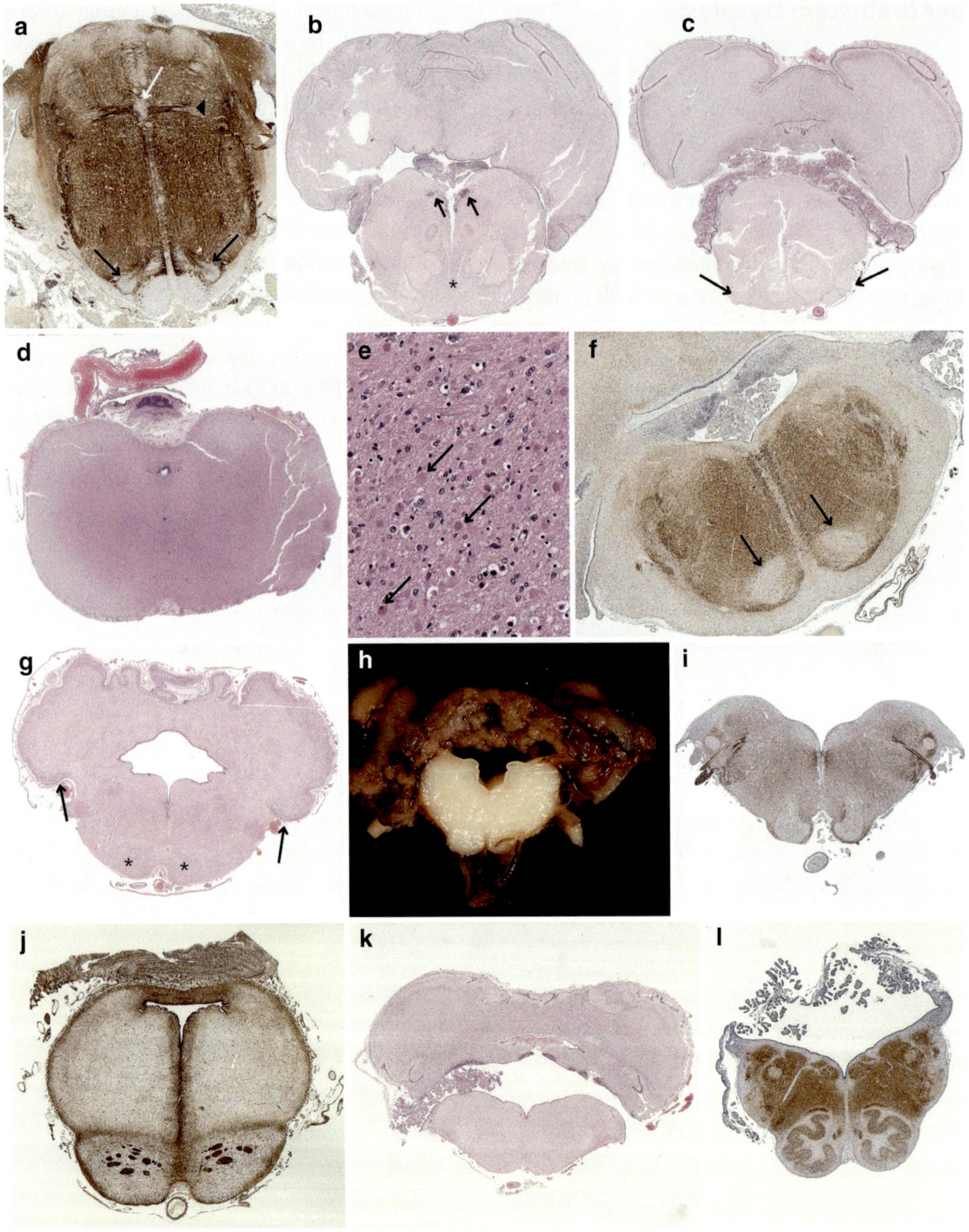

Fig. 7.11 Brainstem dysplasia—others. (**a**) Dysplastic brainstem in a case of anencephaly; the open neural tube defect is dorsal to the brainstem. Ventrally, there are small structures resembling the inferior olivary nuclei (black arrows), and the nuclei of the medullary tegmentum are not discernible. In the dorsal part, there are aberrant transverse axonal tracts (arrowhead). The central canal is not seen, and there are rudimentary ependymal cells (white arrow). (**b**) Hypoplastic pontomedullary junction and cerebellum in a case of caudal regression. The nucleus basis pontis is caudally displaced (asterisk), and there are calcifications in the dorsal tegmentum (arrows). (**c**) There are aberrant tracts in the ventrolateral aspect of the medulla (arrows). (**d**) Midbrain in a case of neuroaxonal dystrophy with osteopetrosis due to a *BORCS5* mutation. The cerebral peduncles are flat, and the aqueduct is reduced to ependymal nests (arrow). (**e**) High magnification reveals numerous swollen dystrophic axons. (**f**) The inferior olivary nuclei are hypoplastic (arrows), and pyramids are absent (neurofilament light chain). (**g**) Hypoplastic pons and cerebellum in Seckel syndrome. The nucleus basis pontis is small, and the corticospinal tracts are absent (asterisks). The fourth ventricle is relatively enlarged, and the cerebellar cortex is irregular. The external granule layer is present only focally (arrows) and degenerated in most of the cortex. (**h**, **i**) The inferior olives are small and simplified, and the pyramids are absent. The tegmental tracts are absent, and the vermis is hypoplastic (neurofilament light chain). (**j**) Hypoplastic pons in Neu–Laxova syndrome. The basis pontis is small, and the corticospinal tracts are severely hypoplastic. The pontine tegmentum is simplified (vimentin). (**k**) The cerebellum is small with reduced foliation, and the fourth ventricle is enlarged. (**l**) The inferior olives are simplified. Other neuronal groups of the medullary tegmentum are present, but the pyramids are absent (synaptophysin)

References

Adle-Biassette H, Saugier-Veber P, Fallet-Bianco C, Delezoide AL, Razavi F, Drouot N, et al. Neuropathological review of 138 cases genetically tested for X-linked hydrocephalus: evidence for closely related clinical entities of unknown molecular bases. Acta Neuropathol. 2013;126(3):427–42. https://doi.org/10.1007/s00401-013-1146-1. Epub 2013 Jul 3. PMID: 23820807

Akman CI, Schubert R, Duran M, Loh J. Gelastic seizure with tectal tumor, lobar holoprosencephaly, and subependymal nodules: clinical report. J Child Neurol. 2002;17(2):152–4. https://doi.org/10.1177/088307380201700215. PMID: 11952080

Arrigoni F, Romaniello R, Peruzzo D, De Luca A, Parazzini C, Valente EM, Borgatti R, Triulzi F. Anterior Mesencephalic Cap Dysplasia: Novel Brain Stem Malformative Features Associated with Joubert Syndrome. AJNR Am J Neuroradiol. 2017;38(12):2385–90. https://doi.org/10.3174/ajnr.A5360. Epub 2017 Aug 24. PMID: 28838911; PMCID: PMC5708532

Barth PG, Majoie CB, Caan MW, Weterman MA, Kyllerman M, Smit LM, Kaplan RA, Haas RH, Baas F, Cobben JM, Poll-The BT. Pontine tegmental cap dysplasia: a novel brain malformation with a defect in axonal guidance. Brain. 2007;130(Pt 9):2258–66. https://doi.org/10.1093/brain/awm188. Epub 2007 Aug 9. PMID: 17690130

Budka H. Intracranial lipomatous hamartomas (intracranial "lipomas"). A study of 13 cases including combinations with medulloblastoma, colloid and epidermoid cysts, angiomatosis and other malformations. Acta Neuropathol. 1974;28(3):205–22. https://doi.org/10.1007/BF00719025. PMID: 4611131

Cauley ES, Hamed A, Mohamed IN, Elseed M, Martinez S, Yahia A, et al. Overlap of polymicrogyria, hydrocephalus, and Joubert syndrome in a family with novel truncating mutations in ADGRG1/GPR56 and KIAA0556. Neurogenetics. 2019;20(2):91–8. https://doi.org/10.1007/s10048-019-00577-2. Epub 2019 Apr 13. PMID: 30982090

Cesmebasi A, Loukas M, Hogan E, Kralovic S, Tubbs RS, Cohen-Gadol AA. The Chiari malformations: a review with emphasis on anatomical traits. Clin Anat. 2015;28(2):184–94. https://doi.org/10.1002/ca.22442. Epub 2014 Jul 25. PMID: 25065525

Chan D, Veltkamp DL, Desai NK, Pfeifer CM. Pontine tegmental cap dysplasia with a duplicated internal auditory canal. Radiol Case Rep. 2019;14(7):825–8. https://doi.org/10.1016/j.radcr.2019.04.009. PMID: 31049119; PMCID: PMC6484283

Chatron N, Cabet S, Alix E, Buenerd A, Cox P, Guibaud L, Labalme A, Marks P, Osio D, Putoux A, Sanlaville D, Lesca G, Vasiljevic A. A novel lethal recognizable polymicrogyric syndrome caused by ATP1A2 homozygous truncating variants. Brain. 2019;142(11):3367–74. https://doi.org/10.1093/brain/awz272. PMID: 31608932

Chiari HJDMW. Ueber veränderungen des kleinhirns infolge von hydrocephalie des grosshirns1. DMW-Deutsche Medizinische Wochenschrift. 1891;17(42):1172–5.

Chiari H. Uber Veranderungen des Kleinhiens, des pons und der medulla oblongata. Folge von congenitaler hydrocephalie des grossherns. Deskschr Akad Wiss Wien. 1895;63:71–116.

Cideciyan D, Rodriguez MM, Haun RL, Abdenour GE, Bruce JH. New findings in short rib syndrome. Am J Med Genet. 1993;46(3):255–9. https://doi.org/10.1002/ajmg.1320460302. PMID: 8488867

Córdova-Fletes C, Becerra-Solano LE, Rangel-Sosa MM, Rivas-Estilla AM, Alberto Galán-Huerta K, Ortiz-López R, et al. Uncommon runs of homozygosity disclose homozygous missense mutations in two ciliopathy-related genes (SPAG17 and WDR35) in a patient with multiple brain and skeletal anomalies. Eur J Med Genet. 2018;61(3):161–7. https://doi.org/10.1016/j.ejmg.2017.11.011. Epub 2017 Nov 23. PMID: 29174089

Cotes C, Bonfante E, Lazor J, Jadhav S, Caldas M, Swischuk L, Riascos R. Congenital basis of posterior fossa anomalies. Neuroradiol J. 2015;28(3):238–53. https://doi.org/10.1177/1971400915576665. PMID: 26246090; PMCID: PMC4757284

Devisme L, Bouchet C, Gonzalès M, Alanio E, Bazin A, Bessières B, et al. Cobblestone lissencephaly: neuropathological subtypes and correlations with genes of dystroglycanopathies. Brain. 2012;135(Pt 2):469–82. https://doi.org/10.1093/brain/awr357. Epub 2012 Feb 9. PMID: 22323514

Ellison D, Lowe JS, Chimelli LMC, et al. Neuropathology. 3rd ed. Elsevier Ltd.; 2013. p. 119–21.

Fallet-Bianco C, Loeuillet L, Poirier K, Loget P, Chapon F, Pasquier L, Saillour Y, Beldjord C, Chelly J, Francis F. Neuropathological phenotype of a distinct form of lissencephaly associated with mutations in TUBA1A. Brain. 2008;131(Pt 9):2304–20. https://doi.org/10.1093/brain/awn155. Epub 2008 Jul 18. PMID: 18669490

Fallet-Bianco C, Laquerrière A, Poirier K, Razavi F, Guimiot F, Dias P, et al. Mutations in tubulin genes are frequent causes of various foetal malformations of cortical development including microlissencephaly. Acta Neuropathol Commun. 2014;2:69. https://doi.org/10.1186/2051-5960-2-69. PMID: 25059107; PMCID: PMC4222268

Fisher Y, Shannon P, Greenberg O, Chitayat D, Chong K, Blaser S, Shinar S. Mesencephalosynapsis and aqueductal stenosis. J Neuropathol Exp Neurol. 2025;84(3):195–209. https://doi.org/10.1093/jnen/nlae128. PMID: 39658320

Fitzgerald B, O'Driscoll M, Chong K, Keating S, Shannon P. Neuropathology of fetal stage Seckel syndrome: a case report providing a morphological correlate for the emerging molecular mechanisms. Brain Dev. 2012;34(3):238–43. https://doi.org/10.1016/j.braindev.2011.05.007. Epub 2011 Jun 12. PMID: 21669506

Fix SE, Nelson J, Schochet SS Jr. Focal leptomeningeal rhabdomyomatosis of the posterior fossa. Arch Pathol Lab Med. 1989;113(8):872–3. PMID: 2757487

Florell SR, Townsend JJ, Klatt EC, Pysher TJ, Coffin CM, Wittwer CT, Viskochil DH. Aprosencephaly and cerebellar dysgenesis in sibs. Am J Med Genet. 1996;63(4):542–8. https://doi.org/10.1002/(SICI)1096-8628(19960628)63:4<542::AID-AJMG6>3.0.CO;2-Q. PMID: 8826432

Fotos J, Olson R, Kanekar S. Embryology of the brain and molecular genetics of central nervous system malformation. Semin Ultrasound CT MR. 2011;32(3):159–66. https://doi.org/10.1053/j.sult.2011.02.011. PMID: 21596273

Friede RL. Surface structures of the aqueduct and the ventricular walls: a morphologic, comparative and histochemical study. J Comp Neurol. 1961;116:229–47. https://doi.org/10.1002/cne.901160210. PMID: 13701951

Friede RL. Developmental neuropathology. Springer-Verlag; 1989.

Gafner M, Garel C, Leibovitz Z, Valence S, Krajden Haratz K, et al. Medullary tegmental cap dysplasia: fetal and postnatal presentations of a unique brainstem malformation. AJNR Am J Neuroradiol. 2023;44(3):334–40. https://doi.org/10.3174/ajnr.A7805. Epub 2023 Feb 23. PMID: 36822823; PMCID: PMC10187821

Glass IA, Dempsey JC, Parisi M, Doherty D. Joubert syndrome. 2003 Jul 9 (updated 2025 Mar 13). In: Adam MP, Feldman J, Mirzaa GM, Pagon RA, Wallace SE, Amemiya A, editors. GeneReviews® (Internet). Seattle: University of Washington, Seattle; 1993–2025. PMID: 20301500; 2025.

Harding B, Vossough A, Goldberg E, Santi M. Pontine tegmental cap dysplasia: neuropathological confirmation of a rare clinical/radiological syndrome. Neuropathol Appl Neurobiol. 2016;42(3):301–6. https://doi.org/10.1111/nan.12281. Epub 2015 Sep 25. PMID: 26331236

Harris SC, Chong K, Chitayat D, Gilmore KL, Jorge AAL, Freire BL, et al. Diagnosis of TBC1D32-associated conditions: expanding the phenotypic spectrum of a complex ciliopathy. Am J Med Genet A.

2023;191(5):1282–92. https://doi.org/10.1002/ajmg.a.63150. Epub 2023 Feb 24. PMID: 36826837; PMCID: PMC10204718

Hevner RF, Dobyns WB, Valente EN, Golden JA, Harding BN, Adle-Biassette H. Joubert Syndrome. In: Developmental neuropathology. United Kingdom: John Wiley & Sons, Incorporated; 2018. p. 151–7. https://doi.org/10.1002/9781119013112.ch14.

Jissendi-Tchofo P, Doherty D, McGillivray G, Hevner R, Shaw D, Ishak G, Leventer R, Barkovich AJ. Pontine tegmental cap dysplasia: MR imaging and diffusion tensor imaging features of impaired axonal navigation. AJNR Am J Neuroradiol. 2009;30(1):113–9. https://doi.org/10.3174/ajnr.A1305. Epub 2008 Oct 8. PMID: 18842761; PMCID: PMC3919876

Joubert M, Eisenring JJ, Robb JP, Andermann F. Familial agenesis of the cerebellar vermis. A syndrome of episodic hyperpnea, abnormal eye movements, ataxia, and retardation. Neurology. 1969;19(9):813–25. https://doi.org/10.1212/wnl.19.9.813. PMID: 5816874

Juric-Sekhar G, Adkins J, Doherty D, Hevner RF. Joubert syndrome: brain and spinal cord malformations in genotyped cases and implications for neurodevelopmental functions of primary cilia. Acta Neuropathol. 2012;123(5):695–709. https://doi.org/10.1007/s00401-012-0951-2. Epub 2012 Feb 14. PMID: 22331178

Kim JY, Lee TJ, Chi JG. Congenital quadrigeminal lipoma with osteocartilaginous element. A case report. J Korean Med Sci. 1996;11(6):537–9. https://doi.org/10.3346/jkms.1996.11.6.537. PMID: 9008105; PMCID: PMC3054263

Laquerriere A, Gonzales M, Saillour Y, Cavallin M, Joyē N, Quēlin C, Bidat L, Dommergues M, Plessis G, Encha-Razavi F, Chelly J, Bahi-Buisson N, Poirier K. De novo TUBB2B mutation causes fetal akinesia deformation sequence with microlissencephaly: an unusual presentation of tubulinopathy. Eur J Med Genet. 2016;59(4):249–56. https://doi.org/10.1016/j.ejmg.2015.12.007. Epub 2015 Dec 28. PMID: 26732629

Lopez E, Thauvin-Robinet C, Reversade B, Khartoufi NE, Devisme L, Holder M, et al. C5orf42 is the major gene responsible for OFD syndrome type VI. Hum Genet. 2014;133(3):367–77. https://doi.org/10.1007/s00439-013-1385-1. Epub 2013 Nov 1. PMID: 24178751

Macferran KM, Buchmann RF, Ramakrishnaiah R, Griebel ML, Sanger WG, Saronwala A, Schaefer GB. Pontine tegmental cap dysplasia with a 2q13 microdeletion involving the NPHP1 gene: insights into malformations of the mid-hindbrain. Semin Pediatr Neurol. 2010;17(1):69–74. https://doi.org/10.1016/j.spen.2010.02.014. PMID: 20434703

Maria BL, Quisling RG, Rosainz LC, Yachnis AT, Gitten J, Dede D, Fennell E. Molar tooth sign in Joubert syndrome: clinical, radiologic, and pathologic significance. J Child Neurol. 1999;14(6):368–76. https://doi.org/10.1177/088307389901400605. PMID: 10385844

Mizuguchi M, Maekawa S, Kamoshita S. Distribution of leptomeningeal glioneuronal heterotopia in alobar holoprosencephaly. Arch Neurol. 1994;51(9):951–4. https://doi.org/10.1001/archneur.1994.00540210125022. PMID: 8080397

Ostrovskaya TI, Lazjuk GI. Cerebral abnormalities in the Neu-Laxova syndrome. Am J Med Genet. 1988;30(3):747–56. https://doi.org/10.1002/ajmg.1320300308. PMID: 3055985

Picker-Minh S, Hartenstein S, Proquitté H, Fröhler S, Raile V, Kraemer N, Apeshiotis S, Leipoldt M, Kalache KD, Morris-Rosendahl D, Boltshauser E, Chen W, Kaindl AM. Pontine tegmental cap dysplasia in an extremely preterm infant and review of the literature. J Child Neurol. 2017;32(3):334–40. https://doi.org/10.1177/0883073816680748. Epub 2016 Dec 20. PMID: 28193110

Pirot N, Crahes M, Adle-Biassette H, Soares A, Bucourt M, Boutron A, Carbillon L, Mignot C, Trestard L, Bekri S, Laquerrière A. Phenotypic and neuropathological characterization of fetal pyruvate dehydrogenase deficiency. J Neuropathol Exp Neurol. 2016;75(3):227–38. https://doi.org/10.1093/jnen/nlv022. Epub 2016 Feb 9. PMID: 26865159

Poretti A, Snow J, Summers AC, Tekes A, Huisman TAGM, Aygun N, Carson KA, Doherty D, Parisi MA, Toro C, Yildirimli D, Vemulapalli M, Mullikin JC, NISC Comparative Sequencing Program; Cullinane AR, Vilboux T, Gahl WA, Gunay-Aygun M. Joubert syndrome: neuroimaging findings in 110 patients in correlation with cognitive function and genetic cause. J Med Genet. 2017;54(8):521–9. https://doi.org/10.1136/jmedgenet-2016-104425. Epub 2017 Jan 13. PMID: 28087721

Raghuveer K, Dikkatwar V, Joshi MV, Shetty DS. Pontine tegmental cap dysplasia: the role of diffusion tensor imaging. BMJ Case Rep. 2023;16(11):e253556. https://doi.org/10.1136/bcr-2022-253556. PMID: 37993144; PMCID: PMC10668148

Ramelli GP, Cortesi C, Boscherini D, Faggin R, Bianchetti MG. Age-dependent presentation of tectal plate tumors: preliminary observations. J Child Neurol. 2011;26(3):377–80. https://doi.org/10.1177/0883073810382141. Epub 2010 Dec 15. PMID: 21160082

Russell DS. Observations on the pathology of hydrocephalus. H.M Stationery Office; 1949.

Sarnat HB. Disorders of segmentation of the neural tube: Chiari malformations. Handb Clin Neurol. 2008;87:89–103. https://doi.org/10.1016/S0072-9752(07)87006-0. PMID: 18809020

Sarnat HB, Flores-Sarnat L. Congenital aqueductal stenosis due to downregulation of a dorsalizing gene. FASEB J. 2008;22:59.4-59.4. https://doi.org/10.1096/fasebj.22.1_supplement.59.4.

Schuhmann MU, Lüdemann WO, Schreiber H, Samii M. Cerebellopontine angle lipoma: a rare differential diagnosis. Skull Base Surg. 1997;7(4):199–205. https://doi.org/10.1055/s--2008-1058596. PMID: 17171031; PMCID: PMC1656654

Shekdar K. Posterior fossa malformations. Semin Ultrasound CT MR. 2011;32(3):228–41. https://doi.org/10.1053/j.sult.2011.02.003. PMID: 21596278

Simonini C, Floeck A, Strizek B, Mueller A, Gembruch U, Geipel A. Fetal ciliopathies: a retrospective observational single-center study. Arch Gynecol Obstet. 2022;306(1):71–83. https://doi.org/10.1007/s00404-021-06265-7. Epub 2021 Oct 1. PMID: 34596737; PMCID: PMC9300526

Tateishi J, Masuda T, Ohmura I, Kirimoto T. (Olivo-ponto-cerebellar atrophy with olivary hypertrophy, binucleated neurons and fibrous gliosis in the cerebral white matter (author's transl)). No To Shinkei. 1979;31(5):523–8. Japanese. PMID: 486270

Ternier J, Wray A, Puget S, Bodaert N, Zerah M, Sainte-Rose C. Tectal plate lesions in children. J Neurosurg. 2006;104(6 Suppl):369–76. https://doi.org/10.3171/ped.2006.104.6.369. PMID: 16776370

Van De Weghe JC, Gomez A, Doherty D. The Joubert-Meckel-Nephronophthisis Spectrum of ciliopathies. Annu Rev Genomics Hum Genet. 2022;31(23):301–29. https://doi.org/10.1146/annurev-genom-121321-093528. Epub 2022 Jun 2. PMID: 35655331; PMCID: PMC9437135

Zakaria RBM, Malta M, Pelletier F, Addour-Boudrahem N, Pinchefsky E, Martin CS, Srour M. Classic "PCH" Genes are a Rare Cause of Radiologic Pontocerebellar Hypoplasia. Cerebellum. 2024;23(2):418–30. https://doi.org/10.1007/s12311-023-01544-2. Epub 2023 Mar 27. PMID: 36971923

8 Cerebellar Malformations

The cerebellum is primarily derived from the embryonic rhombencephalon, with a contribution from the mesencephalon to the formation of the vermis (Otero et al. 1993; Hallonet et al. 1993). It first appears at approximately 32 days post fertilization as a thickening of the alar plate of rhombomere 1 (O'Rahilly 2006). While the mature cerebellar cortex is composed of three layers, the fetal cerebellum demonstrates two to five layers, depending on the stage of development (Rakic et al. 1970).

In the embryonic stage, the cerebellar wall is composed of two layers: a marginal layer and a ventricular layer. Cells from the ventricular layer migrate to form the future Purkinje cells. At 8–10 weeks' gestation, neurons from the rhombic lip—located laterally in the cerebellar primordium—begin to migrate and form the transient external granular layer (EGL), resulting in a three-layered cerebellar cortex consisting of the EGL, a molecular layer, and the future Purkinje cell layer (Rakic et al. 1970, Volpe 2009). Cells from the EGL migrate along Bergmann glia and form the internal granular layer (IGL). At 20–21 weeks' gestation, five layers are visible in the cerebellar cortex with the addition of the lamina dissecans, an acellular band beneath the future Purkinje cell layer, and the IGL underlying it. As migrating neurons continue to populate the cortex, the lamina dissecans disappears by 28–32 weeks' gestation (Volpe 2009, Rakic et al. 1970). At this stage, the Purkinje cells begin to mature and align into a single-cell layer between the molecular layer and the IGL, resulting in a four-layered cortex. The migration of EGL cells into the IGL persists until approximately 1 year after birth, when the mature three-layered cerebellar cortex is established (Volpe 2009). The neurons of the dentate nuclei originate from both the ventricular layer and the rhombic lip. Initially emerging as thick band of cells, they begin forming convolutions at 22 weeks' gestation, assuming their mature structure by term gestation (Shannon et al. 2019).

Lobulation of the cerebellum begins at 12 weeks' gestation with the formation of the posterolateral fissure, delineating the flocculonodular lobe. This is followed by the appearance of the primary fissure that separates the anterior and posterior lobes (Garel et al. 2011). By 4 months of gestation, all nine lobules of the cerebellum are recognizable (Garel et al. 2011). From 24 weeks' gestation, cerebellar development is accelerated, initially driven by an increased foliation and, after 30 weeks' gestation, mainly by proliferation of EGL cells and their migration into the IGL (Rakic et al. 1970; ten-Donkelaar et al. 2003; Sidman et al. 1973). By term, the cerebellar volume increases five-fold, and the surface area expands 30-fold (Gano et al. 2019; Chang 2000).

The fourth ventricle forms from the thinning and widening of the rhombencephalic roof plate. At 10 weeks of gestation, the tissue that will subsequently develop into the choroid plexus creates the plica choroidalis, an indentation in the thinned roof plate that divides it between the anterior (superior portion) and posterior (inferior portion) membranous areas. Next, the anterior membranous area merges into the choroid plexus, while the posterior membranous area forms Blake's pouch. The accumulation of the cerebrospinal fluid in this area results in the cisterna magna that will later regress to form the foramen of Magendie. The Luschka foramina develop from the lateral angles of the rhomboid fossa (Cotes et al. 2015).

8.1 Cerebellar Hypoplasia

A hypoplastic cerebellum is smaller than expected for gestational age but when isolated usually retains a normal structure. At midgestation, the transcerebellar diameter in millimeter roughly corresponds to the gestational age in weeks. With the acceleration of the cerebellar growth from 24 weeks' gestation onward, the growth in transcerebellar diameter is expected to exceed gestational age. These measurements are more accurately assessed using prenatal imaging (Peñuelas et al. 2024). While cerebellar hypoplasia is well documented in the radiological literature in infants and children, cerebellar hypoplasia is not a common isolated finding in fetal neuropathology.

P. Shannon et al., *Atlas of Neurodevelopmental Pathology*, https://doi.org/10.1007/978-3-032-14148-4_8

Cerebellar hypoplasia may occur in isolation, in association with cervical or occipital encephaloceles, or as part of a broader pattern of neuropathological anomalies (e.g., pontocerebellar hypoplasia, mitochondrial disease, microlissencephaly with cerebellar hypoplasia, and others, as described below). The hypoplasia may be global and involve one cerebellar hemisphere or just the vermis. It can range from mild hypoplasia with no other morphologic changes to severe hypoplasia (Fig. 8.1). Histologically, the cerebellum may be normal or show features of dysplasia, migration anomalies, or encephaloclastic injury.

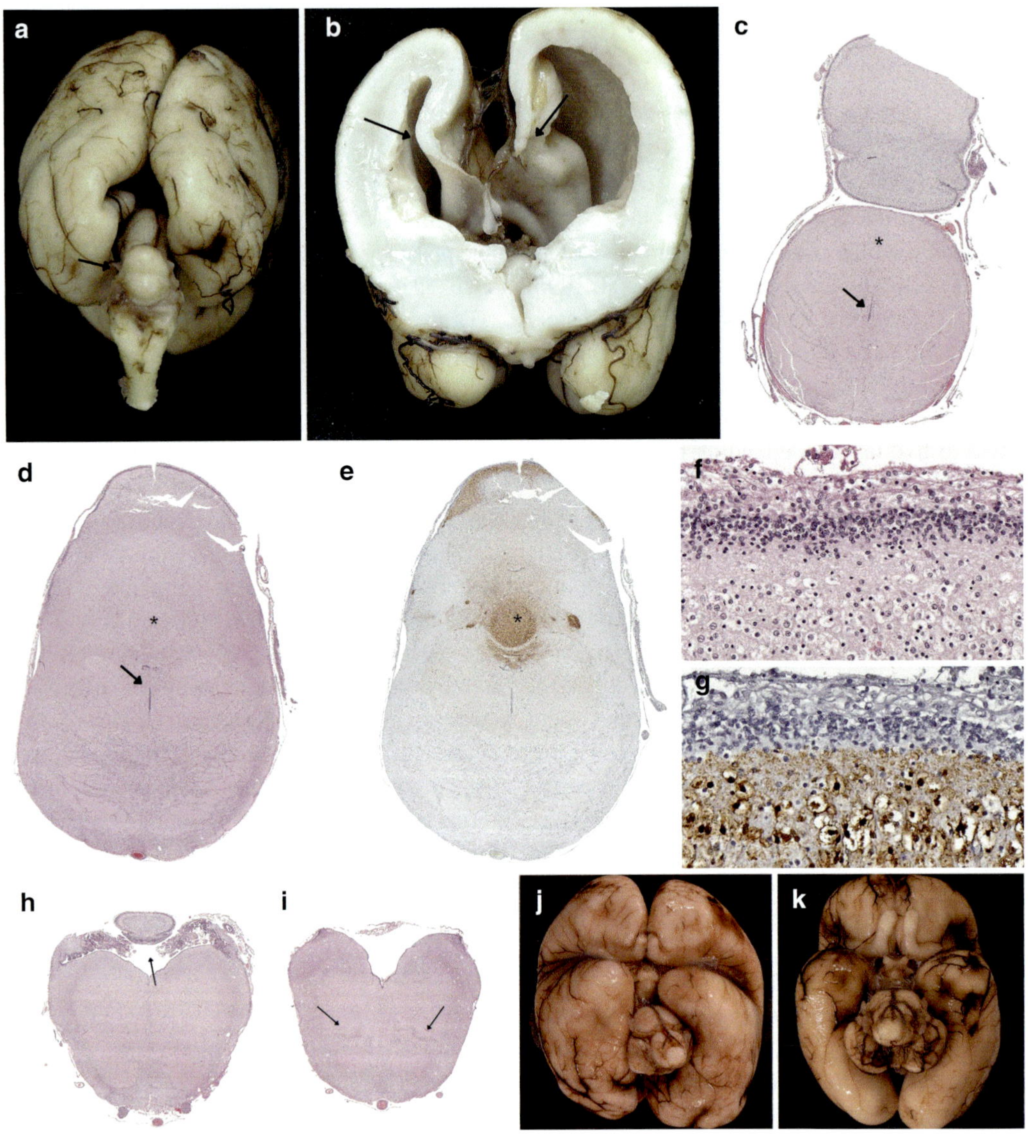

Fig. 8.1 Cerebellar hypoplasia. (**a**) The brain of a female fetus, gestational age of 20 weeks, with severe hypoplasia of the cerebellum, which is reduced to a minute nodule (arrow). (**b**) It was accompanied by severe hydrocephalus and agenesis of the corpus callosum (arrows). (**c**) At the level of the pontomesencephalic junction, there is rudimentary cerebellar tissue without lobulation, the vermis is absent, and the hemispheres are fused, suggestive of RES (see below). Dentate nuclei are not seen. The aqueduct is replaced by ependymal nests (arrow), and there is mesencephalosynapsis (asterisk see Chap. 7). (**d**) At the level of rostral pons, there is rudimentary cerebellar tissue at the top of the figure, the rostral fourth ventricle is replaced by ependymal nests, and at the floor of the fourth ventricle, there is a rounded cluster of heterotopic cells (asterisk). (**e**) Immunohistochemical staining for calbindin highlights the heterotopic cells, as well as a few smaller cell clusters on both sides (arrows), which may represent heterotopic nodules or rudimentary nuclei interpositi (arrows). (**f**) The cortex of the rudimentary cerebellum exhibits an EGL, molecular layer, and IGL. (**g**) Purkinje cells are interspersed with the IGL, in a disorganized multilayered pattern [calbindin]. (**h**) The caudal cerebellum is reduced to a small nodule dorsal to the open medulla (arrow). (**i**) The inferior olivary nuclear complexes are present but hypoplastic and dysplastic (arrows). (**j**) Another case of cerebellar hypoplasia at 20 weeks' gestation. This female fetus had an occipital meningocele, hydrocephalus, and multiple nodular periventricular heterotopias. The cerebellum is hypoplastic, and the hemispheres are poorly developed when compared to (**k**) a normal fetal brain at the same gestational age

8.2 Cerebellar Hemihypoplasia

Hemihypoplasia of the cerebellum ranges from subtle asymmetry between the cerebellar hemispheres with unclear clinical significance to aplasia of one cerebellar hemisphere (Poretti et al. 2010). It is mostly attributed to a hemorrhagic event (Fig. 8.2) but has also been associated with PHACE syndrome, Goldenhar syndrome (Fig. 8.3a–d), and congenital cytomegalovirus (CMV) infection (Robins et al. 1998; Malinger et al. 2006; Massoud et al. 2014; Martinelli et al. 2004). The PHACE syndrome is a neurocutaneous vascular disorder associated with posterior fossa malformations, hemangioma, arterial anomalies, cardiac defects, and ocular anomalies. It lacks a known

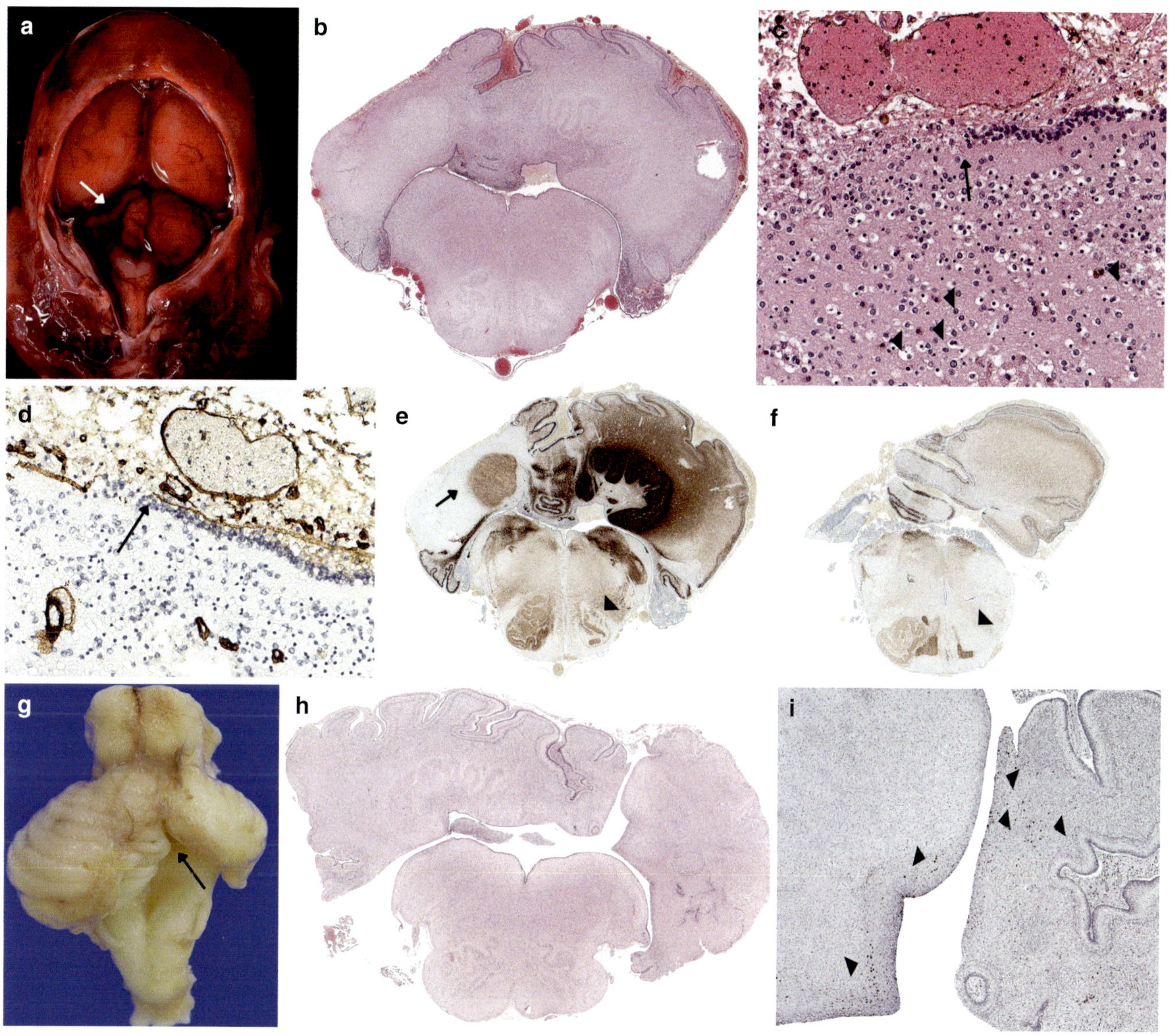

Fig. 8.2 Cerebellar hemihypoplasia—ischemic. (**a**) Posterior fossa of a 24-week-gestation fetus with atrophy of the left cerebellar hemisphere and agenesis of the corpus callosum. The cerebellum is asymmetric with a small left hemisphere. (**b**) The folia on the left hemicerebellum are poorly developed. (**c**) There is an abrupt transition (arrow) between the normal cortex and atrophic cortex. Hemosiderin-laden macrophages (arrowheads) are seen in the affected area, suggestive of a hemorrhagic etiology. (**d**) The pia limitans overlying the normal cortex is intact, and at the point of transition (arrow), it is lost (immunohistochemical staining for collagen IV). (**e**, **f**) The left dentate nucleus is very simplified and appears as a mass of cells without structure (arrow), and the contralateral inferior olivary nuclear complex is severely hypoplastic (arrowheads) (calbindin immunohistocheimstry). (**g**) Cerebellar hemihypoplasia from another case of a 23-week-gestation fetus with widespread chronic histiocytic intervillositis in the placenta. The cerebellum is asymmetric, and the right hemisphere is small and smooth with a paramedian cleft (arrow), while the left hemisphere and vermis are relatively preserved. (**h**) The cleft is seen histologically splaying the right cerebellar hemisphere. (**i**) CD68+ activated microglia are seen on both sides of the cleft (arrowheads)

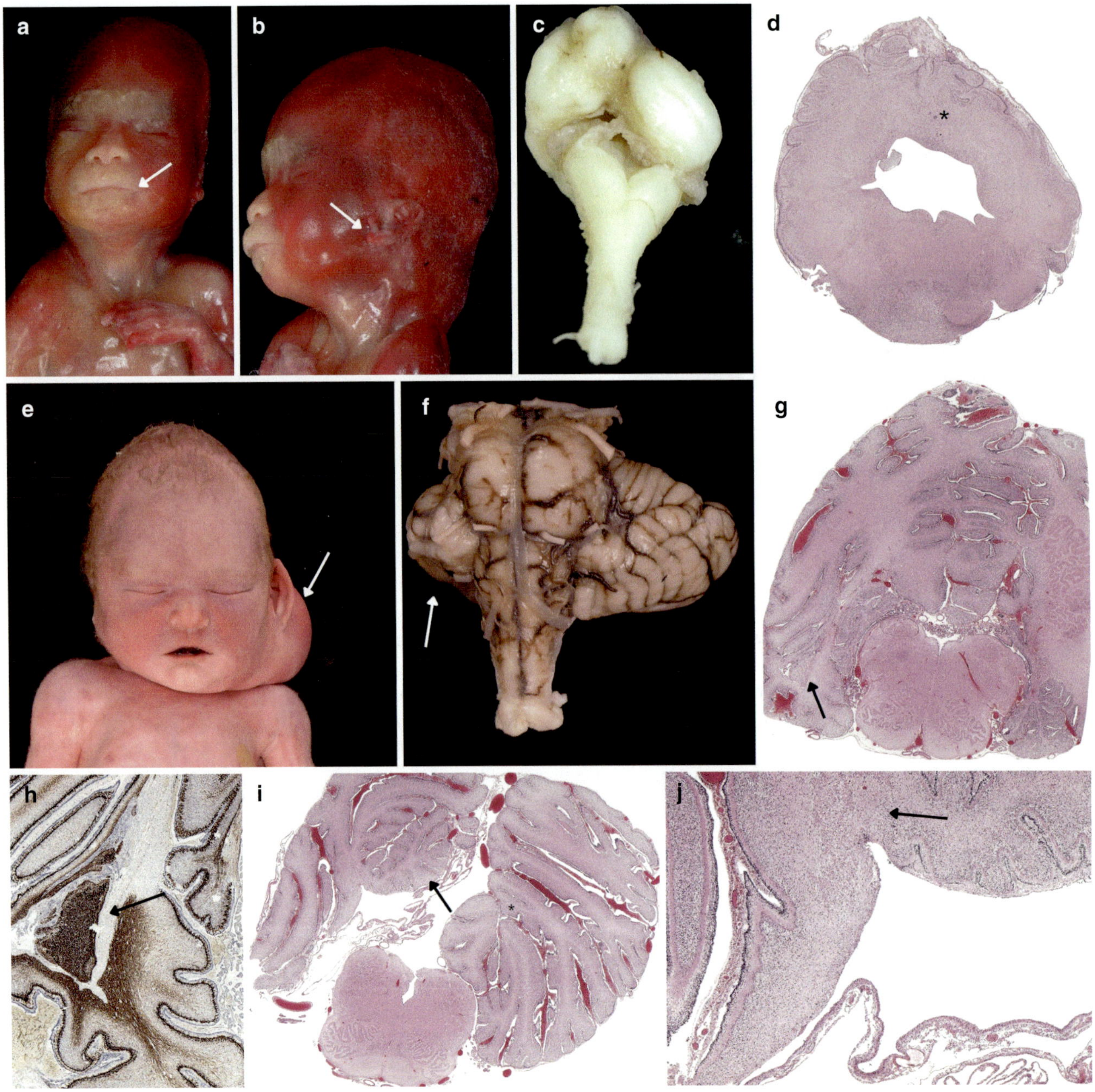

Fig. 8.3 Cerebellar hemihypoplasia—other. (**a**) A 20-week-gestation fetus with Goldenhar syndrome and cerebellar hemihypoplasia. The left lips are tilted upward (arrow), and the left eye appears small. (**b**) The left ear is posteriorly rotated and hypoplastic with a bifid tragus (arrow). (**c**) The cerebellum is smooth and asymmetric, the left hemisphere hypoplastic, and the vermis poorly defined. (**d**) Histologically, there is asymmetric foliation, reduced in the left hemicerebellum, and the vermis is not well formed (asterisk). (**e**) A 31-week-gestation female fetus with a right neck teratoma (arrow) and multiple CNS anomalies, including choroid plexus cysts, bifrontal polymicrogyria, and olivary heterotopia with unknown etiology. (**f**) There is hemihypoplasia of the right cerebellar hemisphere (arrow). (**g**) Histologically, the cerebellum is asymmetric, and there is a heterotopic nodule in the affected hemisphere (arrow) (**h**) seen in a higher magnification staining positive for calbindin (arrow). (**i**) In the caudal cerebellum, the folia are focally malориented (arrow), and there is a choroid plexus cyst (asterisk). (**j**) The heterotopic nodule is adjacent to the choroid plexus cyst (arrow)

genetic cause and is thought to result from an early developmental disruption (Keith 2024). Goldenhar syndrome, also known as hemifacial microsomia, is a disorder of the first and second branchial arches that typically presents as unilateral hypoplasia of facial structures including the eye, ear, maxilla, and mandible (Paradowska-Stolarz et al. 2024). It is frequently associated with additional central nervous system malformations, such as hydrocephalus, occipital and frontal encephaloceles, hypoplasia of the corpus callosum, and rhombencephalosynapsis (RES), as well as cardiac anomalies and vertebral anomalies (Fisher et al. 2025; Gorlin et al. 2023).

Macroscopically, cerebellar hemihypoplasia presents as an asymmetry of the cerebellar hemispheres, with one hemisphere appearing small (Figs. 8.2a, g and 8.3c, f). The affected hemisphere often exhibits absent (Figs. 8.2a, b, g, h and 8.3c, d) or abnormal foliation (Fig. 8.3g–i). Microscopically, findings may include cortical atrophy (Fig. 8.2c), polymicrogyria, or dysplasia in the affected hemisphere (Fig. 8.3g–j). The presence of hemosiderin-laden macrophages or defects in the pia limitans suggests an underlying hemorrhagic etiology (Fig. 8.2c, d). The dentate nucleus may be hypoplastic or dysplastic, and as expected in cerebellar lesions involving the Guillain–Mollaret triangle, the contralateral inferior olivary nuclear complex may show degeneration (Fig. 8.2e, f) (Khoyratty et al. 2013; Uchino et al. 1993).

8.3 Cerebellar Vermian Hypoplasia

In the normal cerebellum, the vermis is a median ridge of foliated cerebellar cortex delimited from the lateral cerebellum by a sulcus on each side, marked anteriorly by a shallow sulcus containing the paravermal vein and posteriorly by the paramedian sulcus (Voogd and Glickstein 1998; Chen et al. 2002). The terms "absent" and "hypoplastic" vermis in the clinical literature are not consistently defined and can refer to at least three distinct pathological states: (1) the vermis as defined above can be present but is smaller and usually simplified (e.g., Dandy–Walker), (2) a central ridge of foliated cerebellar cortex can be present but undemarcated from the cerebellar hemispheres (i.e., RES), and (3) the area usually occupied by a ridge of tissue in the midline is instead a groove (e.g., as observed in Walker–Warburg).

Hypoplasia of the cerebellar vermis typically involves the posterior lobe. In a median section, the arborization of the posterior vermian lobules is reduced relative to gestational age (Kapur et al. 2009). The fastigial angle remains acute, distinguishing this entity from Dandy–Walker malformation (DWM) (Haldipur et al. 2021). Axial sections show an indentation between the hemispheres in the area of the vermis (Fig. 8.4). Both cerebellar vermian hypoplasia and the Dandy–Walker spectrum are attributed to disruptions to the rhombic lip development; however, in vermian hypoplasia, this disruption likely occurs at a later stage of development (Haldipur et al. 2021).

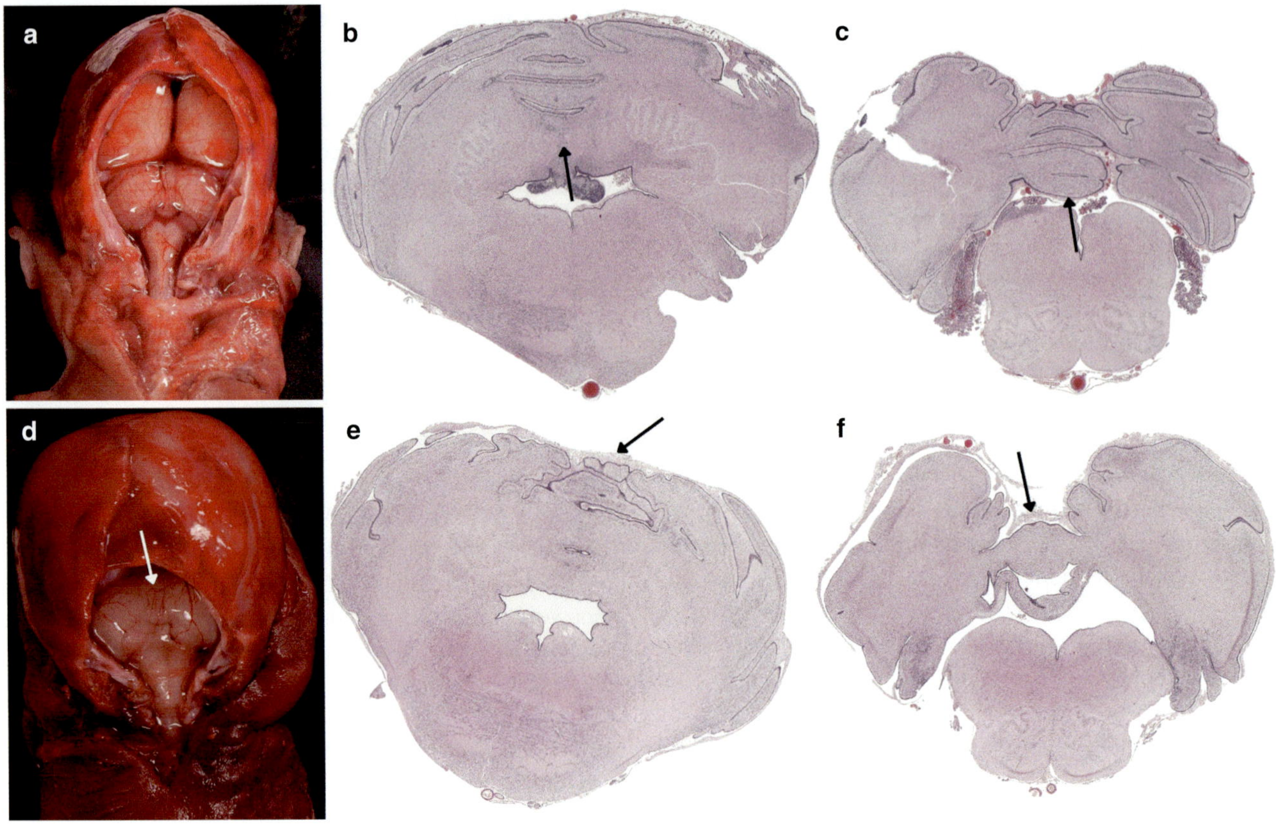

Fig. 8.4 Vermian hypoplasia. (**a**) View of the posterior fossa of a 22-week-gestation fetus with a normal central nervous system. (**b**, **c**) Normal cerebellar vermis (arrows) at the level of the middle cerebellar peduncles and foramina of Luschka (respectively). (**d**) Posterior fossa of a fetus with vermian hypoplasia of the same gestational age and weight; the vermis is poorly defined. (**e**) The dorsal part of the vermis at the level of the middle cerebellar peduncles is mildly hypoplastic (arrow). (**f**) The caudal vermis forms a deep groove between the hemispheres and is significantly smaller compared to the normal control

8.4 Dandy–Walker Malformation

The DWM encompasses a spectrum of cerebellar malformations characterized by (1) agenesis or dysgenesis of the cerebellar vermis, (2) cystic dilation of the fourth ventricle, and (3) upward displacement of the tentorium and torcula (confluence of sinuses). Although early descriptions attributed DWM development to atresia of Magendie foramen (Benda 1954), later studies found evidence of a primary disruption to the development and internalization of the germinal trigone prior to 14 post-conception weeks (Haldipur et al. 2021). The vermian agenesis or dysgenesis is best appreciated on median sections where the fastigial angle is obtuse and the vermis is elongated, attenuated, and rotated superiorly, creating the "tail sign" seen in imaging (Fig. 8.5) (Kapur et al. 2009).

The DWM can occur in isolation or as part of a more pervasive syndrome (Ulm et al. 1999). It is commonly associated with ventriculomegaly, cerebellar dysplasia or hypoplasia, or other neuropathologic anomalies including occipital encephalocele, abnormal gyration, callosal anomalies, heterotopia, syringomyelia, and aqueductal stenosis (Lerman-Sagie et al. 2018; Baro et al. 2018; Fisher et al. 2025). Most cases of the DWM are sporadic, although familial recurrence has been reported. Various segmental chromosomal aberrations were reported in select cases of the DWM, including loss or gain of 6p25.3 encompassing *FOXC1*, loss of chromosome 3q2 encompassing *ZIC1* and *ZIC4*, partial trisomy 12p, 12p deletion, 15q deletion, partial trisomy 9p, and 13q deletion (Aldinger et al. 2009; Grinberg et al. 2004; Sun et al. 2021; Chen et al. 2002; Alanay et al. 2005).

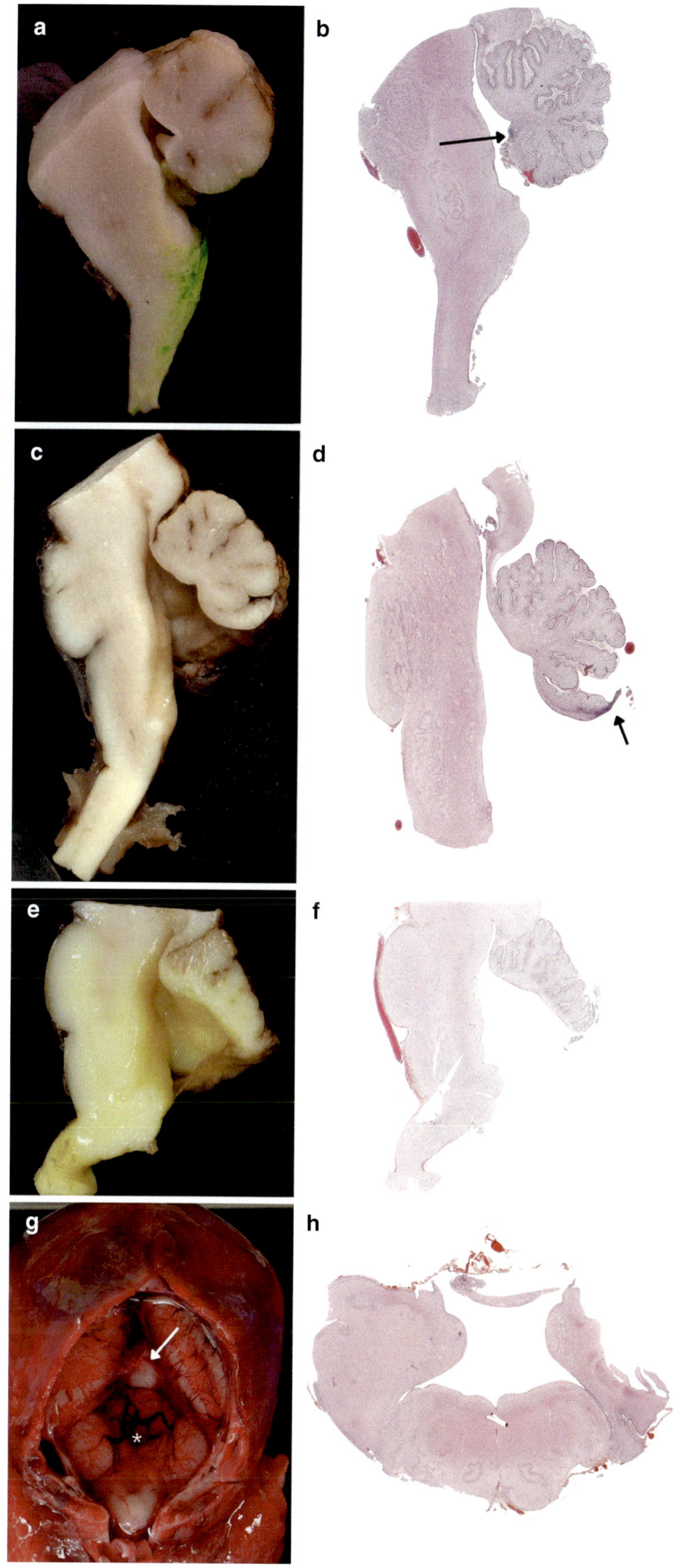

Fig. 8.5 Dandy–Walker malformation. (**a**) Median view of a normal cerebellum and brainstem of a 22-week-gestation fetus. (**b**) The vermis is completely formed, the fastigial angle is acute, and the germinal trigone is internalized (arrow). (**c**) Median view of the brainstem and cerebellum from a fetus with Dandy–Walker spectrum; pregnancy was terminated at 23 weeks. The cerebellum appears roughly appropriate for gestational age, but the vermis is rotated superiorly, and the fourth ventricle is enlarged. (**d**) The fastigial angle is obtuse, and the germinal trigone is outside of the fourth ventricle (arrow). (**e**) Brainstem and cerebellum of the sibling of the prior case, terminated at 21 weeks' gestation for isolated DWM. The cerebellum is hypoplastic, the vermis is rotated upward, and the fourth ventricle is wide. (**f**) The fastigial angle is nearly flat, and the tail of the vermis is not internalized into the fourth ventricle. No genetic alterations were found in this family. (**g**) Posterior fossa of a 23-week-gestation fetus with the DWM; the tentorium and torcula are elevated (arrow), the vermis is not seen (asterisk), and the opening of the fourth ventricle is enlarged. (**h**) The cerebellar vermis is absent at the level of the foramina of Luschka, and the cerebellar hemispheres are splayed

8.5 Rhombencephalosynapsis

Rhombencephalosynapsis is characterized by agenesis or hypoplasia of the cerebellar vermis, resulting in the fusion of the cerebellar hemispheres. It may be complete with vermian aplasia or partial with vermian hypoplasia (Fig. 8.6). Rhombencephalosynapsis is best appreciated on an axial section, where the cerebellum appears rounded due to the absence of the vermis (Fig. 8.6a). The dentate nuclei are closely opposed and may be fused (Fig. 8.6b, c). Partial RES can be anterior or, less commonly, posterior with loss of the vermis rostral or caudal to the primary fissure, respectively (Fig. 8.6d–f) (Pasquier et al. 2009; Krajden Haratz et al. 2021). The fourth ventricle is typically small, and in 18–25%, there are clusters of heterotopic Purkinje cells located in the anterior medullary velum (Fig. 8.6g–i) (Fisher et al. 2025; Pasquier et al. 2009). Rhombencephalosynapsis is commonly associated with ventriculomegaly and aqueductal stenosis, often in conjunction with mesencephalosynapsis (failure of dorsal brainstem colliculi to separate into distinct lateral masses) (Fisher et al. 2025; Pasquier et al. 2009; Krajden Haratz et al. 2021; Ishak 2012). The third ventricle can be dilated or atretic with thalamic fusion (Krajden Haratz et al. 2021; Pasquier et al. 2009). Rarely, RES is associated with aplasia or dysplasia of the inferior olivary nuclear complexes (Pasquier et al. 2009). Other associated abnormalities include agenesis, dysgenesis, or dysplasia of the corpus callosum, holoprosencephaly, and neural tube defects (Krajden Haratz et al. 2021; Ishak et al. 2012; Pasquier et al. 2009; Tully et al. 2012).

Rhombencephalosynapsis is linked to the VACTERL-H association (vertebral, anal, cardiac, tracheoesophageal, renal, limb anomalies with hydrocephalus) and Gomez–Lopez–Hernandez syndrome (RES, scalp alopecia, and trigeminal anesthesia) (Tully et al. 2012; Kunpalin et al. 2024; Perrone et al. 2020). Rhombencephalosynapsis is also a feature of several single-gene variant syndromes, including but not limited to *ADGRL2*, *ZIC1*, and MN1 C-terminal truncation syndrome (Vezain et al. 2018; Vandervore et al. 2018; Palma Milla et al. 2021; Mak et al. 2020). Many chromosomal abnormalities were reported in association with RES; these include deletions of 2q, 14q12q21.2, 15q24.1, 16p11.2, and 16p13.11 as well as an unbalanced subtelomeric translocation t(2;10) (Truwit et al. 1991; Démurger et al. 2013; Previdi et al. 2024; Lespinasse et al. 2004). However, in most cases, a genetic etiology for RES is not identified.

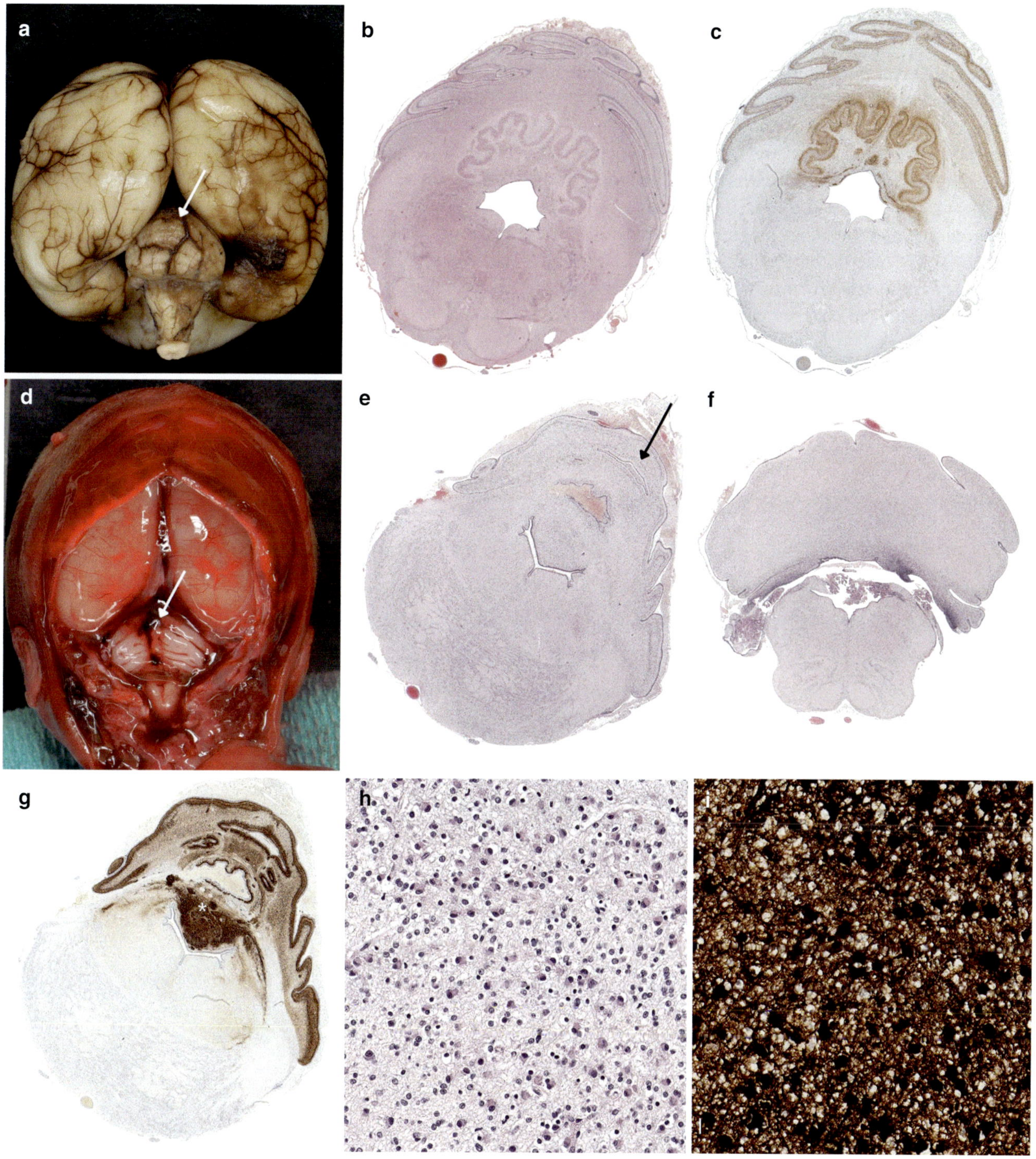

Fig. 8.6 Rhombencephalosynapsis. (**a**) Complete RES at 23 weeks' gestation. The posterior view of the brain demonstrates a globose cerebellum with no identifiable vermis (arrow). (**b**) An axial section of the brainstem and cerebellum at the level of the pontomedullary junction demonstrates a hypoplastic cerebellum with fused cerebellar hemispheres and the absence of the vermis. The dentate nuclei are vertically displaced and very closely apposed. The fourth ventricle is small and abnormally shaped. (**c**) Immunohistochemistry for calbindin highlights the deep nuclei of the cerebellum and demonstrates the abnormal position of the dentate nuclei. (**d**, **e**) Partial RES at 21 weeks' gestation. A hypoplastic anterior vermis is seen in the rostral (anterior) cerebellum (arrow). (**f**) More caudally, the vermis is not identified, and the hemispheres are fused. (**g**) There is a mass of calbindin-positive cells in the anterior medullary velum protruding into the fourth ventricle (asterisk). (**h**, **i**) In a higher magnification, the calbindin-positive cells appear as magnocellular neurons, resembling Purkinje cells

8.6 Cerebellar Dysplasia

The term cerebellar dysplasia encompasses a heterogeneous group of malformations characterized by an abnormal cerebellar morphology. These malformations can include abnormal cortical maturation, heterotopia, and dysplastic changes in the white matter and the deep nuclei. Some patterns of dysplasia can be attributed to specific genetic syndromes, while in other cases, the etiology may be post-encephaloclastic or unknown. On macroscopic examination, the cerebellum may appear asymmetric, with irregular or abnormally smooth folia. The histological changes can be diffuse or localized and may differ based on the etiology. In this section, we will delineate the different patterns of cerebellar dysplasia and their associations.

8.6.1 Cerebellar Dysplasia in Dystroglycanopathies

Dystroglycanopathies are a group of congenital muscular dystrophies caused by defects in the glycosylation of α-dystroglycan and affect predominantly the brain, muscle, and eyes. The neuropathological hallmark of these conditions is cobblestone lissencephaly (see also Chap. 4). Cerebellar pathology in dystroglycanopathies includes varying degrees of hypoplasia and dysplasia and is most severe in cobblestone lissencephaly type A (Devisme et al. 2012). The external surface of the cerebellum appears smooth (Fig. 8.7a, b). Histologically, the cerebellar cortex exhibits focal to extensive polymicrogyria, and the fusion of the folia creates a lacunar appearance (Fig. 8.7c, d) (Devisme et al. 2012). The pia limi-

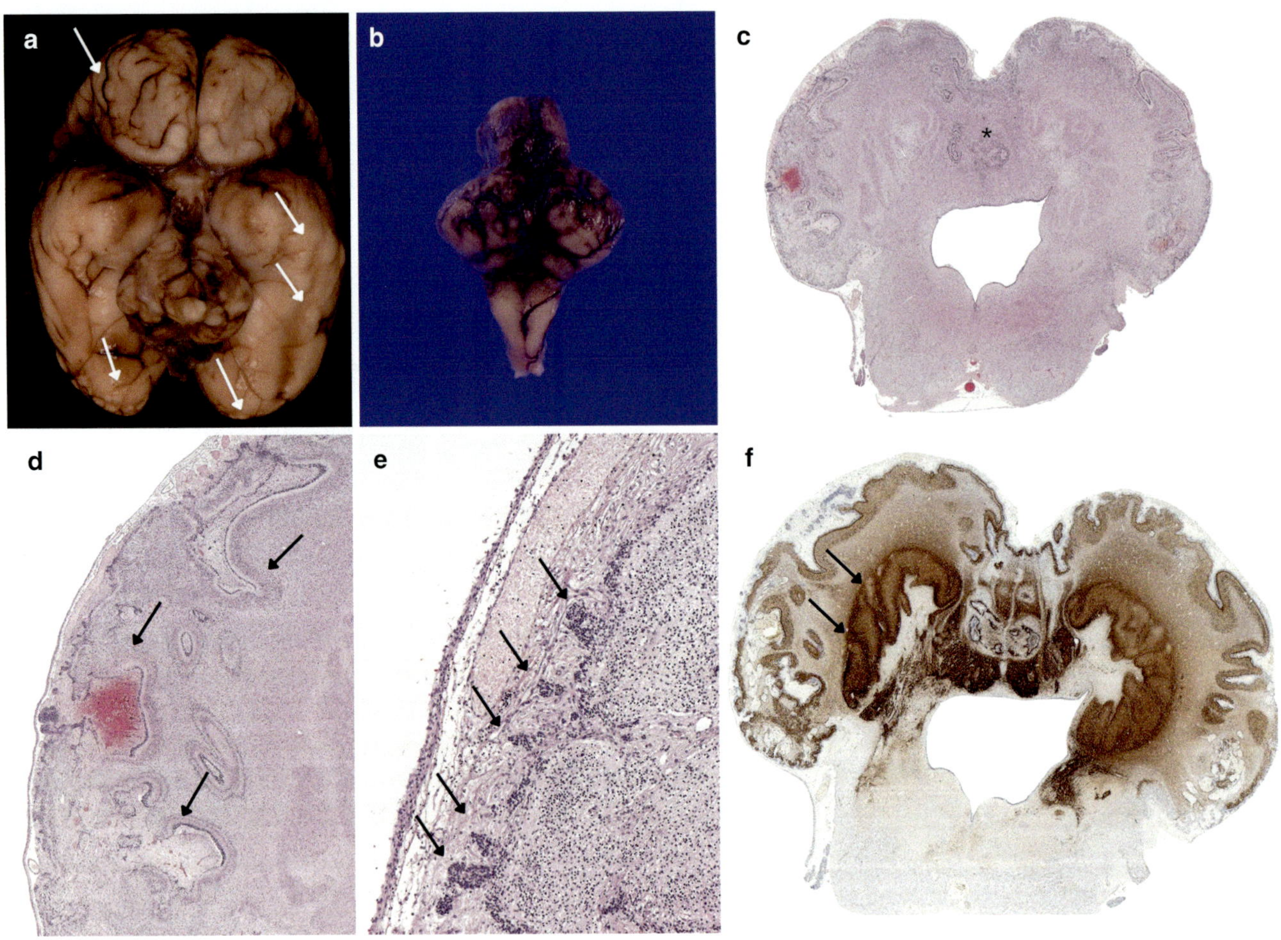

Fig. 8.7 Cerebellar dysplasia in dystroglycanopathies. (**a**) Basal view of the brain of a 23-week-gestation fetus with cobblestone lissencephaly type 2 (dystroglycanopathy). The cerebellum is small, and there are multiple nodules on the external surface of the cerebrum (arrows). (**b**) The cerebellum is smooth, and the vermis is small. (**c**) On the axial section, the fourth ventricle is enlarged on the dorsoventral axis and distorted, the folia are irregular, and the vermis is small and dysplastic. The pons is irregular as well with a disorganized tegmentum and hypoplastic basis pontis. (**d**) The fusion of the folia forms a lacunar appearance (arrows). (**e**) At higher magnification, neuronal overgrowth into the leptomeninges is apparent (arrows). (**f**) The convolutions of the dentate nuclei are thick and irregular, and the right dentate appears fragmented (arrow) [synaptophysin]. The inferior olivary nuclei were dysplastic as well (not seen in this section)

tans is discontinuous with ectopic clusters of granular cells in the pericerebellar leptomeninges (Fig. 8.7e) (Devisme et al. 2012). Often, there is also dentato-olivary dysplasia (Fig. 8.7f).

8.6.2 Cerebellar Dysplasia in Tubulinopathies

Tubulinopathies are neuronal migration anomalies, resulting from defects in microtubule structure caused by mutations in tubulin genes. The brain manifestations are often described as microlissencephaly with cerebellar hypoplasia (see also Chap. 4). Cerebellar involvement includes hypoplasia, dysplasia, and atrophy of the vermis and/or the cerebellar hemispheres (Fig. 8.8a) (Fallet-Bianco et al. 2008; Poirier et al. 2007; Fallet-Bianco et al. 2014).

Histologically, the cerebellar cortex exhibits abnormal lamination (Fig. 8.8b, c). The external granular cell layer is hypoplastic, the molecular layer is nearly absent, Purkinje cells are reduced in numbers, and Bergman glia are misoriented (Fig. 8.8d) (Lecourtois et al. 2010). Purkinje cells appear in clusters and streaks around the fourth ventricle, between the deep nuclei, or in the cerebellar white matter (Fig. 8.8b, c, e) (Fallet-Bianco et al. 2008, 2014; Lecourtois et al. 2010). The dentate nuclei are dysplastic, and the inferior olivary nuclear complexes are frequently absent.

8.6.3 Cerebellar Dysplasia Secondary to Injury

Injury or disruptive processes in the posterior fossa occurring in the post-embryonic phase may result in dysplastic changes in the cerebellum. These injuries may be secondary to old, nonlethal, subpial hemorrhage, old infarcts, congenital CMV infection, or mechanical traction caused by occipital encephaloceles (Figs. 8.9 and 8.10) (Averill et al. 2015). The histologic features of secondary cerebellar dysplasia may resemble those seen in genetic syndromes with polymicrogyria, breaches through the pia limitans, and pericerebellar leptomeningeal neuronal heterotopia (Figs. 8.9c and 8.10c–f). The presence of gliosis, calcifications, and hemosiderin-laden macrophages suggests post-

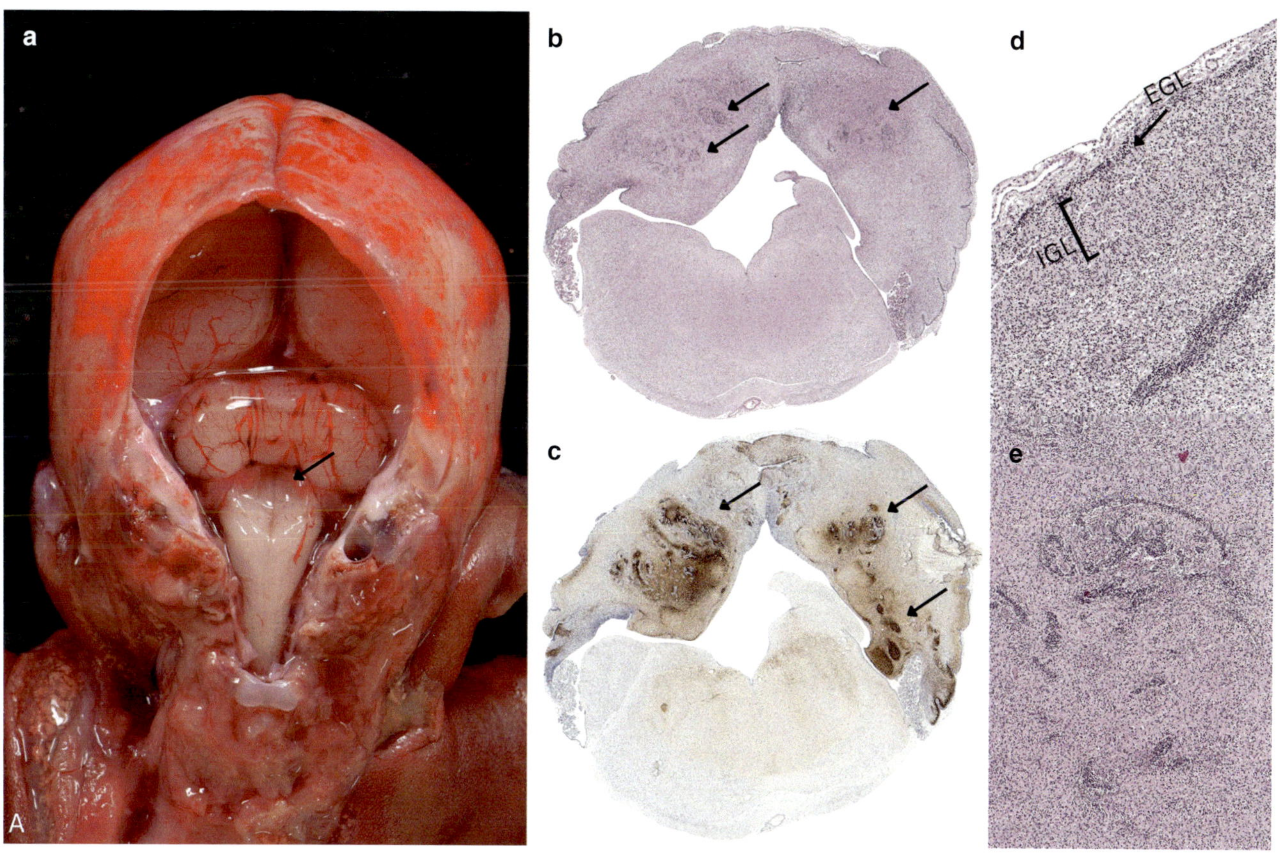

Fig. 8.8 Cerebellar dysplasia in tubulinopathies. (**a**) Posterior fossa of a fetus with microlissencephaly and cerebellar hypoplasia, suggestive of a tubulinopathy. The cerebellum is small and discoid, and the vermis is small, exposing a generous opening of the fourth ventricle. (**b**, **c**) The cerebellum displays dysplastic folia with numerous calbindin-positive neuronal heterotopias (arrows), some of which may represent fragmented nuclei interpositi. (**d**) The cerebellar cortex shows a hypoplastic and irregular EGL, the molecular layer is nearly absent, and the IGL is effaced. Purkinje cells cannot be distinguished in H&E sections. (**e**) In the white matter, there are disorganized streaks of neuronal cells

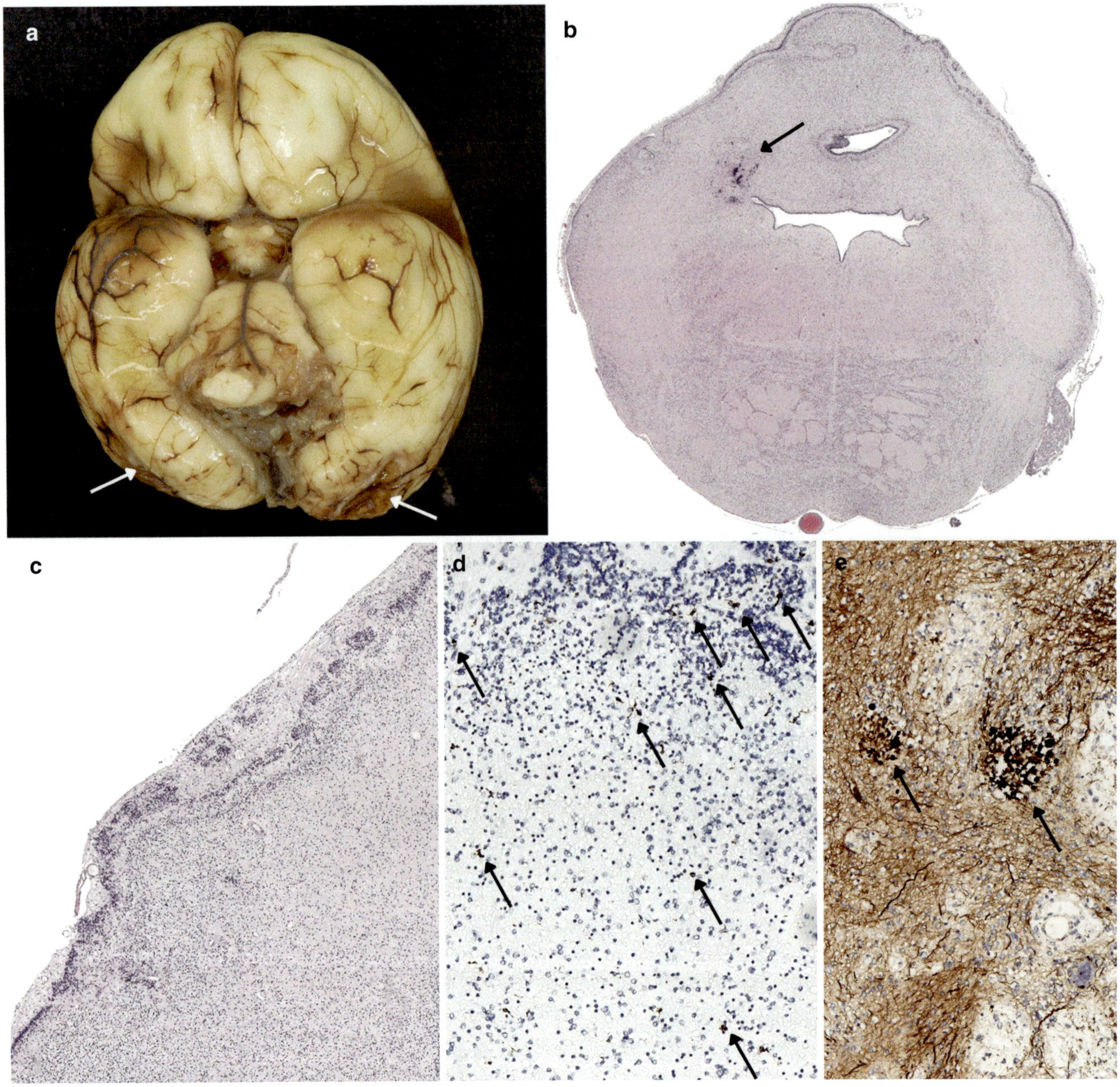

Fig. 8.9 Secondary cerebellar dysplasia due to ischemia. (**a**) The brain of a 21-week-gestation fetus with bilateral cerebral porencephaly (arrows). The cerebellum is small and flat. (**b**) The cerebellar foliation is shallow, and there is a large calcification in the middle cerebellar peduncle (arrow). (**c**) There are multiple areas of neuronal overgrowth into the leptomeninges and underlying cortical dysplasia. (**d**) CD68+ activated microglia are present in the dysplastic cortex and the underlying white matter (arrows). (**e**) There are clusters of swollen axons in the area of calcification in the middle cerebellar peduncle (arrows) [neurofilament light chain]. The constellation of findings in the cerebellum and cerebrum points toward injuries secondary to an ischemic insult

encephaloclastic injury (Fig. 8.9a, b). Activated microglia, however, may also be present in the cerebellar cortex in dystroglycanopathies (e.g., Walker–Warburg syndrome), so the mere presence of these cells does not necessarily indicate a prior injury (Ulfig et al. 2008). Other features of CNS and systemic malformations, as well as placental pathology, should be carefully assessed to determine the underlying etiology.

8.6.4 Dentato-Olivary Dysplasia

Dysplasia of the dentate nuclei can be an isolated finding, but it is often accompanied by dysplasia of the inferior olivary nuclear complex of the ventral medulla. Dentato-olivary dysplasia may occur in isolation or as part of a broader CNS phenotype in many genetic syndromes, such as trisomies, neuroaxonal dystrophy, and metabolic disorders, or in associa-

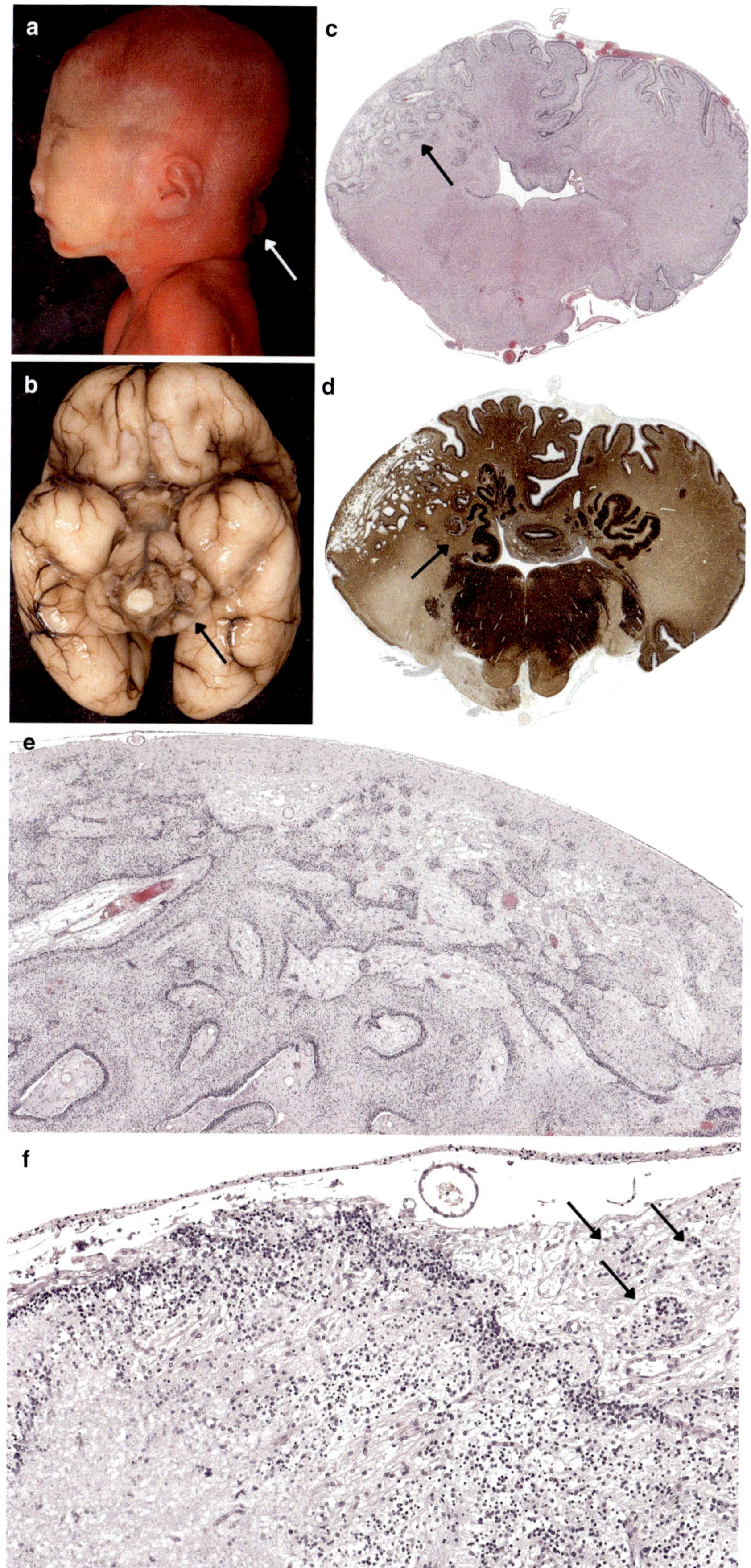

Fig. 8.10 Secondary cerebellar dysplasia—encephalocele. (**a**) A 23-week-gestation fetus with an occipital encephalocele (arrow). (**b**) The cerebellum is asymmetrical, and the left hemicerebellum is smooth (arrow). (**c**) The left cerebellar cortex is dysplastic, and (**d**) the left dentate nucleus is fragmented (synaptophysin). (**e**) There is a lacunar appearance to the cerebellar cortex, similar to that seen in dystroglycanopathies (see Fig. 8.7). (**f**) Clusters of neurons are present in the leptomeninges (arrows)

tion with other CNS malformations (Martland et al. 1997; Kobori et al. 1987; Singh et al. 2004; Saito et al. 2006). These two structures are both of rhombic lip origin, and their development is closely related. They begin developing to their mature structure at 20–22 weeks of gestation, with the development of the olives predating the development of the dentate nuclei by 3–4 weeks (Murofusi 1974). This should be kept in mind when assessing these structures earlier in gestation.

Dysplastic dentate nuclei may appear fragmented (Figs. 8.7f and 8.10d), thick, and hypoconvoluted (Figs. 8.2e and 8.11a) or exhibit abnormal neuronal layering (Friede 1989). Dysplastic olives typically assume a hook-like simplified configuration (Fig. 8.11a). A distinct form of dentato-olivary dysplasia has been described in trisomy 18, with a thick dorsal limb of the inferior olive (Fig. 8.11b, c) and, in a subset of cases, hyperconvolution of the dentate nucleus with cerebellar heterotopia (Norman 1995).

8.6.5 "Trivial" Cerebellar Dysplasia

Focal minor dysplasia is a common finding in the fetal and neonatal cerebellum, and its significance—if any—should be carefully considered. These include small heterotopia around the dentate nuclei or in the cerebellar white matter and focal cortical dysplasia near the cerebellar peduncles or in the nodulus, flocculus, tonsils, and lingula (Friede 1989; Rorke et al. 1968).

8.6.6 Cerebellar Vermian Dysplasia

Although vermian dysplasia has been described in many CNS malformation syndromes, its diagnostic criteria remain poorly defined, and its clinical significance is often uncertain. In the absence of clear criteria, many patterns have been described as vermian dysplasia. We tend to use this term to describe a structural or cytological disorganization of the cerebellar vermis (Fig. 8.11d–f). These changes are a hallmark of Joubert syndrome (see also Chap. 6) and have been described in other genetic syndromes, i.e., Pallister–Killian syndrome and Zellweger syndrome (see also Chap. 12) (Maria et al. 1999; Barkovich et al. 2018; Adiyapatham et al. 2023). Vermian dysplasia may also be a sporadic finding; however, given the poorly defined boundaries of normal variation, the term should be applied with caution.

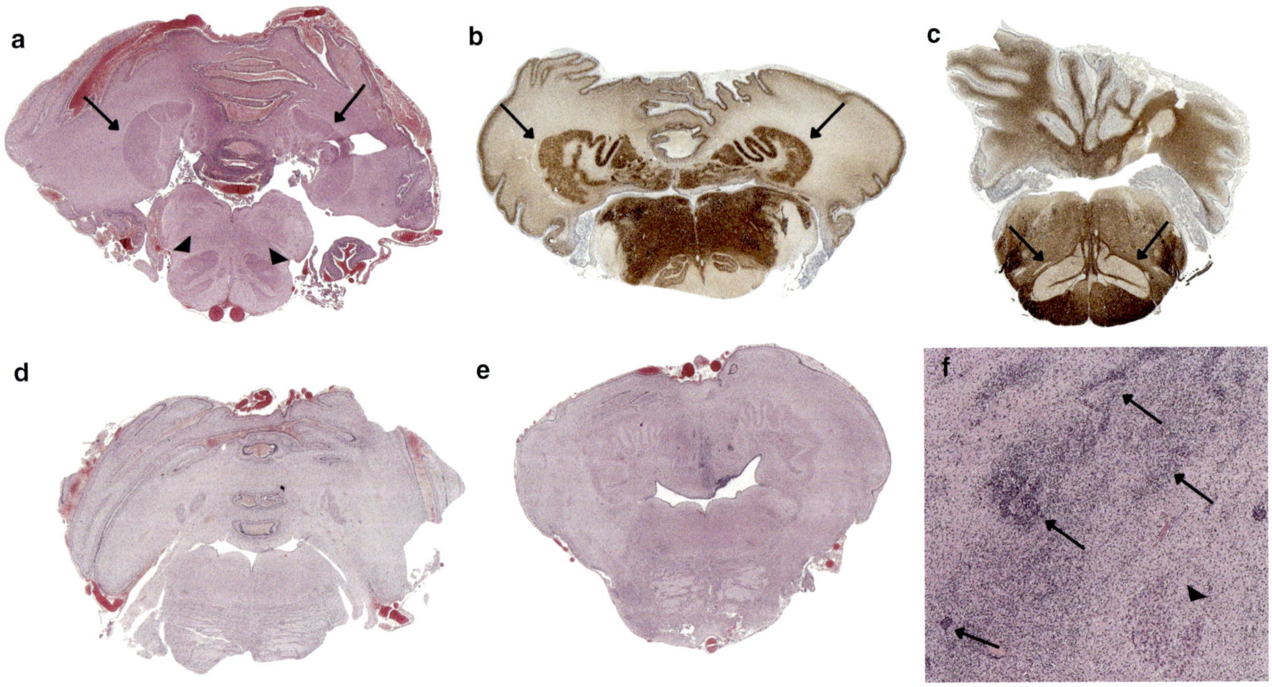

Fig. 8.11 Dentato-olivary dysplasia and vermian dysplasia. (**a**) Thick and hypoconvoluted dentates (arrows) in a case of adenylosuccinate lyase deficiency; pregnancy was terminated at 26 weeks of gestation (see also Chap. 12). The inferior olives are hook-like and hypoconvoluted as well (arrowheads). (**b**, **c**) Dentato-olivary dysplasia in a 23-week-gestation fetus with trisomy 18. The dentates are irregular (B, arrows) [synaptophysin], and the inferior olives demonstrate simplification with a thick dorsal limb (arrows) [neurofilament light chain]. (**d**) The cerebellum of a 23-week-gestation fetus with heterotaxy. There is an abnormal structural organization of the vermis (arrow). (**e**) Between the dentate nuclei, there are excess and delayed streams of apparently migrating cells. (**f**) In higher magnification, these streams include streaks of primitive cells (arrows) and clusters of more mature Purkinje-like heterotopic cells (arrowhead)

8.6.7 Other Cerebellar Dysplasia

Cerebellar dysplasia may be a feature of many other genetic and non-genetic syndromes affecting the CNS. It has been reported with mutations in *PICK3CA*, *COL3A1*, and *GPR56* (Di Stasi et al. 2021; Vandervore et al. 2017; Bahi-Buisson et al. 2010). It can also occur as part of a constellation of multiple congenital anomalies, with or without a genetic explanation. The macroscopic and histologic findings in these cases are similar to those seen with other etiologies described above.

References

Adiyapatham S, Murugesan A. Novel mutation causing Zellweger syndrome. BMJ Case Rep. 2023;16(3):e252014. https://doi.org/10.1136/bcr-2022-252014. PMID: 36931687; PMCID: PMC10030475

Alanay Y, Aktaş D, Utine E, et al. Is Dandy-Walker malformation associated with "distal 13q deletion syndrome"? Findings in a fetus supporting previous observations. Am J Med Genet A. 2005;136(3):265–8.

Aldinger KA, Lehmann OJ, Hudgins L, Chizhikov VV, Bassuk AG, Ades LC, Krantz ID, Dobyns WB, Millen KJ. FOXC1 is required for normal cerebellar development and is a major contributor to chromosome 6p25.3 Dandy-Walker malformation. Nat Genet. 2009;41(9):1037–42. https://doi.org/10.1038/ng.422. Epub 2009 Aug 9. PMID: 19668217; PMCID: PMC2843139

Averill LW, Kandula VV, Akyol Y, Epelman M. Fetal brain magnetic resonance imaging findings in congenital cytomegalovirus infection with postnatal imaging correlation. Semin Ultrasound CT MR. 2015;36(6):476–86. https://doi.org/10.1053/j.sult.2015.04.001. Epub 2015 Apr 3. PMID: 26614131

Bahi-Buisson N, Poirier K, Boddaert N, Fallet-Bianco C, Specchio N, Bertini E, Caglayan O, Lascelles K, Elie C, Rambaud J, Baulac M, An I, Dias P, des Portes V, Moutard ML, Soufflet C, El Maleh M, Beldjord C, Villard L, Chelly J. GPR56-related bilateral frontoparietal polymicrogyria: further evidence for an overlap with the cobblestone complex. Brain. 2010;133(11):3194–209. https://doi.org/10.1093/brain/awq259. Epub 2010 Oct 7.PMID: 20929962

Barkovich EJ, Lateef TM, Whitehead MT. Neuroimaging findings in Pallister-Killian syndrome. Neuroradiol J. 2018;31(4):403–11. https://doi.org/10.1177/1971400917744798. Epub 2017 Dec 20. PMID: 29260614; PMCID: PMC6111437

Baro V, Manara R, Denaro L, d'Avella D. Dandy-Walker malformation and syringomyelia: a rare association. Childs Nerv Syst. 2018;34(7):1401–6. https://doi.org/10.1007/s00381-018-3773-2. Epub 2018 Mar 12. PMID: 29532167

Benda CE. The Dandy-Walker syndrome or the so-called atresia of the foramen Magendie. J Neuropathol Exp Neurol. 1954;13(1):14–29. https://doi.org/10.1093/jnen/13.1.14. PMID: 13118372

Chang CH, Chang FM, Yu CH, Ko HC, Chen HY. Assessment of fetal cerebellar volume using three-dimensional ultrasound. Ultrasound Med Biol. 2000;26(6):981–8. https://doi.org/10.1016/s0301-5629(00)00225-8. PMID: 10996698

Chen CP, Chang TY, Shih JC, Lin SP, Lin CJ Wangm W, Lee CC, Town DD, Pan CW, Tzen CY. Prenatal diagnosis of the Dandy-Walker malformation and ventriculomegaly associated with partial trisomy 9p and distal 12p deletion. Prenat Diagn. 2002;22(12):1063–6. https://doi.org/10.1002/pd.v22:1210.1002/pd.459

Cotes C, Bonfante E, Lazor J, et al. Congenital basis of posterior fossa anomalies. Neuroradiol J. 2015;28(3):238–53.

Démurger F, Pasquier L, Dubourg C, Dupé V, Gicquel I, Evain C, et al. Array-CGH analysis suggests genetic heterogeneity in rhombencephalosynapsis. Mol Syndromol. 2013;4(6):267–72. https://doi.org/10.1159/000353878. Epub 2013 Aug 1. PMID: 24167461; PMCID: PMC3776394

Devisme L, Bouchet C, Gonzalès M, Alanio E, Bazin A, Bessières B, et al. Cobblestone lissencephaly: neuropathological subtypes and correlations with genes of dystroglycanopathies. Brain. 2012;135(Pt 2):469–82. https://doi.org/10.1093/brain/awr357. Epub 2012 Feb 9. PMID: 22323514

Di Stasi M, Izzo G, Cattaneo E, Baraldini V, et al. Cerebellar dysplasia related to PIK3CA mutation: a three-case series. Neurogenetics. 2021;22(1):27–32.

Fallet-Bianco C, Loeuillet L, Poirier K, Loget P, Chapon F, Pasquier L, Saillour Y, Beldjord C, Chelly J, Francis F. Neuropathological phenotype of a distinct form of lissencephaly associated with mutations in TUBA1A. Brain. 2008;131(Pt 9):2304–20. https://doi.org/10.1093/brain/awn155. Epub 2008 Jul 18. PMID: 18669490

Fallet-Bianco C, Laquerrière A, Poirier K, Razavi F, Guimiot F, Dias P, et al. Mutations in tubulin genes are frequent causes of various foetal malformations of cortical development including microlissencephaly. Acta Neuropathol Commun. 2014;2:69. https://doi.org/10.1186/2051-5960-2-69. PMID: 25059107; PMCID: PMC4222268

Fisher Y, Shannon P, Greenberg O, Chitayat D, Chong K, Blaser S, Shinar S. Mesencephalosynapsis and aqueductal stenosis. J Neuropathol Exp Neurol. 2025;84(3):195–209. https://doi.org/10.1093/jnen/nlae128. PMID: 39658320

Friede RL. Developmental neuropathology. Springer-Verlag; 1989.

Gano D, Barkovich AJ. Cerebellar hypoplasia of prematurity: causes and consequences. Handb Clin Neurol. 2019;162:201–16.

Garel C, Falley-Bianco C, Guibard L. The fetal cerebellum: development and common malformation. J Child Neurol. 2011;26(12):1483–92.

Gorlin RJ, Cohen MM Jr, Hennekam RCM. Branchial arch and oral-acral disorders. Syndromes of the head and neck (New York, 2001; online edn, Oxford Academic, 31 Oct 2023), https://doi.org/10.1093/oso/9780195118612.003.0019. Accessed 3 Feb 2025

Grinberg I, Northrup H, Ardinger H, Prasad C, Dobyns WB, Millen KJ. Heterozygous deletion of the linked genes ZIC1 and ZIC4 is involved in Dandy-Walker malformation. Nat Genet. 2004;36(10):1053–5. https://doi.org/10.1038/ng1420. Epub 2004 Aug 29. PMID: 15338008

Haldipur P, Bernardo S, Aldinger KA, Sivakumar T, Millman J, Sjoboen AH, et al. Evidence of disrupted rhombic lip development in the pathogenesis of Dandy-Walker malformation. Acta Neuropathol. 2021;142(4):761–76. https://doi.org/10.1007/s00401-021-02355-7. Epub 2021 Aug 4. PMID: 34347142; PMCID: PMC8544025

Hallonet MER, Le Douarin NM. Tracing neuroepithelial cells of the mesencephalic and metencephalic alar plates during cerebellar ontogeny in quail—chick chimaeras. Eur J Neurosci. 1993;5(9):1145–55.

Ishak GE, Dempsey JC, Shaw DW, Tully H, Adam MP, Sanchez-Lara PA, Glass I, Rue TC, Millen KJ, Dobyns WB, Doherty D. Rhombencephalosynapsis: a hindbrain malformation associated with incomplete separation of midbrain and forebrain, hydrocephalus and a broad spectrum of severity. Brain. 2012;135(Pt 5):1370–86. https://doi.org/10.1093/brain/aws065. Epub 2012 Mar 26. PMID: 22451504; PMCID: PMC3338925

Kapur RP, Mahony BS, Finch L, Siebert JR. Normal and abnormal anatomy of the cerebellar vermis in midgestational human fetuses. Birth Defects Res A Clin Mol Teratol. 2009;85(8):700–9. https://doi.org/10.1002/bdra.20589. PMID: 19441098

Keith L. PHACE syndrome: a review. Semin Pediatr Neurol. 2024;51:101152. https://doi.org/10.1016/j.spen.2024.101152. Epub 2024 Sep 11. PMID: 39389654

Khoyratty F, Wilson T. The dentato-rubro-olivary tract: clinical dimension of this anatomical pathway. Case Rep Otolaryngol. 2013;2013:934386. https://doi.org/10.1155/2013/934386. Epub 2013 Apr 11. PMID: 23662232; PMCID: PMC3639700

Kobori JA, Herrick MK, Urich H. Arhinencephaly. The spectrum of associated malformations. Brain. 1987;110(Pt 1):237–60. https://doi.org/10.1093/brain/110.1.237. PMID: 3801853

Krajden Haratz K, Oliveira Szejnfeld P, Govindaswamy M, Leibovitz Z, Gindes L, Severino M, et al. Prenatal diagnosis of rhombencephalosynapsis: neuroimaging features and severity of vermian anomaly. Ultrasound Obstet Gynecol. 2021;58(6):864–74. https://doi.org/10.1002/uog.23660. PMID: 33942916

Kunpalin Y, Miller E, Raghuram K, Shannon P, Fisher Y, Chau V, et al. Associations and outcomes of prenatally detected rhombencephalosynapsis. Prenat Diagn. 2024;44(10):1159–69. https://doi.org/10.1002/pd.6620. Epub 2024 Jun 5. PMID: 38840304

Lecourtois M, Poirier K, Friocourt G, Jaglin X, Goldenberg A, Saugier-Veber P, Chelly J, Laquerrière A. Human lissencephaly with cerebellar hypoplasia due to mutations in TUBA1A: expansion of the foetal neuropathological phenotype. Acta Neuropathol. 2010;119(6):779–89. https://doi.org/10.1007/s00401-010-0684-z. Epub 2010 Apr 8. PMID: 20376468

Lerman-Sagie T, Prayer D, Stöcklein S, Malinger G. Fetal cerebellar disorders. Handb Clin Neurol. 2018;155:3–23. https://doi.org/10.1016/B978-0-444-64189-2.00001-9. PMID: 29891067

Lespinasse J, Testard H, Nugues F, Till M, Cordier MP, Althuser M, Amblard F, Fert-Ferrer S, Durand C, Dalmon F, Pourcel C, Jouk PS. A submicroscopic unbalanced subtelomeric translocation t(2p;10q) identified by fluorescence in situ hybridization: fetus with increased nuchal translucency and normal standard karyotype with later growth and developmental delay, rhombencephalosynapsis (RES). Ann Genet. 2004;47(4):405–17. https://doi.org/10.1016/j.anngen.2004.07.005. PMID: 15581840

Mak CCY, Doherty D, Lin AE, Vegas N, Cho MT, Viot G, et al. MN1 C-terminal truncation syndrome is a novel neurodevelopmental and craniofacial disorder with partial rhombencephalosynapsis. Brain. 2020;143(1):55–68. https://doi.org/10.1093/brain/awz379. Erratum in: Brain 2020;143(3):e24. doi: 10.1093/brain/awaa007. PMID: 31834374; PMCID: PMC7962909

Malinger G, Zahalka N, Kidron D, et al. Fatal outcome following foetal cerebellar haemorrhage associated with placental thrombosis. Eur J Paediatr Neurol. 2006;10:93–6.

Maria BL, Quisling RG, Rosainz LC, Yachnis AT, Gitten J, Dede D, Fennell E. Molar tooth sign in Joubert syndrome: clinical, radiologic, and pathologic significance. J Child Neurol. 1999;14(6):368–76. https://doi.org/10.1177/088307389901400605. PMID: 10385844

Martinelli P, Maruotti GM, Agangi A, Mazzarelli LL, Bifulco G, Paladini D. Prenatal diagnosis of hemifacial microsomia and ipsilateral cerebellar hypoplasia in a fetus with oculoauriculovertebral spectrum. Ultrasound Obstet Gynecol. 2004;24(2):199–201. https://doi.org/10.1002/uog.1118. PMID: 15287060

Martland T, Harding BN, Morton RE, Young I. Dentato-olivary dysplasia in sibs: an autosomal recessive disorder? J Med Genet. 1997;34(12):1021–3. https://doi.org/10.1136/jmg.34.12.1021. PMID: 9429148; PMCID: PMC1051157

Massoud M, Cagneaux M, Garel C, Varene N, Moutard M-L, Billette T, Benezit A, Rougeot C, Jouannic J-M, Massardier J, Gaucherand P, Desportes V, Guibaud L. Prenatal unilateral cerebellar hypoplasia in a series of 26 cases: significance and implications for prenatal diagnosis. Ultrasound Obstet Gynecol. 2014;44:447–54. https://doi.org/10.1002/uog.13217.

Murofushi K. Normalentwicklung und Dysgenesien von Dentatum und Oliva inferior (Normal development and dysgenesias of the dentate nucleus and inferior olive (author's transl)). Acta Neuropathol. 1974;27(4):317-328. https://doi.org/10.1007/BF00690696. German. PMID: 4407534.

Norman MG. Congenital malformations of the brain: pathologic, embryologic, clinical, radiologic, and genetic aspects. New York: Oxford University Press; 1995.

O'Rahilly R, Müller F. The embryonic human brain an atlas of developmental stages. 3rd ed. Hoboken: Wiley-Liss; 2006.

Otero RA, Sotelo C, Alvarado-Mallart RM. Chick/quail chimeras with partial cerebellar grafts: An analysis of the origin and migration of cerebellar cells. J Comp Neurol. 1993;333(4):597–615.

Palma Milla C, Patricia PM, Lezana JM, Cruz J, Quesada JF, Vila S, Álvarez-Mora I, Arteche-López A, Gómez-Manjón I, Sánchez MT, Gómez-Rodríguez MJ, Sánchez J, Moreno-García M. A novel pathogenic variant in the MN1 gene in a patient presenting with rhombencephalosynapsis and craniofacial anomalies, expanding MN1 C-terminal truncation syndrome. J Pediatr Genet. 2021;12(3):254–7. https://doi.org/10.1055/s-0041-1728650. PMID: 37575653; PMCID: PMC10421676

Paradowska-Stolarz AM, Ziomek M, Sluzalec-Wieckiewicz K, Duś-Ilnicka I. Most common congenital syndromes with facial asymmetry: a narrative review. Dent Med Probl. 2024;61(6):925–32. https://doi.org/10.17219/dmp/186086. PMID: 39496100

Pasquier L, Marcorelles P, Loget P, Pelluard F, Carles D, Perez MJ, Bendavid C, de La Rochebrochard C, Ferry M, David V, Odent S, Laquerrière A. Rhombencephalosynapsis and related anomalies: a neuropathological study of 40 fetal cases. Acta Neuropathol. 2009;117(2):185–200. https://doi.org/10.1007/s00401-008-0469-9. Epub 2008 Dec 5. PMID: 19057916

Peñuelas N, Saco A, Marimón L, Diez-Ahijado L, Nadal A, Sisuashvili L, Darecka K, Gratacós E, Crispi F, Monterde E, García-Otero L, Arca G, Bassat Q, González R, Menéndez C, Ordi J, Rakislova N. Gestational age assessment by ultrasound cerebellar measurements in fetal and perinatal deaths. Am J Obstet Gynecol. 2024;19:S0002-9378(24)01155-4. https://doi.org/10.1016/j.ajog.2024.11.016. Epub ahead of print. PMID: 39571773

Perrone E, D'Almeida V, de Macena Sobreira NL, et al. Gomez-López-Hernández syndrome: a case report with clinical and molecular evaluation and literature review. Am J Med Genet A. 2020;182(7):1761–6.

Poirier K, Keays DA, Francis F, Saillour Y, Bahi N, Manouvrier S, et al. Large spectrum of lissencephaly and pachygyria phenotypes resulting from de novo missense mutations in tubulin alpha 1A (TUBA1A). Hum Mutat. 2007;28(11):1055–64. https://doi.org/10.1002/humu.20572. PMID: 17584854

Poretti A, Limperopoulos C, Roulet-Perez E, et al. Outcome of severe unilateral cerebellar hypoplasia. Dev Med Child Neurol. 2010;52:718–24.

Previdi A, Jordan P, Egloff C, Coussement A, Ahmed-Eli S, Tudal L, Bienvenu T, Picone O, Dupont JM. Prenatal diagnosis of a 15q24.1 microdeletion in a fetus with cerebral and urogenital abnormalities. Clin Genet. 2024;106(5):537–44. https://doi.org/10.1111/cge.14592. Epub 2024 Jul 16. PMID: 39012202

Rakic P, Sidman RL. Histogenesis of cortical layers in human cerebellum, particularly the lamina dissecans. J Comp Neurol. 1970;139(4):473–500.

Robins JB, Mason GC, Watters J, et al. Case report: cerebellar hemihypoplasia. Prenat Diagn. 1998;18:173–7.

Rorke LB, Riggs HE, Fogelson MH. Cerebellar heterotopia in infancy. J Neuropathol Exp Neurol. 1968;27(1):140–1. PMID: 5656557

Saito Y, Hayashi M, Miyazono Y, Shimogama T, Ohno K. Arthrogryposis multiplex congenita with callosal agenesis and dentato-olivary dysplasia. Brain Dev. 2006;28(4):261–4. https://doi.org/10.1016/j.braindev.2005.08.009. Epub 2005 Dec 20. PMID: 16368213

Shannon P, Carreon CK, Ernst LM, Huff DS, Ruchelli ED. Brain and spinal cord. In: Color atlas of human fetal and neonatal histology. Cham: Springer International Publishing; 2019. p. 291–310. https://doi.org/10.1007/978-3-030-11425-1_29.

Sidman RL, Rakic P. Neuronal migration, with special reference to developing human brain: a review. Brain Res. 1973;62(1):1–35.

Singh V, Boesel CP, Baker P. Septo-optic dysplasia and dentato-olivary dysplasia in a case of 18q deletion/3p trisomy. Clin Neuropathol. 2004;23(1):28–33. PMID: 14986931

Sun Y, Zhang N, Tian H, et al. Prenatal diagnosis of the Dandy-Walker malformation associated with partial trisomy 12p and distal 15q deletion. J Genet. 2021;100:40.

ten-Donkelaar HJ, Lammens M, Wesseling P, Thijssen HOM, Renier WO. Development and developmental disorders of the human cerebellum. J Neurol. 2003;250(9):1025–36.

Truwit CL, Barkovich AJ, Shanahan R, Maroldo TV. MR imaging of rhombencephalosynapsis: report of three cases and review of the literature. AJNR Am J Neuroradiol. 1991;12(5):957–65. PMID: 1950929; PMCID: PMC8333516

Tully HM, Dempsey JC, Ishak GE, Adam MP, Curry CJ, Sanchez-Lara P, Hunter A, Gripp KW, Allanson J, Cunniff C, Glass I, Millen KJ, Doherty D, Dobyns WB. Beyond Gómez-López-Hernández syndrome: recurring phenotypic themes in rhombencephalosynapsis. Am J Med Genet A. 2012;158A(10):2393–406. https://doi.org/10.1002/ajmg.a.35561. Epub 2012 Sep 10. PMID: 22965664; PMCID: PMC3448816

Uchino A, Hasuo K, Uchida K, Matsumoto S, Tsukamoto Y, Ohno M, Masuda K. Olivary degeneration after cerebellar or brain stem haemorrhage: MRI. Neuroradiology. 1993;35(5):335–8. https://doi.org/10.1007/BF00588362. PMID: 8327105

Ulfig N, Steinbrecher A, Stoltenburg-Didinger G, Rezaie P. Differential activation of mononuclear phagocytes in cerebellar malformation associated with Walker-Warburg syndrome. Neuropathology. 2008;28(3):333–40. https://doi.org/10.1111/j.1440-1789.2007.00856.x. Epub 2007 Dec 5. PMID: 18069971

Ulm B, Ulm MR, Deutinger J, Bernaschek G. Isolated Dandy-Walker malformation: prenatal diagnosis in two consecutive pregnancies. Am J Perinatol. 1999;16(2):61–3. https://doi.org/10.1055/s-2007-993837. PMID: 10355911

Vandervore L, Stouffs K, Tanyalçin I, Vanderhasselt T, Roelens F, Holder-Espinasse M, Jørgensen A, Pepin MG, Petit F, Khau Van Kien P, Bahi-Buisson N, Lissens W, Gheldof A, Byers PH, Jansen AC. Bi-allelic variants in COL3A1 encoding the ligand to GPR56 are associated with cobblestone-like cortical malformation, white matter changes and cerebellar cysts. J Med Genet. 2017;54(6):432–40. https://doi.org/10.1136/jmedgenet-2016-104421. Epub 2017 Mar 3. PMID: 28258187

Vandervore LV, Schot R, Hoogeboom AJM, Lincke C, de Coo IF, Lequin MH, Dremmen M, van Unen LMA, Saris JJ, Jansen AC, van Slegtenhorst MA, Wilke M, Mancini GMS. Mutated zinc finger protein of the cerebellum 1 leads to microcephaly, cortical malformation, callosal agenesis, cerebellar dysplasia, tethered cord and scoliosis. Eur J Med Genet. 2018;61(12):783–9. https://doi.org/10.1016/j.ejmg.2018.10.018. Epub 2018 Oct 31. PMID: 30391508

Vezain M, Lecuyer M, Rubio M, Dupé V, Ratié L, David V, Pasquier L, Odent S, Coutant S, Tournier I, Trestard L, Adle-Biassette H, Vivien D, Frébourg T, Gonzalez BJ, Laquerrière A, Saugier-Veber P. A de novo variant in ADGRL2 suggests a novel mechanism underlying the previously undescribed association of extreme microcephaly with severely reduced sulcation and rhombencephalosynapsis. Acta Neuropathol Commun. 2018;6(1):109. https://doi.org/10.1186/s40478-018-0610-5. PMID: 30340542; PMCID: PMC6195752

Volpe JJ. Cerebellum of the premature infant: rapidly developing, vulnerable, clinically important. J Child Neurol. 2009;24(9):1085–104.

Voogd J, Glicktein M. The anatomy of the cerebellum Trends in Neurosciences. 1998;21(9):370–375. https://doi.org/10.1016/S0166-2236(98)01318-6.

Vascular Malformations

9

The vasculature of the central nervous system is derived initially from an endothelial plexus in the primitive meninx that coats the surface of the neuraxis. By the end of neurulation, this plexus is drained by a capital venous plexus to a large cardinal vein and supplied by three pairs of aortic arches. Arterial development proceeds by the fusion of the aortic arches proximally to form the future internal carotid arteries, which give rise to the transient trigeminal, otic, and hypoglossal arteries, which in turn anastomose and give rise to longitudinal aortae by Carnegie stage 13. The longitudinal aortae initially carry blood flowing in a caudal to rostral direction and fuse by stage 16 to become the basilar artery. The temporary carotid–basilar anastomoses are replaced in function by posterior communicating arteries by stage 16, and a middle cerebral artery as well as anterior cerebral artery are present, supplying the telencephalic vesicle at stage 17. The circle of Willis is essentially present and closed between Carnegie stages 20 and 23 (Takakuwa et al. 2016; Padget 1948), and the leptomeningeal pattern of major arterial branching is established by 28 weeks' gestation. Radial penetrating arteries are present in the cortical mantle by 13–15 weeks, and basal penetrating arteries with smooth muscle coats are present in the striatum by midgestational age (Padget 1948).

Venous drainage: By Carnegie stage 17, venous drainage occurs via three dural venous plexuses (rostral, middle, and caudal). These drain ventrally to paired ventral sinuses running under the otic capsules to the jugular veins; an interruption of this ventral drainage by an expansion of the otic capsule by stage 19 leads to an expansion of the more dorsal formation of the sigmoid sinuses. Also, by stage 19, marginal veins draining the telencephalic vesicle have met in the midline to form a sagittal plexus, which drains posteriorly to form the median prosencephalic vein of Markowski, a midline longitudinal vein that initially drains the choroid plexus. Cavernous sinus is present by as early as Carnegie stages 22 and 23. As the prosencephalic neuraxis is subsequently penetrated by vessels, the internal cerebral veins develop and start to drain the choroid plexus. The median prosencephalic vein regresses by about 5 weeks' gestation, with a caudal portion becoming the vein of Galen. The anterior and middle venous plexus fuse to form a tentorial plexus and interhemispheric plexus. The expansion of the cerebral vessels leads to a simplification of the superficial meningeal venous plexus with primitive straight sinus, transverse sinus, and marginal sinus present by 24 weeks. Microvascular proliferation continues throughout gestation, first most intensely in the ventricular zone and in deep structures and then in the cortical plate (Padget 1956).

There are a wide variety of variant developmental patterns, but these are rarely of specific pathological interest, although they can point toward specific malformation (e.g., anterior cerebral artery abnormalities in holoprosencephaly or abnormal pericallosal artery trajectory in agenesis of the corpus callosum). We will focus here specifically on vascular lesions.

9.1 Arterial Anomalies

Abnormal fetal arterial histology may accompany the arteriopathies accompanying COL4A1 and COL4A2 mutation where it has been reported to accompany cortical infarction, intracranial hemorrhage and porencephaly (Fig. 9.1a). The pathology is that of a reduction in the smooth muscle coating of small arteries and a vacuolation of the myocytes, particularly at the junction of the adventitia and media (Shannon et al. 2021) (Fig. 9.1b). A more subtle attenuation of the smooth muscle is also found in white matter vessels (Gubana et al. 2022) accompanying the usual pattern of hemorrhage and thrombosis.

Intracranial arterial medial calcification is a non-specific finding that can occasionally be seen in diffuse calcinosis of infancy, a condition in which cardiac valves and large elastic arteries demonstrate extensive calcification; fetal cases may present with hydrops. The histopathology is of medial calcification of penetrating arteries (Fig. 9.1c, d) and intracranial infarction or hemorrhage. Such cases have been linked to

P. Shannon et al., *Atlas of Neurodevelopmental Pathology*, https://doi.org/10.1007/978-3-032-14148-4_9

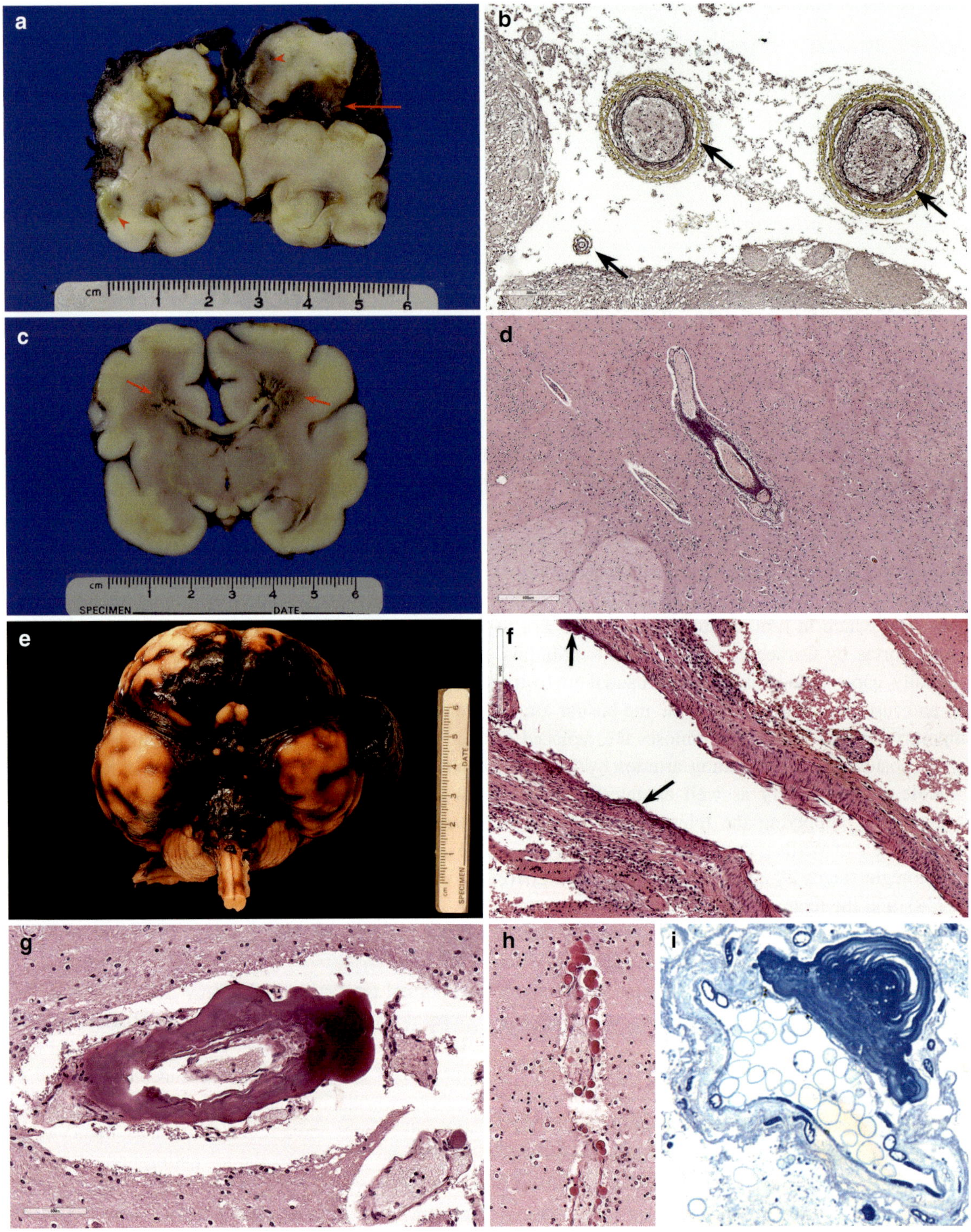

Fig. 9.1 (**a**) A 34-week gestation, with COL4A1 mutation demonstrating porencephaly (arrow) and multiple cortical infarcts (arrowheads), with evidence of old deep hemorrhage microscopically. (**b**) The large and small leptomeningeal arteries demonstrate circumferential vacuolation at the junction of the adventitia and media, giving a distinct bull's-eye impression (Movat Pentachrome). (**c**) A 32-week-gestation hydropic infant with diffuse medial calcinosis of infancy; there is bilateral white matter injury (arrows), most likely due to global circulatory compromise in this case. (**d**) Penetrating artery, the same case as (**c**), demonstrating bland mineralization of the media. This pathology was focal, as compared to the diffuse white matter injury. (**e**) Term gestation, intrapartum death with massive basal subarachnoid and subdural hemorrhage in the neonatal lethal form of osteogenesis imperfecta. (**f**) Careful examination of the internal carotid and its proximal branches showed evidence of rupture with mineralization of the internal elastic laminae. The rupture was possibly due to the distortion of the fragile sphenoid in combination with abnormal rigidity of the elastica. (**g**) Raine syndrome with massive irregular mineralization of the penetrating artery subintima and media. (**h**) Capillaries and venules of the same case demonstrated innumerable spherical mineralizations. (**i**) On plastic-embedded sections, the affected capillaries show laminated mineralization apparently based in the endothelial basal lamina (toluidine blue)

autosomal recessive mutations in ENPP1 or less frequently ABCC6 (Chong and Hutchins 2008; Nitschke 2012). We have also seen calcification of the internal carotid elastica with intrapartum arterial rupture and massive basal subarachnoid hemorrhage in a case of lethal osteogenesis imperfecta (Fig. 9.1e, f).

9.2 Microvascular Disease

9.2.1 Raine Syndrome

Raine syndrome (OMIM 259775, lethal sclerosing osteomalacia with cerebral calcification) may also demonstrate prominent intracranial vascular calcifications in late gestation (Chitayat et al. 2007) that on histology may massively involve penetrating arteries (Fig. 9.1g) and thin-walled vessels (Fig. 9.1h). In the single case of our experience, these appear as laminated mineralization based in the media or capillary basal lamina (vascular, Fig. 9.1l).

9.2.2 Fowler Disease

Fowler disease (OMIM 225790, proliferative vasculopathy and hydranencephaly) (Fig. 9.2a) is a lethal microvascular thrombotic disease of the central nervous system. The pathology demonstrates severe ventriculomegaly (Fig. 9.2a) and a rostral to caudal gradient of severity, with the brain being affected more than the spinal cord. There is a centrifugal pattern of necrosis predominantly affecting the cerebral mantle (Bessieres-Grattagliano et al. 2009; Williams et al. 2010) (Fig. 9.2b). The histology is characterized by a proliferative microvasculopathy demonstrating PAS (+) inclusions (Fig. 9.2c) and forming glomeruloid vascular tufts (Fig. 9.2d). On electron microscopy, the inclusions are intracytoplasmic and fibrillary (Fig. 9.2e), although the number of inclusions may vary substantially in quantity from case to case. The condition is inherited as an autosomal recessive condition and linked to mutations in FLVCR2 (Meyer et al. 2010). Rare microvascular tufts as an occasional finding can be seen in many inflammatory or microvascular diseases of the fetal central nervous system, suggesting that the histology is due to an abnormality in endothelial proliferation and remodeling. On the other hand, we have seen a case of a midgestation fetus with diffuse microvascular disease (Fig. 9.2f) characterized by microvascular dilation and proliferation and lacking large tufts (Fig. 9.2g) but with widespread microvascular thrombosis that lacked large endothelial inclusions or mutations in FLVCR2 (Fig. 9.2h), suggesting that the histology is not simply due to a propensity for thrombosis itself.

Perivascular calcifications may be prominent in severe fetal cytomegalovirus infection and may be post-necrotic in origin (Fig. 9.2i). However, cytomegalovirus may infect the endothelium, and calcification of the neonatal media has been observed (personal observation) (Fig. 9.2j). Perivascular pathology, characterized as amphophilic globules, is often conceived of as a product of local tissue injury. These can be found accompanying fetal white matter injury and telencephalic gliosis (Gilles et al. 1998; Golden et al. 1997) and can also be seen in fetal hydrops, cytogenetic abnormalities (Fig. 9.2k) including Down syndrome, and metabolic abnormalities (Fig. 9.2l) and occasionally as an incidental finding in an otherwise normal brain. They may demonstrate a locally brisk-associated microglial reaction.

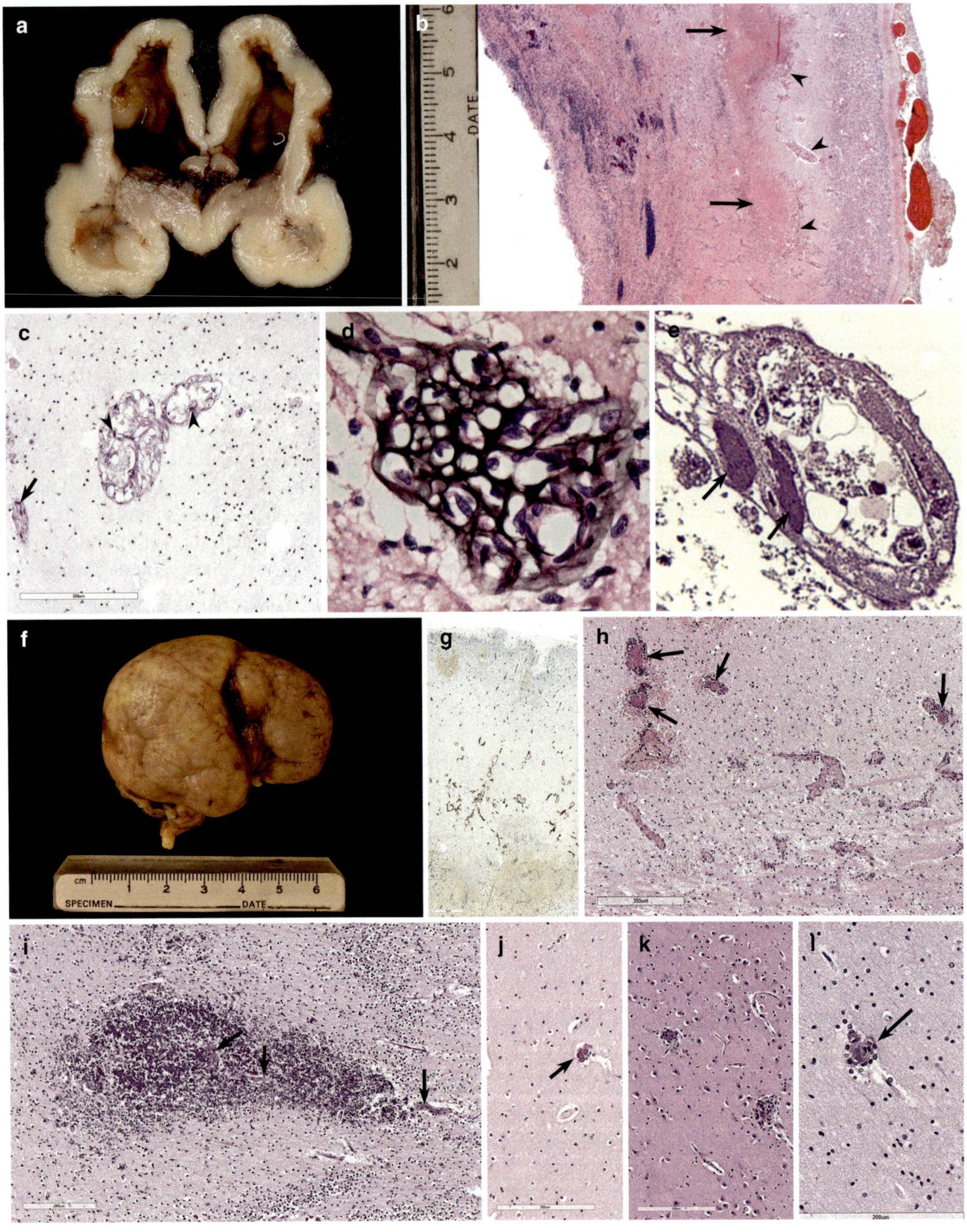

Fig. 9.2 (**a**) Fowler disease demonstrating ventriculomegaly with a shaggy, irregular ventricular lining of the lateral ventricles and marked thinning of the cortical mantle. (**b**) Full-thickness section of the frontal convexity with innumerable deep post-necrotic calcifications and large areas of geographic necrosis (arrows) with adjacent microvascular proliferation (arrowheads) obvious at even low power. (**c**) The microvasculature contains numerous PAS (+) inclusions (arrowheads) that remain even after the affected vessels are occluded and necrotic (arrow, periodic acid–Schiff). (**d**) Staining the basal lamina with PASM demonstrates glomeruloid proliferations of endothelial cells. (**e**) Plastic-embedded tissue demonstrates compact fibrillary intracytoplasmic PAS (+) inclusions. (**f**) Midgestational fetal brain with extensive irregular cortical damage and ventriculomegaly (not shown). (**g**) Cortical mantle of the same case demonstrating thinned subplate with irregularly dilated deep microvasculature (immunohistochemistry for Collagen IV). (**h**) Innumerable microvascular thrombi with local reaction (arrows); these were also numerous in the brainstem and cerebellum with local gliosis, aqueductal gliosis, and mineralization. Trio whole exome sequencing unrevealing. (**i**) Tissue mineralization in midgestational fetal cytomegalovirus encephalitis, surrounding the course of a penetrating cortical vessel (arrows); in this particular case, the perivascular propensity for massive calcification was marked. (**j**) Perivascular amphophilic globule, term stillbirth with pontosubicular necrosis. (**k**) Multiple amphophilic globules, with brisk microglial reaction, in a 30-week-gestation fetus with ventriculomegaly, a small cerebellar vermis, and a terminal microdeletion at Chr. 10p15.3p1 (**k** and **l**) Perivascular amphophilic globule in fetus with glutamine synthetase deficiency with a microglial reaction (arrow). These were a widespread finding

9.3 Infantile Hemangiomas

Infantile hemangioma may be intracranial or spinal, often with extracranial extension. They can form a soft tissue or dural mass that can occupy basal or posterior basal cisterns and which may involve the fourth ventricle. Hydrocephalus, transverse sinus thrombosis, and cerebellar hemihypoplasia may accompany the lesion, as well as malformations including polymicrogyria, Dandy–Walker malformation, and cerebral heterotopias as well as congenital heart disease, anomalies of the large basal arteries, and PHACE syndrome (Fig. 9.3a, b). Histologically, these are masses of thin-walled dilated capillaries with plump endothelium and GLUT1 reactivity (Fig. 9.3c) (Viswanathan et al. 2009; Feygin et al. 2021).

9.3.1 Venous and Capillary Angiomas

We have seen two cases of capillary–venous (non-infantile) angiomas: a venous angioma in the atrial choroid plexus (Fig. 9.3d, e), presenting with third-trimester intracranial hemorrhage and hydrocephalus, both of which are recorded due to in utero development of cavernous angiomas (e.g., Lerner et al. 2006; Goyal et al. 2023; Henrich et al. 2002), and a capillary angioma, which may be more generally benign (Guibaud et al. 2003) (Fig. 9.3f).

Mixed arterial and venous masses: A wide variety of venous developmental anomalies are recorded, predominantly in the radiological literature (Jaimes et al. 2025). We will focus on those that usually prompt diagnostic evaluation at autopsy.

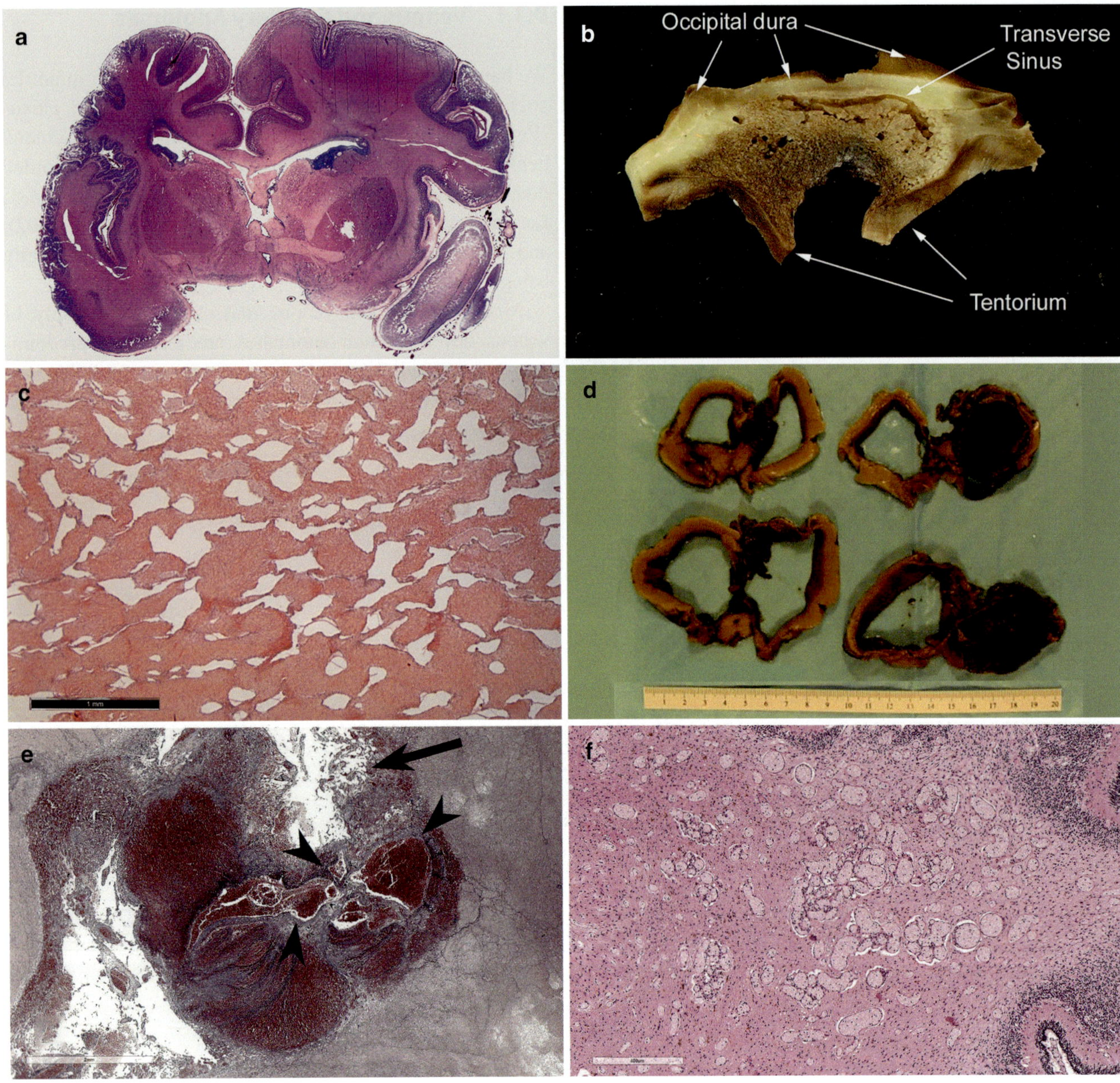

Fig. 9.3 (**a**) Whole mount of a 34-week gestation with left-sided peri-Sylvian polymicrogyria. (**b**) Axial section through the occipital dura and tentorium, the same case in (**a**), demonstrating massive spongy hypertrophy of the dura, with large irregular intradural channels. (**c**) Histology of the affected dura, from (**a**), demonstrating dilated and anastomosing vascular channels, lined with CD34 and Glut1 (+) endothelium. (**d**) Third-trimester hydrocephalic brain, with massive ventriculomegaly, extensive hemosiderin staining, and a large hematoma centered on the right ventricular trigone (*Case courtesy of Dr. G Schauer, Kaiser Permanente, California*). (**e**) The same case as (**d**). In the center of the hematoma is a compact collection of fibrotic thin-walled vessels (arrowheads), with surrounding laminated thrombohematoma that is undergoing organization by granulation tissue. (**f**) Incidental finding, term stillbirth secondary to placental disease; the cerebellum demonstrates a unilateral compact tangle of thin-walled capillary venous channels, without local hemorrhage or tissue injury

9.4 Dural Sinus Malformation

Dural sinus malformation (DSM) consists of dilated dural sinuses, which, in the antenatal form, are usually one or more of the sagittal, confluens sinuum (Latin for confluence of sinuses), or transverse sinuses (Fig. 9.4a). Sometimes, DSM is attributed to a failure of the confluens sinuum to regress in size relative to brain growth, but this does not strike the authors as so much an explanation as a simple morphological description. Many such sinus malformations at autopsy drain dural or pial arteriovenous fistulas (Fig. 9.4b), which may themselves be important in maintaining the relative size of the dilated sinus, and in at least one case, dilation of the confluens sinuum and regres-

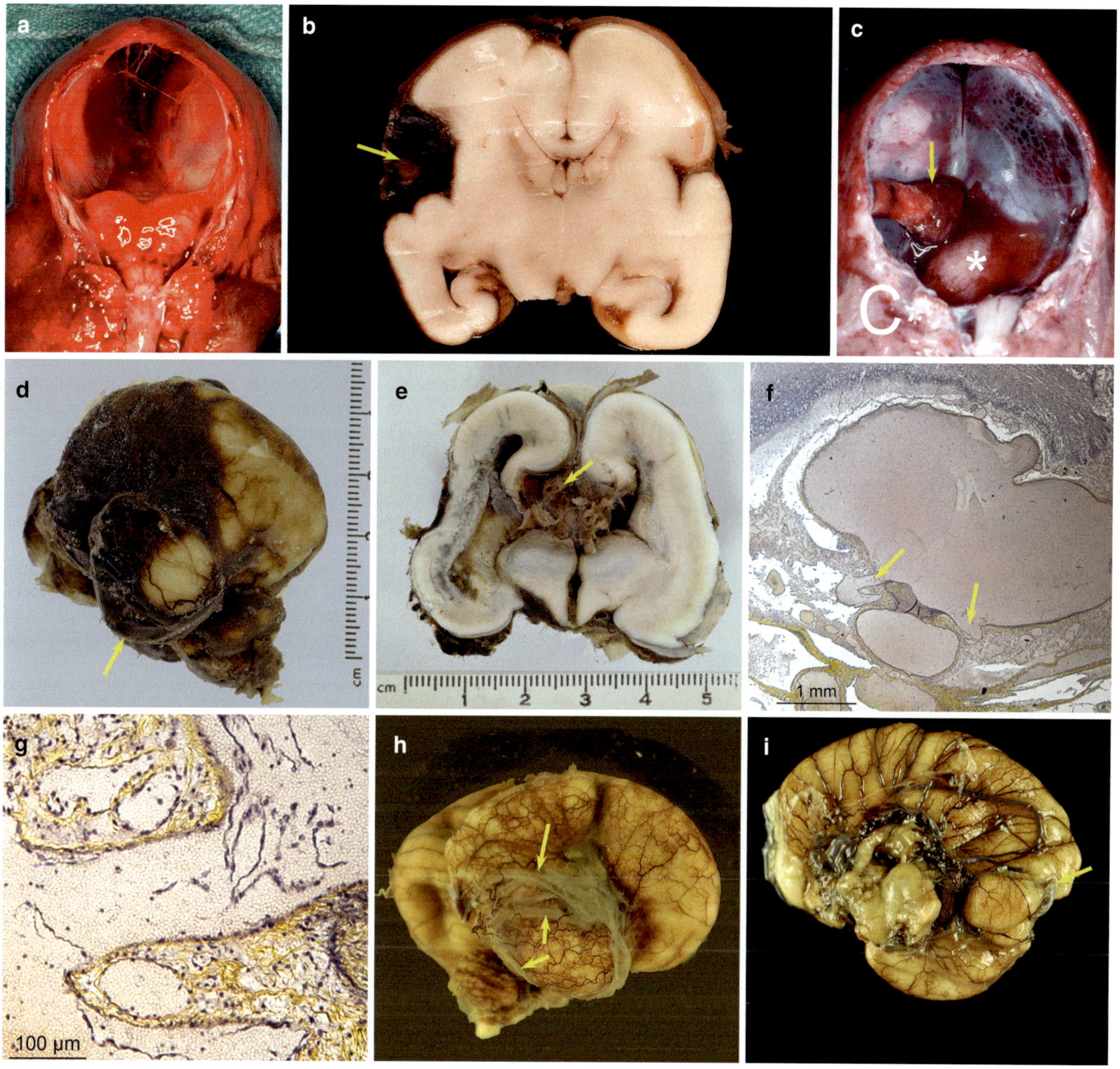

Fig. 9.4 (**a**) Massively dilated confluens sinuum in midgestation fetus, with fine fibrous trabeculae extending between the lateral and superior walls. (**b**) The same case as (**a**), demonstrating dural arteriovenous fistula with acute thrombosis (arrow) occupying the Sylvian fissure. (**c**) Similar case as (**a**) but demonstrating a developing thrombus adherent to the left wall of the confluens sinuum, impinging on the tentorium and mildly displacing the subjacent cerebellum (asterisk). (**d**) A 22-week-gestation brain with hypoplastic left frontal lobe and large tortuous and engorged veins (arrow) over the anterior and inferior temporal lobe. (**e**) Coronal section, same case as (**d**), demonstrating congested left hemisphere with an underlying discoloration and volume loss due to tissue injury in the cerebral mantle. The vein of Galen (arrow) is dilated and tortuous. (**f**) Section through leptomeninges of the left inferior frontal lobe, demonstrating an ectatic artery, leading to multiple thin-walled channels (arrows) (Movat Pentachrome). (**g**) Higher power of lower left-hand field of (**f**), demonstrating direct connection of arterial channel into a thin-walled venous channel (Movat Pentachrome). (**h**) Midgestation fetal brain with multiple grossly dilated arteries (arrows) originating basally and coursing posteriorly over the right hemisphere (*Case courtesy of Dr. L. Hamilton, University of Ottawa*). (**i**) Medial aspect of (**h**) demonstrating a tangle of paramedian veins anteriorly and grossly dilated arteries coursing toward the straight sinus (transected at arrow and removed with dura and reflections)

sion of a dilated sagittal sinus over time with serial imaging have been observed to accompany a large pial arteriovenous fistula (McInnes et al. 2009). However, one can encounter an isolated dilated confluens sinuum without any obvious fistula (personal observation); whether a small fistula gave rise to such a malformation and resolved and whether small fistulas are caused by the elevated venous pressure of an abnormally large dural sinus are alternative hypotheses. Thrombosis of a fetal DSM (Fig. 9.4c) with good outcome is common, particularly in those with no or minimal arterialization. Parenchymal injury and ventriculomegaly are adverse risk factors (Yang et al. 2018).

9.5 Arteriovenous Fistula and Vein of Galen Malformation

Arteriovenous fistulas (i.e., direct connection of muscular arteries to thin-walled veins without an intervening capillary bed) themselves may be encountered in the leptomeninges in the absence of DSM. In angiodysgenetic necrotizing encephalopathy, there is a variably diffuse collection of superficial small arteries and dilated venous channels (Fig. 9.4d), in which abnormal arteries are apparently connected to widely dilated venous channels of the pia or arachnoid. This vascular anomaly is accompanied by underlying ischemic injury or hemorrhage in the brain, non-aneurysmal dilation of the vein of Galen, and dilated cardiomyopathy with apparent high output failure and fetal hydrops (Fig. 9.4e, f, g) (Arvantis et al. 1996; Bloxham 1992). An association with renal agenesis has been recorded (2011). We have in addition seen a pial fistula characterized by multiple arteries draining into a dilated and muscularized straight sinus (Fig. 9.4h, i).

Vein of Galen malformations by contrast are a subset of fistulas in which drainage is via a midline vein recalling in its anatomy the median prosencephalic vein of Markowski and may be associated with RASA1 mutations. These may be an anterior network supplied by choroidal, pericallosal, and thalamoperforating arteries (choroidal type) or a direct artery-to-vein fistula to the draining vein (mural type) (Grillner et al. 2016; Raybaud et al. 1989).

References

Arvanitis DL, Apostolidou IA, Routsis PV, Biskini EI, Kalpoyannis NS. Angiodysgenetic necrotizing encephalopathy or diffuse meningocerebral angiomatosis. Pediatr Neurol. 1996;14(2):155–7.

Bessieres-Grattagliano B, Foliguet B, Devisme L, Loeuillet L, Marcorelles P, Bonniere M, Laquerriere A, Fallet-Bianco C, Martinovic J, Zrelli S, Leticee N, Cayol V, Etchevers HC, Vekemans M, Attie-Bitach T, Encha-Razavi F. Refining the clinicopathological pattern of cerebral proliferative glomeruloid vasculopathy (Fowler syndrome): report of 16 fetal cases. Europ J Med Genet. 2009;52:386–92.

Bloxham CA. Angiodysgenetic necrotising encephalopathy: presentation as an intrauterine death. Acta Neuropathol. 1992;84(2):221–4.

Chitayat D, Shannon P, Keating S, Toi A, Blaser S, Friedberg T, Superti-Furga A, Chong K, Unger S. Raine syndrome: a rare lethal osteosclerotic bone dysplasia: prenatal diagnosis, autopsy, and neuropathological findings. Am J Med Genet. 2007;143A:3280–5.

Chong CR, Hutchins GM. Idiopathic infantile arterial calcification: the spectrum of clinical presentations. Pediatr Dev Pathol. 2008;11(5):405–15.

Feygin T, Goldman-Yassen AE, Licht DJ, Schmitt JE, Mian A, Vossough A, Castelo-Soccio L, Treat JR, Bhatia A, Pollock AN. Neuroaxial infantile hemangiomas: imaging manifestations and association with hemangioma syndromes. AJNR Am J Neuroradiol. 2021;42(8):1520–7.

Gilles FH, Leviton A, Golden JA, Paneth N, Rudelli RD. Groups of histopathologic abnormalities in brains of very low birthweight infants. J Neuropathol Exp Neurol. 1998;57(11):1026–34.

Golden JA, Gilles FH, Rudelli R, Leviton A. Frequency of neuropathological abnormalities in very low birth weight infants. J Neuropathol Exp Neurol. 1997;56(5):472–8.

Goyal A, Fernandes-Torres J, Flemming KD, Williams LN, Daniels DJ. Clinical presentation, natural history, and outcomes for infantile intracranial cavernous malformations: case series and systematic review of the literature. Childs Nerv Syst. 2023;39(6):1545–54.

Grillner P, Soderman M, Holmin S, Rodesch G. A spectrum of intracranial vascular high-flow arteriovenous shunts in RASA1 mutations. Childs Nerv Syst. 2016;32(4):709–15.

Gubana F, Christov C, Coste T, Tournier-Lasserve E, Benachi A, Fallet-Bianco C, Encha-Razavi F, Martinovic J. Prenatal diagnosis of COL4A1 mutations in eight cases: further delineation of the neurohistopathological phenotype. Pediatr Dev Pathol. 2022;25(4):435–46.

Guibaud L, Garel C, Annie B, Pascal G, François V, Vavasseur C, Oury JF, Pracros JP. Prenatal diagnosis of capillary telangiectasia of the cerebellum—ultrasound and MRI features. Prenat Diagn. 2003;23(10):791–6.

Henrich W, Stupin JH, Bühling KJ, Bührer C, Bassir C, Dudenhausen JW. Prenatal sonographic findings of thalamic cavernous angioma. Ultrasound Obstet Gynecol. 2002;19(5):518–22.

Jaimes C, Ferraciolli SF, Orbach DB. Cerebrovascular anomalies in the fetus. Am J Neuroradiol. 2025;46(2):231–9.

Lerner A, Gilboa Y, Gerad L, Malinger G, Kidron D, Achiron R. Sonographic detection of fetal cerebellar cavernous hemangioma with in-utero hemorrhage leading to cerebellar hemihypoplasia. Ultrasound Obstet Gynecol. 2006;28(7):968–71.

McInnes M, Fong K, Grin A, ter Brugge K, Blaser S, Halliday W, Shannon P. Malformations of the fetal dural sinuses. Can J Neurol Sci. 2009;36(1):72–7.

Meyer E, Ricketts C, Morgan NV, Morris MR, Pasha S, Tee LJ, et al. Mutations in FLVCR2 are associated with proliferative vasculopathy and hydranencephaly-hydrocephaly syndrome (Fowler syndrome). Am J Hum Genet. 2010;86:471–8.

Nitschke Y, Baujat G, Botschen U, Wittkampf T, du Moulin M, Stella J, et al. Generalized arterial calcification of infancy and pseudoxanthoma elasticum can be caused by mutations in either ENPP1 or ABCC6. Am J Hum Genet. 2012;90(1):25–39. https://doi.org/10.1016/j.ajhg.2011.11.020. Epub 2011 Dec 29

Padget DH. The development of the cranial arteries in the human embryo. Contrib Embryol Carnegie Instn. 1948;32:205–61.

Padget DH. The cranial venous system in man in reference to development, adult configuration, and relation to the arteries. Am J Anat. 1956;98:307–55.

Raybaud CA, Strother CM, Hald JK. Aneurysms of the vein of Galen: embryonic considerations and anatomical features relating to the pathogenesis of the malformation. Neuroradiology. 1989;31:109–28.

Shannon P, Hum C, Parks T, Schauer GM, Chitayat D, Chong K, Shinar S, Blaser S, Gaea Moore G, Van Mieghem T. Brain and placental pathology in fetal COL4A1 related disease. Pediatr Dev Pathol. 2021;24(3):175–86.

Takakuwa T, Koike T, Muruanaka T, et al. Formation of the circle of Willis during human embryonic development. Congenit Anom (Kyoto). 2016;56(5):233–6.

Viswanathan V, Smith ER, Mulliken JB, Fishman SJ, Kozakewich HPW, Burrows PE, Orbach DB. Infantile Hemangiomas Involving the Neuraxis: Clinical and Imaging Findings. AJNR Am J Neuroradiol. 2009;30(5):1005–13.

Williams D, Patel C, Fallet-Bianco C, Kalyanasundaram K, Yacoubi M, Dechelotte P, Scott R, Bazin A, Bessieres B, Marton T, Cox P. Fowler syndrome—a clinical, radiological, and pathological study of 14 cases. Am J Med Genet. 2010;152A:153–60.

Yang E, Storey A, Olson HE, JS, Estroff JA, Trenor CC, Cooper BK, Smith ER, Orbach DB. Imaging features and prognostic factors in fetal and postnatal torcular dural sinus malformations, part II: synthesis of the literature and patient management. J Neurointerv Surg. 2018;10(5):471–5.

10 Congenital Cystic Lesions

A malformative cyst is defined as a non-tumoral fluid-filled collection exerting a mass effect on the brain. Most such cysts are detectable after 15 weeks of gestation. The cysts associated with cerebellar malformation complexes will be discussed in this chapter. The designation of the different types of cysts is based predominantly on the lining of the cyst wall.

10.1 Arachnoid Cysts

These most commonly occur in the middle cranial fossa, Sylvian fissure, interhemispheric fissure, posterior fossa, and suprasellar cisterns but can occur over the convexity, quadrigeminal plate, cerebellopontine angle, or midline posterior fossa (Fig. 10.1a). Histologically, they consist of a layer of arachnoid fibroblasts and collagen and result from an anomalous splitting or duplication of the arachnoid membrane into a distinct inner and outer leaflet during folding of the neural tube and the formation of normal subarachnoid cisterns. The cerebrospinal fluid accumulates between the two layers and exerts chronic mass effect. They may accompany aqueductal stenosis and when interhemispheric may accompany agenesis or dysgenesis of the corpus callosum or more unusually temporal lobe agenesis (Fig. 10.1b). Intraventricular arachnoid cysts are recorded and have been postulated to arise from choroid plexus mesenchyme (Yeates and Enzmann 1979).

10.1.1 Genetics and Syndromes

Familial arachnoid cysts in some families may be linked to chromosome 6q22.31–23.2 (Bayrakli et al. 2012). They can accompany mutations in FOXC2 (Qin et al. 2019); SPG4, accompanying hereditary spastic paraplegia (Orlacchio et al. 2004); and GPSM2, in the Chudley–McCullough syndrome, with frontal polymicrogyria, gray matter heterotopia, cerebellar dysplasia, and ventriculomegaly (Doherty et al. 2012), and Kallmann syndrome (Massimi et al. 2016).

10.2 Choroid Plexus Cysts

The choroid plexus develops as an organ of the neuroepithelium in the lateral ventricles, the roof of the third ventricle, and at the fourth ventricular outflow. In the seventh week of development, the neuroepithelium invaginates into the ventricles and is penetrated by the first intra-axial blood vessels and a loose mesenchymal stroma. From the 9th to the 11th week of post conception, the stroma expands, and the plexus reaches its maximal relative extent, filling 75% of the lateral ventricles; the stroma becomes loose in about 16 weeks and from about 17 weeks on starts to decrease in relative volume, and the connective tissue becomes more prominent. After roughly 29 weeks, the stroma is increasingly fibrotic (Shuangshoti and Netsky 1970).

Choroid plexus cysts are neuroepithelial in origin; most that are diagnosed clinically are asymptomatic, do not interfere with brain development, are diagnosed in the early second trimester, and resolve by 32 weeks' gestation. They are generally conceived of as true epithelial cysts lined by choroid plexus epithelium with an underlying fibrovascular stroma (Fig. 10.1c). The majority of these are diagnosed in the lateral ventricles by ultrasound in the second trimester and resolve by 32 weeks' gestation and are usually asymptomatic (Dziegielewska et al. 2001; Yang et al. 2021; Filardi et al. 2009) but may occasionally interfere with CSF flow. Occasionally one encounters unlined cystic spaces in the choroid plexus stroma (Fig 10.1h, i), which we term cisternae.

10.2.1 Genetics and Syndromes

Choroid plexus cysts are increased in prevalence in aneuploidies (trisomy 18, 21, and 9) (Reinsch et al. 1997, Walkinshaw 2000, Geary et al. 1997, Beke et al. 2008) and

P. Shannon et al., *Atlas of Neurodevelopmental Pathology*, https://doi.org/10.1007/978-3-032-14148-4_10

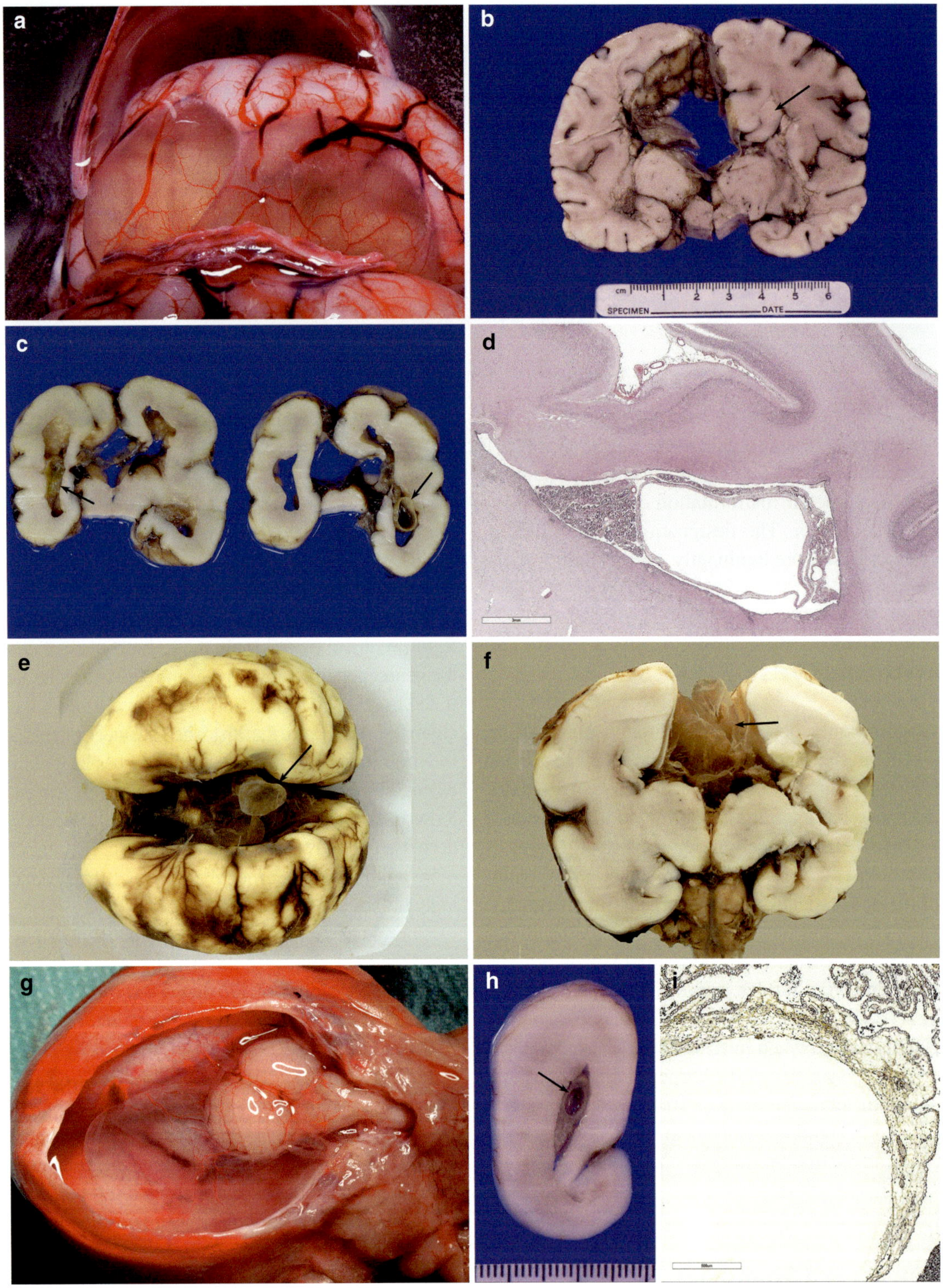

Fig. 10.1 (**a**) Large interhemispheric arachnoid cyst at autopsy: the large veins in this case travel superficially, while the arteries maintain their course close to the brain surface. (**b**) Term infant with distortion of the left medial hemisphere by arachnoid cyst, with agenesis of the corpus callosum and Probst bundle formation (arrow). (**c**) Fetal brain 26 weeks' gestation with multiple anomalies, including coarse premature sulcation, agenesis of the corpus callosum, and periventricular nodular heterotopias, with large bilateral choroid plexus cysts in the ventricular trigone (arrows). (**d**) The same case, section on the right, demonstrating a large thick-walled uniloculate cyst. (**e**) Aicardi syndrome, 26 weeks with large multiloculate interhemispheric cyst. (**f**) The same case, demonstrating cystic choroid plexus (arrow) with associated agenesis of the corpus callosum. (**g**) An 18-week-gestation fetus with massive left infratentorial paracerebellar choroid plexus cyst arising near the foramen of Luschka and accompanied by obstructive hydrocephalus (not shown). (**h**) A 22-week-gestation fetus: the left ventricular trigone demonstrates an apparent cyst (arrow). (**i**) Histology demonstrates a large interstitial space or cistern in the choroid plexus stroma, unlined by the endothelium or epithelium

MECP2 duplication. Midline choroid plexus cysts in particular are also associated with agenesis of the corpus callosum, hydrocephalus, ventriculomegaly (Fu et al. 2014), cortical migrational anomalies and Aicardi syndrome (Herman et al. 2007) (Fig. 10.1e, f). The fourth ventricular outflow cysts may be associated with hydrocephalus (Fig. 10.1g). Occasionally, one sees cisterns in the choroid plexus mesenchyme that radiologically are called cysts but are not really lined by the epithelium or endothelium (Fig. 10.1h, i). The proportion of such cisterns or even simply hydropic fronds of the choroid plexus among "cysts" that are only ever seen on imaging is unclear, but in our experience a non-trivial proportion of cases thought to have early second-trimester choroid plexus cysts on ultrasound, do not show true cysts on histology.

10.3 Ventricular Diverticula

These are evaginations of a ventricular cavity into a subdural space or cistern. In the perinatal state, they consist of attenuated neuroglial tissue with its associated arachnoid, usually arising from a massively distended choroidal fissure in the medial wall of the lateral ventricular trigone or ballooned corpus callosum (Fig. 10.2), although they may rarely originate from the third or fourth ventricle, and in later life, they may rupture. As such, they are generally secondary phenomena arising from hydrocephalus and can accompany other features of hydrocephalus including a ruptured septum pellucidum. Ventricular diverticula may also accompany holoprosencephaly, as they can form the posterior and dorsal cyst wall common in alobar holoprosencephaly.

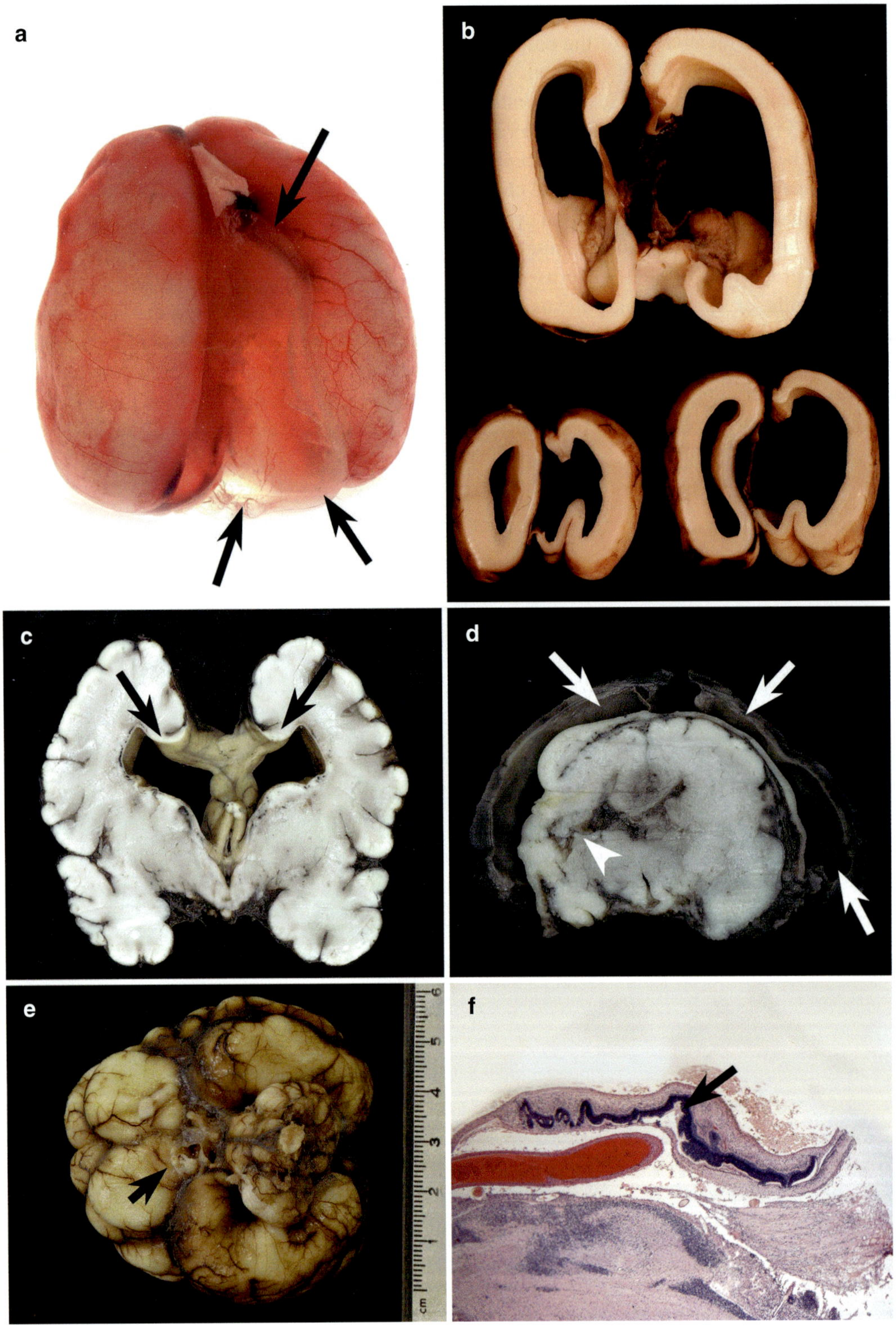

Fig. 10.2 (**a**) A 22-week-gestation fetus: the posterior choroidal fissure on the right is ballooned medially (arrows) to form a thin-walled apparently interhemispheric cyst. (**b**) On coronal section, it is a delicate membrane, easily torn, which on histology is composed of the arachnoid and attenuated brain. Such medial cysts may be asymmetric or symmetric. (**c**) Term brain, in which the corpus callosum is attenuated and balloons dorsally (arrows) as an interhemispheric cyst, in the context of congenital aqueductal stenosis. (**d**) Post-encephaloclastic diverticulum, 27 weeks' gestation: there is a porus, extending from the ventricle toward the hemispheric surface (arrowhead). The adjacent brain is extending as a thin-walled diverticulum of the cortical mantle across the surface of the brain even over the interhemispheric fissure to the contralateral hemisphere (arrows). Such a porencephalic cyst is exceptional in its extent. (**e**) Inferior surface of the brain with multiple leptomeningeal, cortical, and subcortical heterotopias at 24 weeks, with one olfactory bulb expanded as a disrupted cystic structure. (**f**) On histology, the cyst appears to be a collapsed vesicle lined in part by the neuroepithelium and germinal matrix

10.4 Porencephalic Cysts

After encephaloclastic events, porencephalic cysts and diverticula with similarly composed but usually more obviously reactive and scarred walls with irregular remnants of the brain adherent to arachnoid may form extensive and unusually shaped cystic diverticula, even herniating under dural reflections (Fujita et al. 2001; Hori et al. 1984; Wakai and Nagai 1984).

10.5 Neurenteric Cysts

These are cysts lined by endoderm and mostly located along the spine, often at the cervical and cervicothoracic levels. Intracranial examples are generally in the posterior fossa. These are discussed under spinal malformations (see Chap. 11).

10.6 Other Neuroepithelial Cysts

An enlarged olfactory bulb ventricle may form an unusual neuroepithelial cyst that is presumably derived from the so-called olfactory ventricle within the olfactory bulb and tract. We have seen one case accompanying multiple brain anomalies, especially cerebral cortical migrational anomalies. Cerebellar vermian cysts (Chanclud et al. 2023) are unusual midline cysts located in the cerebellar vermis. Neuroimaging of these cysts suggests that they arise in the primary fissure, but in our personal experience, although limited to two cases, similar entities can be cleft-like intraparenchymal cavities containing fluid and occasional macrophages (Fig. 10.3) associated in one case with extensive cerebral leptomeningeal heterotopias syndrome and in another with glutamine mtRNA synthetase deficiency. The radiological literature suggests a clinically benign course when these are isolated.

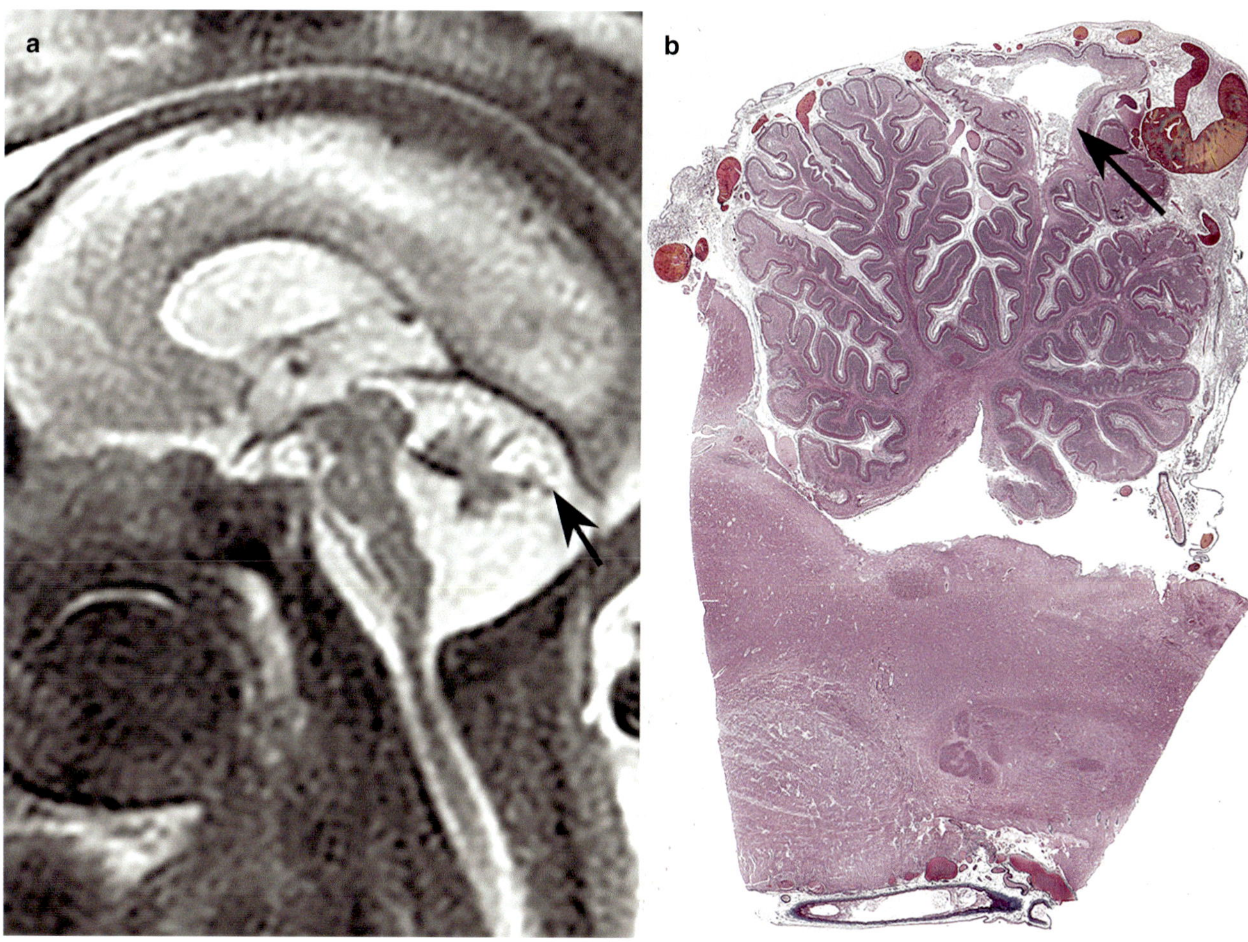

Fig. 10.3 A 22-week-gestation fetus, pregnancy interrupted for extensive leptomeningeal heterotopias. (**a**) Midline MRI shows apparent cystic structure within the vermis (arrow). (**b**) On whole mount, this was a fluid- and macrophage-filled cleft in the substance of the white matter of the folium (*MRI courtesy of* Dr. S. Blaser, The Hospital for Sick Children, Toronto)

Ependymal cysts are uncommon, generally subarachnoid cysts with a wall of reactive glia and lined at least partially by ependyma. These are well recorded in the pediatric and adult literature, but while they would clearly seem to be of maldevelopmental origin, they are uncommon in our experience of fetal remains. It may be that in fetal life, they are small and overshadowed by other pathologies (Morigaki et al. 2011; Williams et al. 2000).

References

Bayrakli F, Okten AI, Kartal U, et al. Intracranial arachnoid cyst family with autosomal recessive trait mapped to chromosome 6q22.31–23.2. Acta Neurochir. 2012;154(7):1287–92.

Beke A, Barakonyi E, Belics Z, et al. Risk of chromosome abnormalities in the presence of bilateral or unilateral choroid plexus cysts. Fetal Diagn Ther. 2008;23(3):185–91.

Chanclud J, Valence S, Vande Perre S, Guilbaud L, Moutard ML, Jouannic JM, Le Pointe HD, Blondiaux E, Garel C. Prenatal diagnosis of vermian cyst: a new type of posterior fossa cyst. Pediatr Radiol. 2023:461–9.

Doherty D, Chudley AE, Coghlan G, et al. GPSM2 mutations cause the brain malformations and hearing loss in Chudley-McCullough syndrome. Am J Hum Genet. 2012;90(6):1088–93.

Dziegielewska KM, Ek J, Habgood MD, Saunders NR. Development of the choroid plexus. Microsc Re Tech. 2001;52(1):5–20.

Filardi TZ, Finn L, Gabikian P, et al. Treatment of intermittent obstructive hydrocephalus secondary to choroid plexus cyst. 2009;4(6):571–4.

Fu F, Liu HL, Li R, et al. Prenatal diagnosis of foetuses with congenital abnormalities and duplication of the MECP2 region. Gene. 2014;546(2):222–5.

Fujita K, Enomoto T, Yanaka K, Nose T. Ventricular diverticulum at the posterior horn of the lateral ventricle presenting as aplasia cutis congenita. Childs Nerv Syst. 2001;17(12):750–3.

Geary M, Patel S, Lamont R. Isolated choroid plexus cysts and association with fetal aneuploidy in an unselected population. Ultrasound Obstet Gynecol. 1997;10(3):171–3.

Herman TE, Lee BC, Siegel MJ. Aicardi syndrome choroid plexus cysts. J Perinatol. 2007;27(5):323–4.

Hori A, Eubel R, Ulbrich R. Congenital ventricular diverticulum in the brainstem. Report of four cases. Acta Neuropathol. 1984;63(4):330–3.

Massimi L, Isso A, Paternoster G, et al. Arachnoid cyst: a further anomaly associated with Kallmann syndrome? Childs Nerv Syst. 2016;32(9):1607–14.

Morigaki R, Shinno K, Pooh KH, Nakagawa Y. Giant glioependymal cyst in an infant. J Neurosurg Pediatr. 2011;7(2):175–8.

Orlacchio A, Gaudiello F, Totaro A, et al. Neurology A new SPG4 mutation in a variant form of spastic paraplegia with congenital arachnoid cysts. 2004;62(10):1875–8.

Qin X, Wang Y, Xu S, Hong X. Familial arachnoid cysts: a review of 35 families. Childs Nerv Syst. 2019;35(4):607–12.

Reinsch RC. Choroid plexus cysts--association with trisomy: prospective review of 16,059 patients. Am J Obstet Gynecol. 1997;176(6):1381–3.

Shuangshoti S, Netsky MG. Human choroid plexus: morphologic and histochemical alterations with age. Am J Anat. 1970;128(1):73-95. https://doi.org/10.1002/aja.1001280107. PMID: 4193921.

Wakai S, Nagai M. Ventricular Diverticulum. J Neurol Neurosurg Psychiatry. 1984;47(5):514–7.

Walkinshaw SA. Fetal choroid plexus cysts: are we there yet? Prenat Diagn. 2000;20(8):657–62.

Williams Z, Herrick MK, Tse V. Ependyma-lined cysts. Clin Neuropathol. 2000 May-Jun;19(3):138–41.

Yang R, Yan H, Dewan MC, et al. Giant choroid plexus cysts with calvarial erosion: a case report and literature review. Childs Nerv Syst. 2021;37(7):2381–5.

Yeates A, Enzmann D. An intraventricular arachnoid cyst. Case report. J Comput Assist Tomogr. 1979;3:697–700.

Spinal Cord and Spinal Column Malformations

11

At roughly 17 days post fertilization, the embryo is a trilaminar disk: underneath the ectoderm, the notochordal process arises from the primitive node and extends rostrally to the prechordal plate and caudally as a notochordal plate. At 23 days, the primitive node is hollowed out to form a primitive pit, which extends obliquely and caudally as the notochordal canal. The floor of the notochordal canal breaks down and communicates with the endoderm, and the canal forms a communication with the amniotic cavity dorsally and the umbilical vesicle ventrally so that locally the site of the future neurectoderm is in continuity with the endoderm. This communication initially localizes to what will become the future cervical level, and as the notochord extends caudally, the canal is displaced more caudally to the future T6 by 28 days, and the notochordal–endodermal connection is lost after 2–8 days. The notochordal plate then becomes the cylindrical notochord, which is complete by day 30 (O'Rahilly and Muller 2006).

Starting at 25 days post fertilization, the paraxial mesoderm forms paired condensations of epithelioid cells (the somites) on either side of the neuraxis. Eventually, 38 or 39 pairs form in a rostral to caudal order, and not all are present at any point. The medioventral and core cells of each somite form the sclerotome, while the dorsolateral cells give rise to the dermatomyotome, which will form the skeletal muscle and dermis. The sclerotome will contribute cells to form a perinotochordal sheath. The dorsal sclerotome will contribute cells to surround the spinal cord dorsally and give rise to rostral hypocellular areas and caudal cell dense areas that develop into the neural arch and ribs; chondrification is thought to be induced by the notochord and neural tube at around 6 weeks' gestation. The anterior and posterior longitudinal ligaments form from mesenchymal elements during the chondrification phase.

The perinotochordal sheath also develops a segmented architecture with loose and dense zones, although these are out of step with the dorsal sclerotomal elements. The loose areas become the paired centra on either side of the notochord, which fuse to form the vertebral bodies and chondrify. Cell dense areas contribute to the annulus fibrosus and the nucleus pulposus. Toward the end of the embryonic period, the notochord itself becomes segmented; the narrow aspects are replaced by the vertebral centra, while expansions contribute to the nucleus pulposus, and in fetal life, notochordal remnants are generally present in the intervertebral disks. Concurrent with the development of the dermatomyotome, the neural crest forms and gives rise to the dorsal root ganglia among other peripheral structures. Neurogenesis and gliogenesis of the central gray matter in the spinal cord proceed from the central neuroepithelium, while the ingrowth of dorsal root ganglia axons forms the dorsal columns. Descending axonal tracts arrive at variable rates, with bulbospinal tracts mostly established by the end of the embryonic period in cervical levels, and corticospinal tracts, which innervate alpha motor neurons, extend to the lumbar cord by midgestation and distal sacral levels by term. After the embryonic period, spinal cord elongation is slower than vertebral column growth, so the conus relatively ascends to the level of the third lumbar vertebra by term (O'Rahilly and Muller 2001).

Clearly, spinal cord and spinal column abnormalities are closely linked, and many spinal cord and soft tissue anomalies are linked to neural tube defects, which are covered in Chap. 3.

11.1 Split Cord Malformations

Split cord malformations (SCMs) are multiple neural tubes in the same fetus, extending for variable lengths of the neural canal, and may be fused rostrally or caudally. Generally, there are two spinal cord structures, but triplications have been recorded (e.g., Sandberg et al. 2007).

P. Shannon et al., *Atlas of Neurodevelopmental Pathology*, https://doi.org/10.1007/978-3-032-14148-4_11

11.1.1 Neuropathology and Pathogenesis of SCM

There are multiple embryological explanations for split cord malformations. One suggestion is localized twinning: in this conception during primary neurulation the dorsal folds over converge on each side to form two neural tubes, around each of which forms a neural arch, and the midline bone spur forms from the fusion of the medial pedicles of the opposing neural arches (Herren and Edwards 1940).

Alternatively, the notochord might split, and a duplicated overlying neural tube forms; each hemi-notochord induces a medial and lateral neural arch fused in the midline, and a dorsal diverticulum from the underlying yolk sac herniates between the hemi-notochords to differentiate into mesodermal elements.

Under another conception that unifies many ideas, SCMs result from the persistence of an abnormal connection or communication between the endoderm and the notochord, in the manner of a notochordal canal. The persistent neurenteic canal connecting the neurectoderm and the endoderm results in a local splitting of the notochord, the mesenchymal elements, and the neural plate. The surrounding mesenchyme condenses around the connecting canal and results in a split notochord and possibly a split spinal cord, and the abnormal neurenteric connection, with its mesenchymal sheath, can persist as a split vertebral body (Fig. 11.1a, b), a neurenteric cyst, or a persistent neurenteric canal (Pang et al. 1992). Such connections may be multiple.

In diastematomyelia, two hemi-cords are present, either within the same dural sac or in separate sacs separated by a bony or cartilaginous spur or connective tissue splitting the neural canal (Fig. 11.1c, d). In diplomyelia, there are two complete cords in a single dural sac, possibly tethered by the fibrous midline septum to the adjacent dura. One of the cords does not supply nerve roots and is therefore considered an accessory. In dimyelia (Fig. 11.1e, f), there is complete duplication, with complete nerve roots that may be separated by a bony or cartilaginous septum. The reader is referred to Hori et al. (1982) for a detailed illustration. In a hemimyelocele, one duplicated cord is incorporated into an open neural tube defect (Duckworth et al. 1968).

Split cord malformations may be associated with neural tube defects, lipomas, dermoid cysts, or ventral abnormalities, including a midline vertebral body track, a sagittal cleft, and neurenteric cysts or a persistent neurenteric canal.

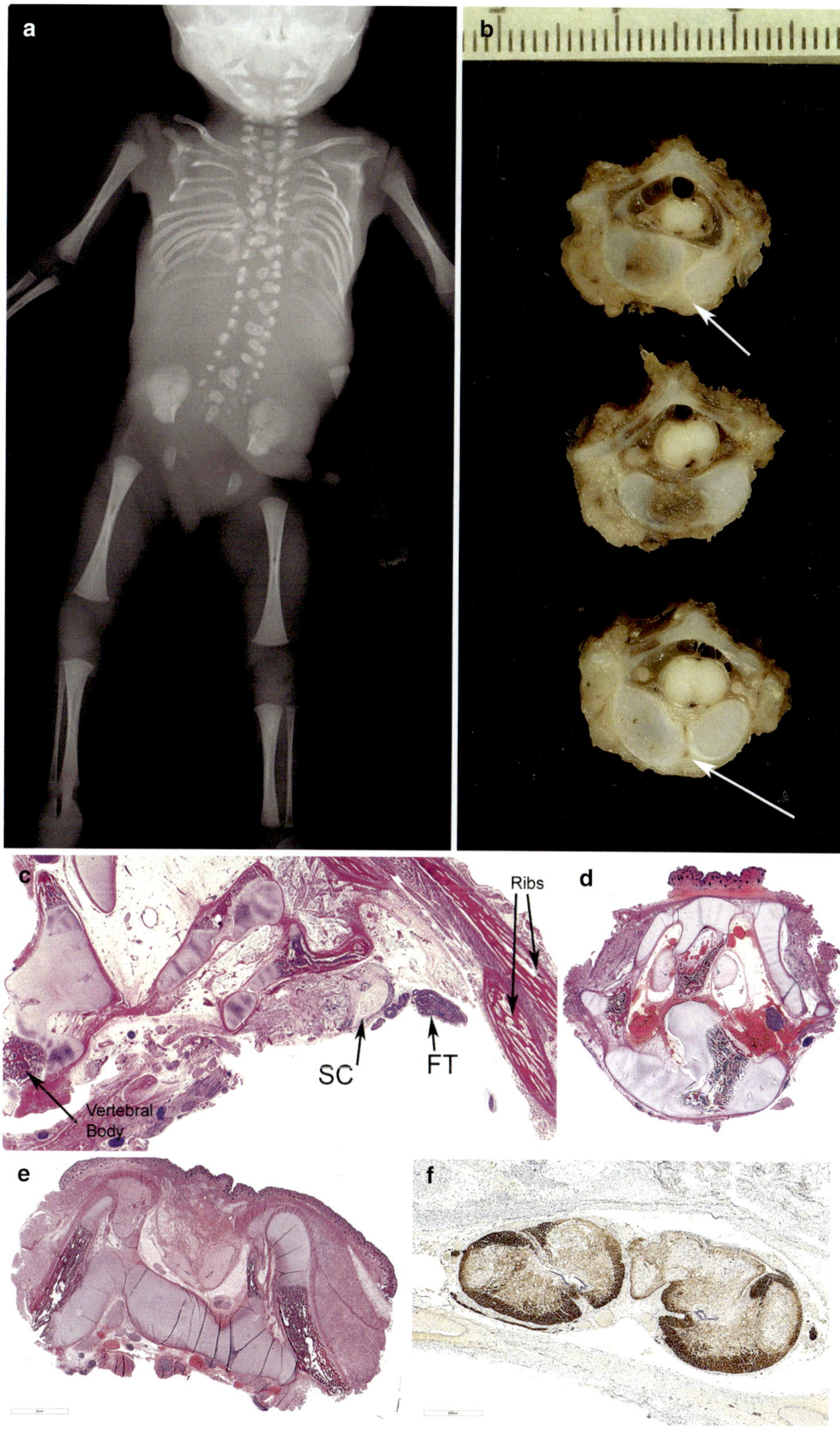

Fig. 11.1 (**a**) Fetus with extensive segmentation anomalies, with fused and irregular ribs, hemivertebrae, and irregular fusion of vertebral bodies. (**b**) Axial sections through the spine demonstrating median and paramedian clefts formed by fibrous tissue extending through the cartilaginous anlage of the vertebral bodies (arrows). (**c**) The same case as (a): with paraspinal duplication of the spinal cord (SC) in the thoracic spine with adjacent heterotopic fallopian tube (FT) (**d**). Diastematomyelia: two hemi-cords, each in its own dural sac and separated by chondro-osseous septum. (**e**) Low-lying duplicated cord (dimyelia) in sacral spina bifida. Note the dysmorphic subjacent sacral vertebral body. (**f**) The same case as (**e**), with immunohistochemistry for neurofilament light chain demonstrating complete albeit dysmorphic complement of neural elements in each cord with associated nerve roots

11.2 Klippel–Feil Syndrome

The Klippel–Feil anomaly describes a segmentation defect in the rostral cervical spine, resulting in fused vertebral segments: this may be associated with spinal cord abnormalities (Fig. 11.2a, b) and neurenteric cysts (Can et al. 2015). This anomaly may be a component of a wide variety of malformations and syndromes (Frikha 2020), including heterotaxy and neural tube defects, but may also be inherited as either an autosomal dominant (KFS1 or KFS3) or recessive monogenic defect (KFS2 or KFS4).

11.3 Neurenteric Cysts

These may also be referred to as enterogenous or endodermal cysts. These are cysts lined by the endoderm and mostly located along the spine. Intracranial examples are generally in the posterior fossa and ventral in position. They are thought to arise from a persistent or abnormal neurenteric canal—a transient connection between the developing notochord and the endoderm (Fig. 11.2c, d) (Prasad et al. 1996)—or from a split notochord (Agnoli et al. 1984; Emerson and Azzarelli 2004). Histologically, they are a fibrous or smooth muscle capsule lined by endodermal epithelium of foregut, midgut, or hindgut derivation and may have mucoid or liquid contents. The cyst wall may have associated neuroglial tissue and can be highly organized, resembling the gut wall, or may be attenuated. The cyst is generally extra-axial and partially intradural. If they are paravertebral, they may extend into the neural canal through one of the neural foramina (Fig. 11.2e, f, g) or through a defective or split vertebral body (Can et al. 2015). Local segmentation disorders of the spinal column are frequent. Occasionally, the gut itself is in continuity with the cyst (Ogulnick et al. 2021; Worell et al. 2021). These cysts are thought to arise by the persistence of a neurenteric connection, either of the neurenteric canal itself or of an abnormal accessory canal, or by the displacement of endodermal cells by neurenteric adhesion. In persistent neurenteric canal, the gut itself communicates with the neural canal and may be continuous with the central canal of the spinal cord (Fig. 11.3a, b) (Shukla et al. 2015).

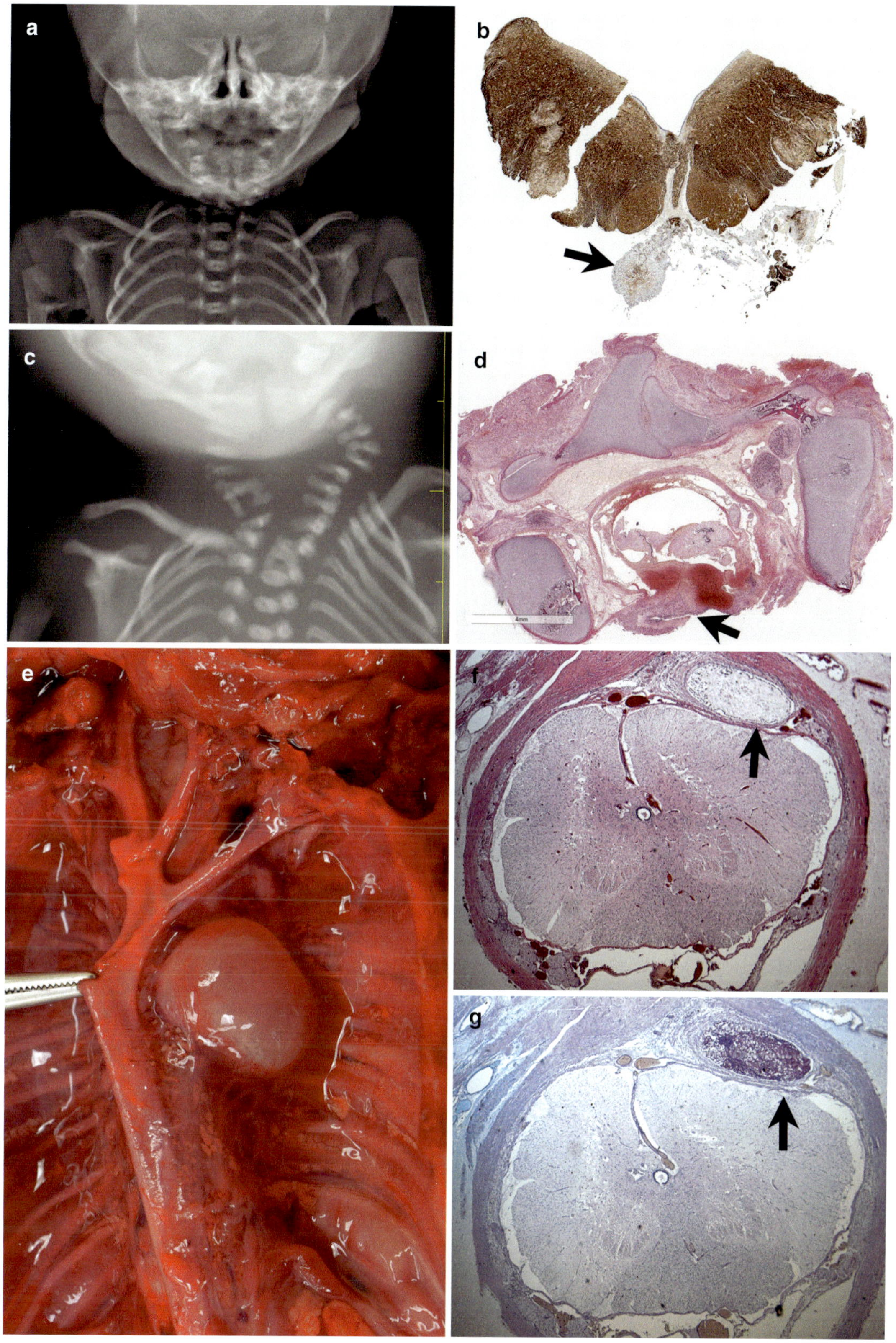

Fig. 11.2 (**a**) Cervical spine radiology at 23 weeks' gestation, with prominent median clefts in vertebral bodies together with a reduction in the number of cervical segments. The case demonstrated hydrocephalus, aqueductal stenosis, and central doublet abnormalities in the motile cilia. (**b**) Lower medulla of case (**a**), demonstrating an elongated caudal extent of the floor of the fourth ventricle, an absence of the medial lemniscus system, and a tangle of axons ventrally embedded in fibrous tissue. (**c**) Cervical spine radiology at 22 weeks' gestation with absent vertebral bodies and irregularly fused left lateral elements. (**d**) The same case as (**c**) with absent vertebral body and esophagus (arrow) adjacent to cervical dura; dorsally, there is dimyelia. (**e**) Large paraspinal neurenteric cyst in a 26-week-gestation fetus with congenital heart disease. (**f**) The same case as (**e**) with intradural extension of cyst (arrow) through neural foramen. (**g**) The same case as (**e**) and (**f**), stained with PAS/Alcian blue, demonstrating inspissated gastrointestinal mucin

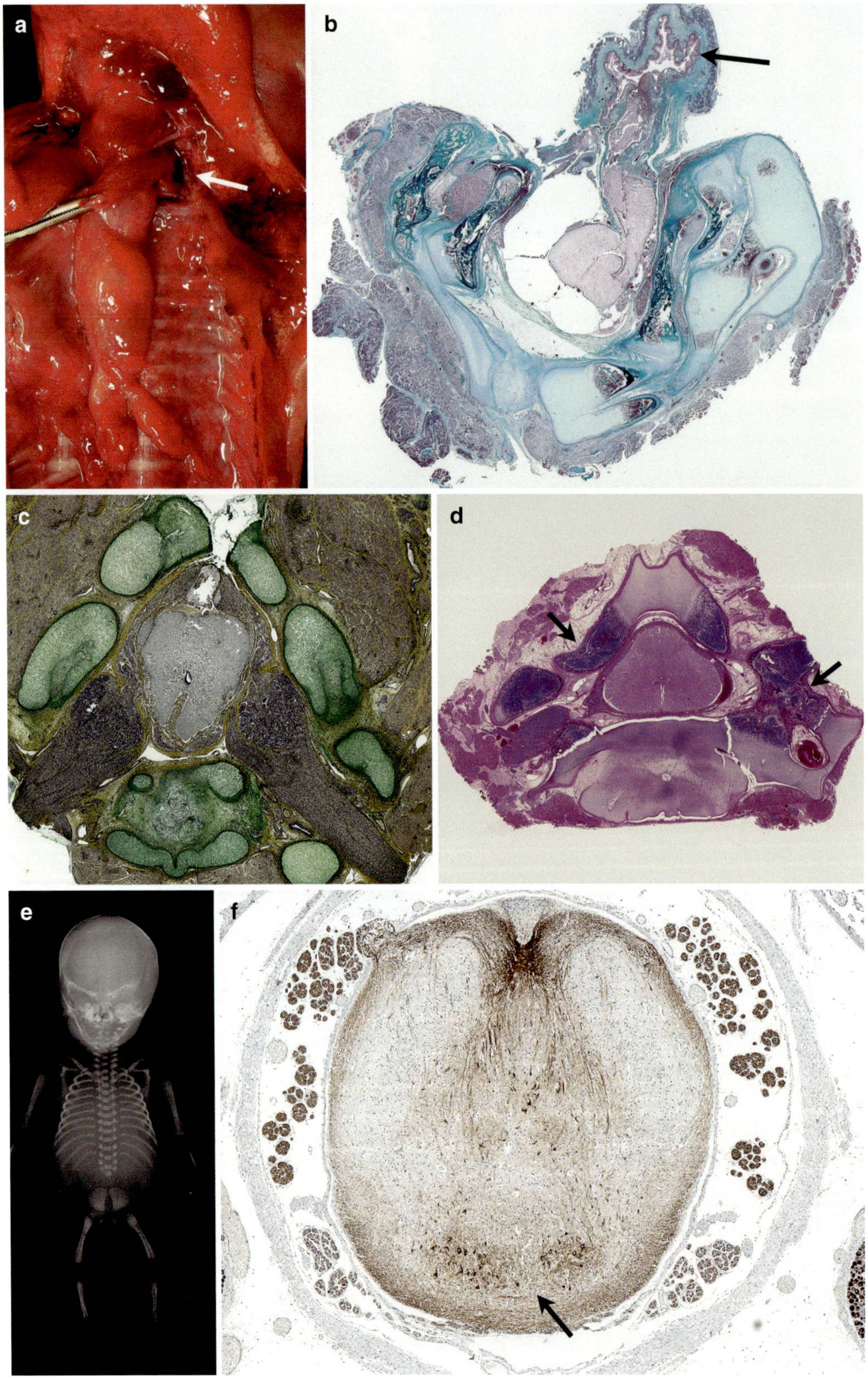

Fig. 11.3 (**a**) Persistent neurenteric canal, with the esophagus extending from an intrathoracic stomach through an anterior defect in the lower cervical spinal column (arrow). (**b**) Histological preparation, same case as (**a**) showing the esophagus (arrow) in direct communication with the central canal of the spinal cord through an anteriorly defective and dysmorphic cervical vertebra. A spinal cord duplication was present more rostrally. (**c**) Cervical cord in achondrogenesis type 2, 24 weeks' gestation: the vertebral body is hypoplastic, and the neural canal is narrowed, impinging on and distorting the spinal cord. (**d**) Cervical cord at term, perinatal lethal osteogenesis imperfecta, with deformation and microscopic callus formation indicating healing fracture in pedicles and laminae (arrows). (**e**) Caudal regression with short spinal column and absent sacrum. (**f**) Lower spinal cord stained with immunohistochemistry for neurofilament light chain, with almost complete fusion of ventral elements (arrow)

11.4 Congenital Spinal Stenosis

This is a congenital narrowing of the neural canal. In our experience, it is most commonly seen in the context of skeletal dysplasia accompanying platyspondyly (e.g., achondrogenesis, thanatophoric dysplasia, campomelic dysplasia, achondroplasia [Fano et al. 2022; Legare 1998]), in which the vertebral bodies are flat and generally narrowed and may lack the cervical and lumbar enlargements. The pedicles are consequently close together, but it may also be seen where there is severe hypoplasia of the neural arch (McDowell et al. 2017; Faye-Petersen and Knisely 1991) (Fig. 11.3c). In fetal remains, it is usually most obvious in the lumbar or cervical spine where the cord is largest and is difficult to appreciate without en bloc removal of the cord and vertebral column. The fundamental problem generally seems to be poor growth of the vertebral body cartilaginous anlage (Fig. 11.3d).

11.5 Caudal Regression

Caudal regression refers to aplasia or hypoplasia and simplification of the distal spinal column, often with accompanying hypomobility or malformation of the lower limbs. Caudal regression in morphology ranges from simple coccygeal agenesis without functional repercussions to lumbosacral agenesis with the fusion or absence of the iliac bones and sirenomelia. It may accompany anal atresia and a wide variety of genitourinary tract abnormalities, including renal agenesis. Caudal regression can be classified according to the laterality or symmetry of sacral agenesis as well as the degree and type of lumbar cord involvement (Renshaw 1978). However, sirenomelia involves fusion of the lower limbs or reduction into a single limb, which may be markedly simplified or hypoplastic, and is probably better thought of as a defect in mediolateral patterning.

11.5.1 Neuropathology

The neuropathology of caudal regression is poorly described. The spinal cord is often short, and the abnormalities are predominantly terminal in caudal regression (Fig. 11.4e, f). The affected cord may be atrophic. The ventral horns may be fused, hypoplastic, or depleted of motor neurons with thin ventral nerve roots and peripheral nerves. The dorsal horns are relatively broad and flat, and the dorsal columns may be gliotic or hypoplastic, and the affected leg muscle may show maturational delay (Price et al. 1970). A variety of central nervous system anomalies are described, including microcephaly, hydrocephalus, ventriculomegaly, spinal neural tube defects, and SCM. In sirenomelia, the caudal cord may show simple hydromyelia or complex patterns of spina bifida, spinal cord duplication, and heterotopic tissue elements in the neural canal (Fig. 11.4a–d).

11.5.2 Pathogenesis

There may be a defect in secondary neurulation, and the caudal mesoderm in general is affected (Duesterhoeft et al. 2007). The major risk factor seems to be maternal diabetes, affecting 15–20% of fetuses (Lynch et al. 2000). Distal sacral agenesis is a well-recognized component of Currarino syndrome (OMIM #17650) related to heterozygous mutations in MNX1. Caudal dysgenesis with sacral spina bifida may be linked to VANGL1 mutations (OMIM #600145) and may be a component of the VACTERL association. Sirenomelia has been linked in some families to mutations in CDX2 as an autosomal dominant trait with variable expressivity (Lecoquierre et al. 2020).

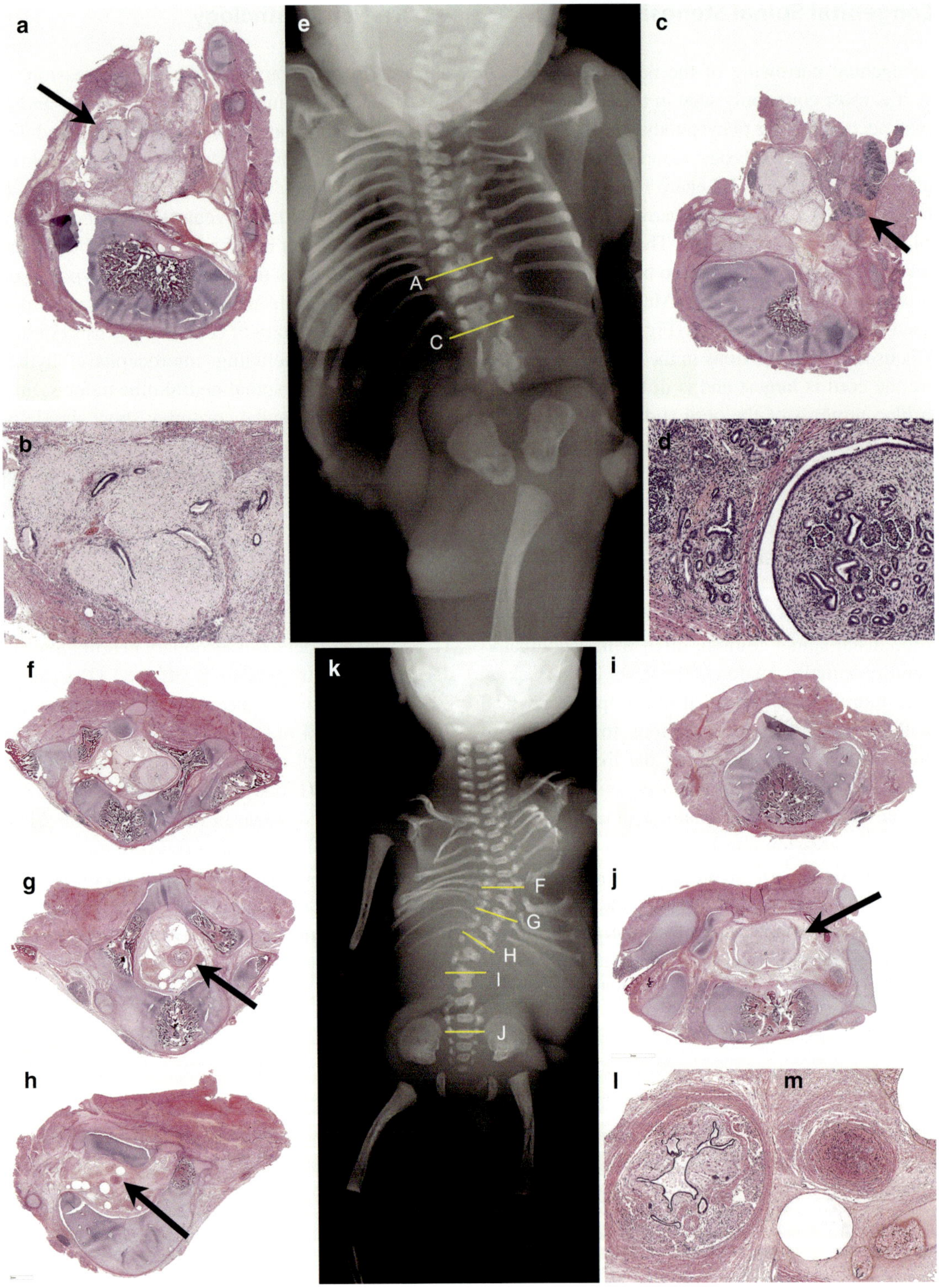

Fig. 11.4 (**a**) Sirenomelia at 23 weeks gestation, with caudal closed spina bifida and irregular neural mass embedded in fibroadipose tissue (arrow). (**b**) Irregularly branched central canal and cord in neural mass. (**c**) More caudal section, same case as (**a**), with absent posterior elements and renal tissue (arrow) embedded adjacent to neural mass. (**d**) The same case as (**a**), demonstrating well-formed glomeruli and dysplastic tubules. (**e**) The same case as (**a**), showing approximate levels of sections sampled. (**f**) Interrupted cord, 22 weeks' gestation: at mid-thoracic levels, the cord is unremarkable albeit placed eccentrically in the canal as is common in fetal scoliosis. (**g**) More caudal section, the same case as (**f**); the spinal cord is hypoplastic with a dilated central canal, but the vertebral structure is relatively preserved. (**h**) More caudal section, the same case as (**f**); the cord is reduced to a stenotic dural sac; the dorsal and lateral aspects are simplified and hypoplastic. (**i**) More caudal section, the same case as (**f**). The cord and dura are absent, and the neural canal is replaced by a lump of cartilage fused to the vertebral body. (**j**) Sacral section, the same case as (**f**). Histology is very nearly normal, although dorsal elements are missing. (**k**) Radiology, the same case as (**f**), demonstrating levels of sections. (**l**) Higher power of cord remnant from (**g**). The cord is reduced to a thin-walled tube with a few neurons in it. (**m**) Higher power of cord remnant from (**h**). The dura is recognizable as such by its layered structure but is clearly narrow and contains only minute fragments of neural tissue

11.6 Segmental Spinal Dysgenesis

This represents a segmental vertebral abnormality that is accompanied by paraplegia and an underlying hypoplasia of the spinal cord. This naturally has some overlap with sacral agenesis/caudal regression (Valdez Quintana et al. 2016) (type 1 segmental dysgenesis as per Tortori-Donati et al. 1999), but in type 2, there is a segmental narrowing or atrophy of the cord accompanying the dysgenic vertebrae (Fig. 11.4f–m).

11.7 Congenital Motor Neuron Disease

This is a group of diseases leading to a paucity of fetal motor neurons, resulting in fetal akinesia and often arthrogryposis congenita. Probably, the most well-documented cause of this type of congenital disease is spinal muscular atrophy type 1 (Werdnig–Hoffmann disease), in which there is early programmed cell death of the generated motor neurons secondary to homozygous mutations in SMA1, but this disease rarely presents with fetal akinesia. A variety of other genes have been implicated in primary deficiency of motor neurons, including IGHMBP2 (SMARD1, OMIM #604320), LAS1L (Butterfield et al. 2014), BICD2 (Rossor et al. 2015), and GLE1 mutation (Paakkola et al. 2018), although pathologic description is unusual. In SMARD1, the principal abnormality is a bland paucity of neurons with chromatolysis of the remaining motor neurons and occasional ventral and peripheral displacement (Fig. 11.5a). Motor neuron disease may also be a feature of lysosomal storage disease and neuroaxonal dystrophy, although in these conditions, the principal abnormality is mild to moderate loss, and the diagnostic features of the underlying disease are most prominent (Fig. 11.5b). Hypoxic ischemic injury to the spinal cord is an important cause of fetal arthrogryposis and is usually marked by local cord atrophy and gliosis with a brisk microglial and astrocytic response (Fig. 11.5c, d); the injury may vary considerably from level to level and in our experience can be diagnosed when there are other patterns of hypoxic ischemic injury in the neuraxis (e.g., tegmental injury, hydranencephaly, and cerebral polymicrogyria).

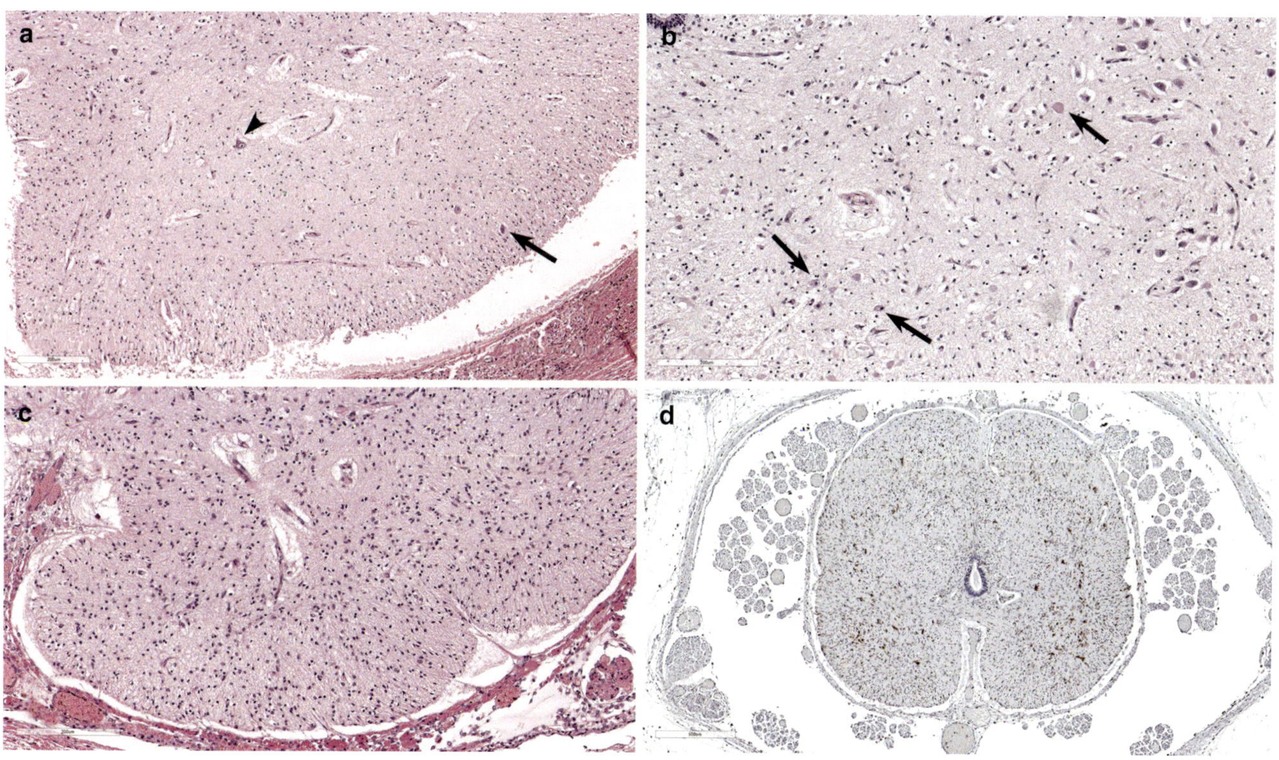

Fig. 11.5 (**a**) Ventral lumbar spinal cord, SMARD1 at 36 weeks gestation with hypoplasia of the ventral gray matter and a bland paucity of motor neurons (arrowhead), some of which (arrow) are peripherally displaced. (**b**) Ventral lumbar spinal cord in a case of arthrogryposis in neuroaxonal dystrophy (20 weeks' gestation), with mild paucity of motor neurons, which are small (arrows) and variably chromatolytic. (**c**) Ventral lumbar spinal cord, 23 weeks' gestation; spinal cord hypoxic ischemic injury, with dense gliosis, atrophy, and almost complete absence of motor neurons. (**d**) The same case as (**c**), with CD68 immunohistochemistry demonstrating brisk proliferation and hypertrophy of microglia, especially in the ventral gray matter

References

Agnoli AL, Laun A, Schönmayr R. Enterogenous intraspinal cysts. J Neurosurg. 1984;61(5):834–40.

Butterfield RJ, Stevenson TJ, Xing L, et al. Congenital lethal motor neuron disease with a novel defect in ribosome biogenesis. Neurology. 2014;82(15):1322–30.

Can A, Dos Santos Rubio EJ, Jasperse B, et al. Spinal neurenteric cyst in association with Klippel-Feil syndrome: case report and literature review. World Neurosurg. 2015;84(2):592.e9–14.

Duckworth T, Sherrard WJ, Lister J, Seymour N. Hemimyelocele. Dev Med Child Neurol.1968: Suppl 16:69+

Duesterhoeft SM, Ernst LM, Siebert JR, Kapur RP. Five cases of caudal regression with an aberrant abdominal umbilical artery: further support for a caudal regression-sirenomelia spectrum. Am J Med Genet. 2007;143A:3175–84.

Emerson RE, Azzarelli B. Enterogenous cysts of the spinal canal and cerebellopontine angle. Appl Immunohistochem Mol Morphol. 2004;12(3):230–3.

Fano V, Kim CA, Rosselli P, Dib RE, Shediac R, Magalhães T, Mesojedovas D, Llerena J Jr. Impact of achondroplasia on Latin American patients: a systematic review and meta-analysis of observational studies. Orphanet J Rare Dis. 2022;17(1):4.

Faye-Petersen OM, Knisely AS. Neural arch stenosis and spinal cord injury in thanatophoric dysplasia. Am J Dis Child. 1991;145(1):87–9.

Frikha R. 2020 Klippel-Feil syndrome: a review of the literature. Clin Dysmorphol. 2020;29(1):35–7.

Herren RY, Edwards JE. Diplomyelia (duplication of the spinal cord). Arch Pathol. 1940;30:1203–13.

Hori A, Fischer G, Dietrich-Schott B, Ikeda K. Dimyelia, diplomyelia, and diastematomyelia. Clin Neuropathol. 1982;1:23–30.

Lecoquierre F, Brehin AC, Coutant S, Coursimault J, Bazin A, Finck W, Benoist G, Begorre M, Beneteau C, Cailliez D, Chenal P, De Jong M, Degré S, Devisme L, Francannet C, Gérard B, Jeanne C, Joubert M, Journel H, Laurichesse Delmas H, Layet V, Liquier A, Mangione R, Patrier S, Pelluard F, Petit F, Tillouche N, van Ravenswaaij-Arts C, Frebourg T, Saugier-Veber P, Gruchy N, Nicolas G, Gerard M. Exome sequencing identifies the first genetic determinants of sirenomelia in humans. Hum Mutat. 2020;41(5):926–33.

Legare JM. 1998 Oct 12 (updated 2023 May 11). Achondroplasia. In: Adam MP, Feldman J, Mirzaa GM, Pagon RA, Wallace SE, Amemiya A, editors. GeneReviews® (Internet). Seattle: University of Washington; 1998.

Lynch SA, Wang Y, Strachan T, Burn J, Lindsay S. Autosomal dominant sacral agenesis: Currarino syndrome. J Med Genet. 2000;37:561–6.

McDowell MM, Dede O, Bosch P, Tyler-Kabara EC. Absent pedicles in campomelic dysplasia. Childs Nerv Syst. 2017;33(6):987–92.

O'Rahilly R and Muller F. 2001 The skeletal system and limbs in human embryology and teratology Wiley-Liss, pp. 257–391.

O'Rahilly R, Muller F. Stage 8: the first appearance of the nervous system. In: The embryonic human brain: an atlas of developmental stages. 3rd ed. Wiley and Sons Inc.; 2006. p. 25–38.

Ogulnick JV, Kazim SF, Carlson AP, et al. Fenestration of intracranial neurenteric cyst: a case report. Surg Neurol Int. 2021;14(12):287.

Paakkola T, Vuopala K, Kokkonen H, et al. A homozygous I684T in GLE1 as a novel cause of arthrogryposis and motor neuron loss. Clin Genet. 2018;93(1):173–7.

Pang D, Dias M, Ahab-Barmada M. Split cord malformation: part I: a unified theory of embryogenesis for double spinal cord malformations. Neurosurg. 1992;31(3):451–80.

Prasad VS, Reddy DR, Murty JM. Cervico-thoracic neurenteric cyst: clinicoradiological correlation with embryogenesis. Childs Nerv Syst. 1996;12(1):48–51.

Price DL, Dooling EC, Richardson EP Jr. Caudal dysplasia (caudal regression syndrome). Arch Neurol. 1970;23(2):212–20.

Renshaw TS. Sacral agenesis. J Bone Jt Surg. 1978;60(3):373–83.

Rossor AM, Oates EC, Salter HK, et al. Phenotypic and molecular insights into spinal muscular atrophy due to mutations in BICD2. Brain. 2015;138(Pt 2):293–310.

Sandberg GD, Wong K, Horkayne-Szakaly I, Dickey G, Rorke-Adams LB, Rushing EJ. Trimyelia with divergent cord pathways and three foramina magni. Childs Nerv Syst. 2007;23(2):249–53.

Shukla M, Behari S, Guruprasad B, Das KK, Mehrotra A, Srivastava AK, Sahu RN, Awadhesh K, Jaiswal AK, Jain M. Spinal neurenteric cysts: associated developmental anomalies and rationale of surgical approaches. Acta Neurochir. 2015;157(9):1601–10.

Tortori-Donati P, Fondelli MP, Rossi A, Raybaud CA, Cama A. Capra V segmental spinal dysgenesis: neuroradiologic findings with clinical and embryologic correlation. Am J Neuroradiol. 1999;20(3):445–56.

Valdez Quintana M, Michaud J, El-Chaar D, El Demellawy D, Nikkel SM, Miller E. Fetal segmental spinal dysgenesis and unusual segmental agenesis of the anterior spinal artery. Childs Nerv Syst. 2016;32(8):1537–41.

Worrell S, Randall A, O'Donnell B. Cervicothoracic neurenteric cyst with contralateral diaphragmatic hernia: an unusual combination. Pediatr Dev Pathol. 2021;24(5):467–70.

Conjoined Twins

12

Conjoined twins are an extremely rare phenomenon occurring in roughly up to 1.5 per 100,000 births (Mutchinick et al. 2011; Martínez-Frías et al. 2009). The precise etiology and mechanism are unclear, but some authors believe that conjoined twins result from a failure of development of primitive structures at later stages of embryonic development, particularly during Carnegie stage 6 (days 12–15), or the primitive streak stage of human development (Levin et al. 1996; Kaufman 2004a, b; Sadler 2010).

These types of twins are physically connected with each other and may share homologous tissues, organs, and even larger parts of their body. Although rare, the condition is a significant contributor to perinatal mortality and is said to be clinically suspected when the twin fetuses cannot be visualized on ultrasound examination (D'Alton and Simpson 1995).

Conjoined twins are classified by the proposed site of union and divided into two groups depending upon the aspect of the embryonic disk involved. The ventral subgroups are joined over a single yolk sac with a shared abdomen and umbilicus and include those joined rostrally, caudally, and laterally. The dorsal subgroup is conjoined at the neural tube, each with a separate abdomen and umbilical cord (Spencer 2000a, b). Conjoined twins may also be classified as symmetrical, where two more or less equal individuals are fused, or asymmetrical (heteropagus), where one twin has succumbed and been partially resorbed (the "parasite") but remains attached to the surviving twin (Fieggen et al. 2004).

The pathogenesis of conjoined twins is unclear, but some authors presume it to be a result of two embryonic primordia in a single embryoblast, forming two embryonic disks in close proximity of each other (Spencer 2003). The growing disks subsequently interfere with each other's development, the type and severity of which are determined by their mutual position and distance (Boer et al. 2019; Boer et al. 2021). Also described are fission and fusion theories. The former theory suggests that the embryo undergoes incomplete division of the monozygotic embryonic disk around 13–15 days after fertilization (Kaufman 2004a, b). The fusion theory on the other hand suggests that two separate embryos undergo a second fusion 13 days after fertilization (Boer et al. 2019).

This chapter will focus on what little is known regarding the neuropathological anomalies associated with certain types of conjoined twinning.

12.1 Cephalopagus Twins

Cephalopagus twins are characterized as being joined at the head extending down to the umbilicus (Winkler et al. 2008). Essentially, two cerebral hemispheres are each connected to their own eyeball by optic nerve without formation of optic chiasm. There are two brainstems and two spinal cords (Singh et al. 2003). Associated anencephaly or encephalocele may be observed (Lee et al. 2012; Ozkur et al. 2006).

12.2 Craniopagus Twins

These types of twins are joined at the cranium without involvement of the foramen magnum, base of the skull, or face (Mian et al. 2017; Winkler et al. 2008; Spencer 1992) (Fig. 12.1). The union may be classified as partial or total. The former involves a limited surface area (more commonly frontal and less commonly occipital or parietal) that is joined between the two twins with the crania either intact or with cranial defects. Each child of the partial union maintains their own calvarial convexities except at the common area of skull junction, while cerebral deformities and compaction are mild and local. The dura of both children may be intact or deficient, and cortical gyri may interdigitate with one another, but leptomeninges are usually separable (Stone and Goodrich 2006), although they could be fused (Winston 1987) as well. Only rare cases of shared brain tissue with associated leptomeningeal blood vessels have been reported (Baldwin and Dekaban 1958; Campbell et al. 2004). A total

P. Shannon et al., *Atlas of Neurodevelopmental Pathology*, https://doi.org/10.1007/978-3-032-14148-4_12

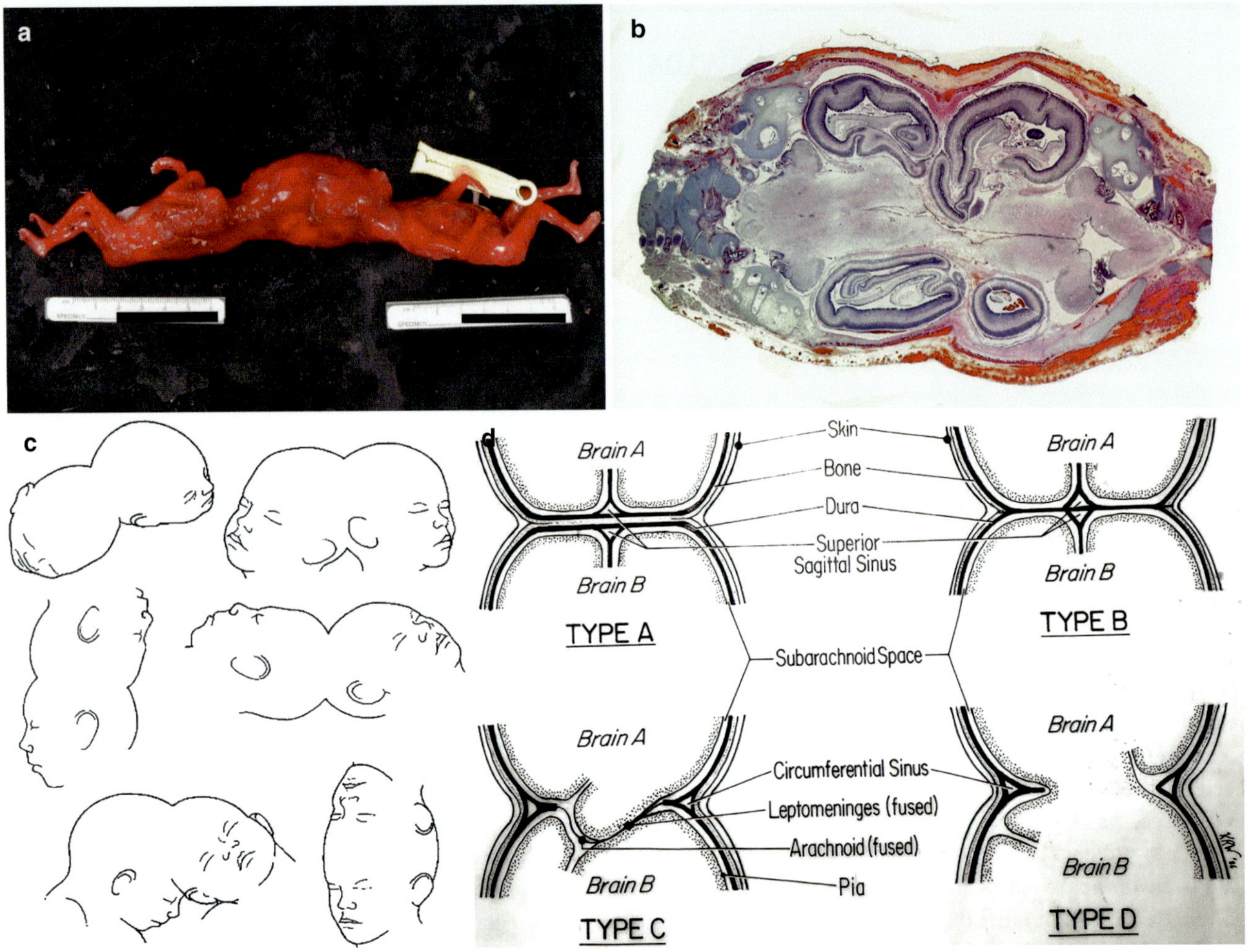

Fig. 12.1 Craniopagus twins. (**a**) Note the two heads joined at the cranium. (**b**) Each twin has two cerebral hemispheres appearing to share the same dura in this example, but with leptomeninges appearing to be split. (**c**) Angles of union in craniopagus twin (*From* Spencer (2000) Part II; *with permission*). (**d**) Types of brain relationships in craniopagus twins (*From* Winston 1987; *with permission*)

union is more extensive with more widely connected cranial cavities. Essentially, the total union gives the appearance of a common cranium housing four cerebral hemispheres (Stone and Goodrich 2006; Walker and Brown 2004; O'Connell 1976). The reader is referred to excellent reviews by both Walker and Brown (2004) and O'Connell (1976) for more details on the classification of craniopagus twins.

Associated neuropathological abnormalities can include fused meninges, cerebrum, and/or spinal cord. The cerebral hemispheres may be simply united or apposed to each other, and the union may or may not involve the cerebellum (Spencer 2000a, b). Extensive union (possibly early stage) may involve the surface of the neural tube with a large defect in the meninges and the cranial vault, whereas less intimate (thought to be later stage) fusion may result in a small bony defect over two separate layers of intact dura mater (Spencer 2003). Anencephaly may also be present (Abrams et al. 1984).

12.3 Pyopagus Twins

These are symmetrical twins joined at rump, which usually involve bony fusion of the sacra (Fieggen et al. 2003, 2004). Pyopagus twins may share the same perineal region, neural cords, vascular structures, and gastrointestinal, urological, and reproductive systems (Spitz 2005). While neuropathological data are limited, reported CNS anomalies include Chiari (types 1 and 2) malformations, spina bifida, fusion of conus, and fused spinal cord with single dural sac, conus, and filum terminale (Fieggen et al. 2003; Hirokazu et al. 2013). Syringes have also been reported in pyopagus twins whereby two cords share a fibrolipomatous sheath within a single dural sac or the spinal cords from each twin may each possess distinct dural sacs within a common neural canal. The central canal may be dilated and/or collapsed. Dorsally elongated central canal lined by the ependyma and extending between the posterior columns has also been described (Guo et al. 2014). Bony abnormalities of the spine (e.g., hemivertebrae) may also be present (Fieggen and Dunn 2004).

12.4 Dicephalus Twins

With dicephalus twins, there are two heads but only two arms, two legs, and one torso (Groner et al. 1996). The fused heads each have their own cerebral hemispheres (Fig. 12.2). These cases when encountered are typically in the context of stillborn fetuses or infants that pass away shortly after birth (Groner et al. 1996). Associated neuropathological anomalies could include anencephaly, two fused spinal cords, myelomeningocele, and/or Chiari malformation (Itoh et al. 1993).

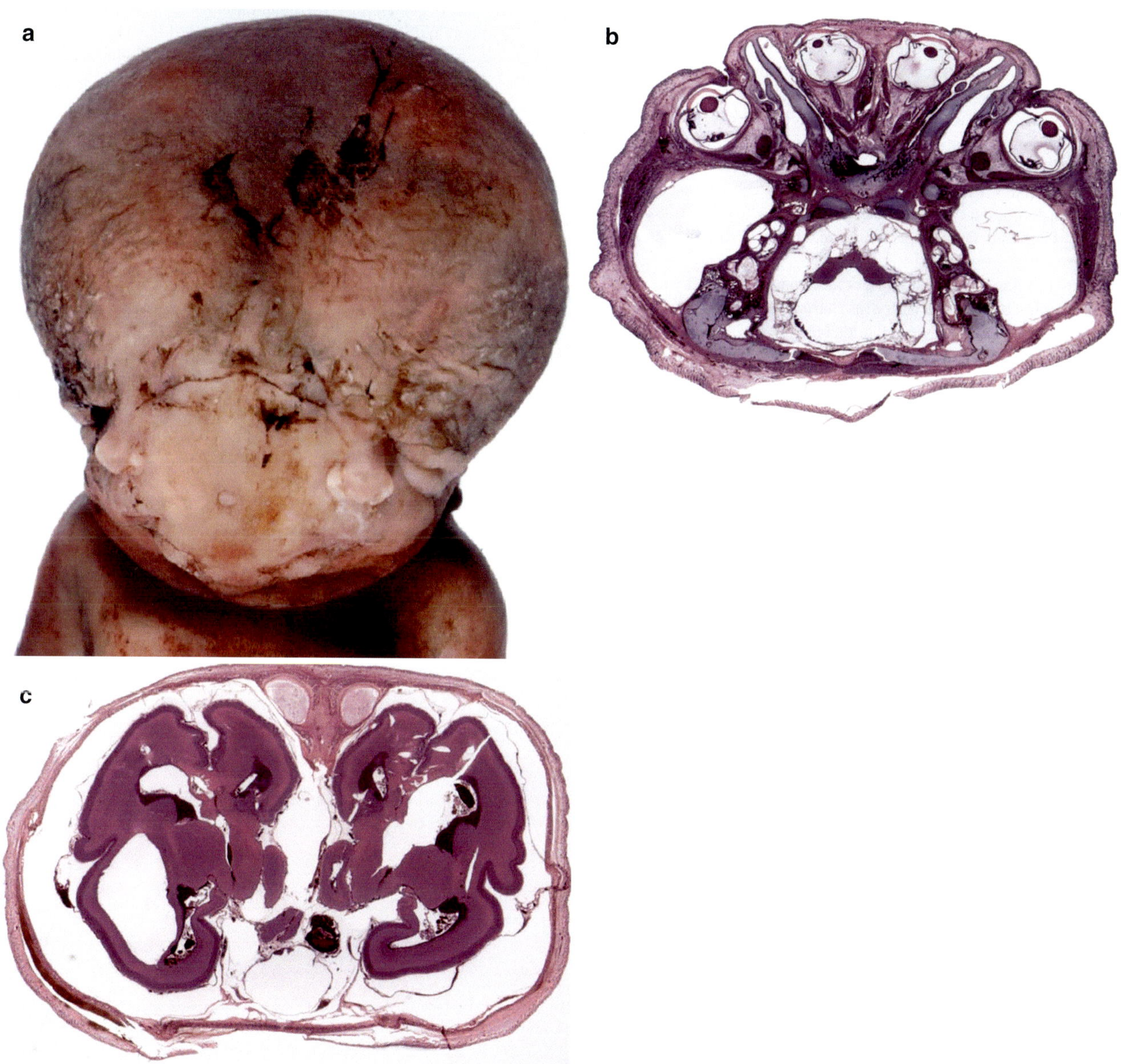

Fig. 12.2 Dicephalus twins. (**a**) Fused heads. Each twin possesses their own pair of eyes (**b**) and cerebral hemispheres (**c**). (*Courtesy of* Dr. Gerard Jansen, *Neuropathologist, University of Ottawa*)

References

Abrams SL, Callen PL, Anderson RL, Stephens JD. Anencephaly with encephalocele in craniopagus twins: prenatal diagnosis by ultrasonography and computed tomography. J Ultrasound Med. 1984;4(9):485–8.

Baldwin M, Dekaban A. The surgical separation of Siamese twins conjoined by the head followed by normal development. J Neurol Neurosurg Psychiatry. 1958;21:195–202.

Boer LL, Schepens-Franke AN, Oostra RJ. Two is a crowd: two is a crowd: on the enigmatic etiopathogenesis of conjoined twinning. Clin Anat. 2019;32(5):722–41.

Boer LL, Schepens-Franke AN, Winter E, Oostra RJ. Characterizing the coalescence area of conjoined twins to elucidate congenital disorders in singletons. Clin Anat. 2021;34(6):848–58.

Campbell S, Theile R, Stuart G et al. Craniopagus: second Brisbane case. Case report. J Neurosurg 2004;100(5 Suppl Pediatrics):519–24.

D'Alton ME, Simpson LL. Syndromes in twins. Semin Perinatol. 1995;19(5):375–86.

Fieggen AG, Dunn RN, Pitcher RD, et al. Ischiopagus and pygopagus conjoined twins: neurosurgical considerations. Childs Nerv Syst. 2004;20(8–9):640–51.

Fieggen G, Millar A, Rode H, et al. Spinal cord involvement in pyopagus conjoined twins: case report and review of the literatures. Childs Nerv Syst. 2003;19:183–7.

Groner JI, Teske DW, Teich S. Dicephalus dipus dibrachius: an unusual case of conjoined twins. J Pediatr Surg. 1996;31(12):1698–700.

Guo A, Chitayat D, Blaser S, et al. Fetal Syringomyelia. Acta Neuropathol Comm. 2014;2:91.

Hirokazu T, Takayuki I, Yoshinori, et al. Separation surgery of pygopagus asymmetrical conjoined twins sharing U-shaped spinal cord: case report and literature review. Childs Nerv Syst. 2013;29:697–706.

Itoh K, Imai Y, Obayashi C, et al. Pathological findings in dicephalus dipus dibrachius: implications for mechanisms in two pairs of lateral conjoined twins. Kobe J Med Sci. 1993;39(3):95–106. PMID:8255077

Kaufman MH. The embryology of conjoined twin. Childs Nerv Syst. 2004a;20(8–9):508–25.

Kaufman MH. The embryology of conjoined twins. Childs Nerv Syst. 2004b;20(8–9):508–25.

Lee AW, Farnquist b, Islam O, et al. Noninvasive investigation of asymmetrically conjoined tripus twins with features of rachipagus, parapagus dicephalus, and cephalopagus. Clin Anat. 2012;2598:1023–9. PMID 21433086

Levin M, Roberts DJ, Holmes LB, Tabin C. Laterality defects in conjoined twins. Nature. 1996;384(6607):321.

Martínez-Frías ML, Bermejo E, Mendioroz J, et al. Epidemiological and clinical analysis of a consecutive series of conjoined twins in Spain. J Pediatr Surg. 2009;44(4):811–20.

Mian A, Gabra NI, Sharma T, et al. Clin Anat. 2017;30(3):385–96. https://doi.org/10.1002/ca.22839. PMID: 2819536

Mutchinick OM, Luna-Munoz L, Amar E, et al. Conjoined twins: a worldwide collaborative epidemiological study of the International Clearinghouse for Birth Defects Surveillance and Research. Am J Med Gent Semin Med Genet. 2011;157(C4):274–87.

O'Connell JE. Craniopagus twins: surgical anatomy and embryology and their implications. J Neurol Neurosurg Psychiatry. 1976;39(1):1–22.

Ozkur A, Karaca M, Gocmen A, et al. Cephalopagus conjoined twins presented with encephalocele: diagnostic role of ultrafast MR imaging. Diagn Interv Radiol. 2006;12(2):90–2.

Sadler TW. Third month to birth: the fetus and placenta. In: Sadler TW, editor. Langman's medical embryology, 11e. Philadelphia: Lippincott Williams & Wilkins; 2010. p. 91–111.

Singh M, Singh KP, Shaligram P. Conjoined twins cephalopagus janiceps monosymmetros: a case report. Birth Defects Res A Clin Mol Teratol. 2003;67(4):268–72. PMID12854662

Spencer R. Theoretical and analytical embryology of con-joined twins. Part I: embryogenesis. Clin Anat. 2000a;13(1):36–53.

Spencer R. Theoretical and analytical embryology of con-joined twins. Part II: adjustments to union. Clin Anat. 2000b;13(2):97–120.

Spencer R. Conjoined twins: theoretical embryologic basis. Teratology. 1992;45(6):591–602.

Spencer. Embryology. In: Spencer. Conjoined twins developmental malformations and clinical implications. Johns Hopkins University Press 2003. p 9–57.

Spitz L. Conjoined twins. Prenat Diagn. 2005;25(9):814–9.

Stone JL, Goodrich JT. The craniopagus malformation: classification and implications for surgical separation. Brain. 2006;129(Pt5):1084–95.

Walker M, Browd SR. Craniopagus twins: embryology, classification, surgical anatomy, and separation. Childs Nerv Syst. 2004;20(8–9):554–66.

Winkler N, Kennedy A, Byrine J, Woodward P. The imaging spectrum of conjoined twins. Ultrasound Q. 2008;24(4):249–55.

Winston KR. Craniopagi: anatomical characteristics and classification. Neurosurgery. 1987;21(6):769–81.

13 Metabolic and Other Genetically Defined Abnormalities

Malformations of the brain and spinal cord may arise from lysosomal disorders, as well as inborn errors of metabolism and axonal function. These genetic defects may result in disruptions of cell proliferation, neuronal migration, and/or organization. This chapter presents the neuropathological abnormalities associated with some of the metabolic and neurodegenerative disorders.

13.1 Lysosomal Storage Diseases

Classically, lysosomal storage diseases result from a deficiency in a lysosomal enzyme activity, resulting in an accumulation of substrate, typically within macrophages or the neural elements generating the substrate. The biochemistry and pathology of these diseases are generally well explored in the larger pediatric literature, which we will not review here, and most lysosomal storage diseases are poorly represented in reports of fetal central nervous system remains (Pollanen and Brody 1990). However, there are striking exceptions to this rule.

Gaucher disease is caused by a deficiency in β-glucocerebrosidase (glucosylceramidase) enzyme activity and has three major clinical presentations (Hughes and Pastores 2023), of which one (type 2) presents in utero or before 2 years of age with progressive neurological disease and hepatosplenomegaly. A perinatal lethal form can also present with ichthyosiform skin disease, pterygia, and hydrops. There are numerous mutations that are lethal early in life in homozygous or compound heterozygous states, with one study of 31 such cases demonstrating 33 different lethal alleles (Stone et al. 2000), sharing an overlap with mutations present in other clinical presentations. The perinatal lethal form often demonstrates homozygosity for recombinant alleles. In fetal remains, hydrops may be prominent. The brain may show delayed development with periventricular hemorrhagic infarction (Eblan et al. 2005; Mignot et al. 2006) (Fig. 13.1a). Histologically, these forms demonstrate accumulation of PAS (+) glucocerebroside in neurons and macrophages (Fig. 13.1b, c) with neuronal loss particularly in the earlier maturing neuronal groups at all levels of the central nervous system.

Although not usually thought of as lysosomal storage diseases in the usual sense of deficiencies of specific degradative enzymes, genetic abnormalities of lysosomal function or transportation should also be considered as a cause of lysosomal storage. Defects of lysosomal acidification or transport may produce fetal pathology. In fetal ATP6V0A1-related disease (Bott et al. 2021), the genetic defect is a sporadic mutation in a transmembrane ATPase protein that results in impaired lysosomal acidification, resulting in a neuroaxonal dystrophy. The brain (Fig. 13.1d–f) demonstrates an axonal dystrophy in the setting of the accumulation of lysosomal material in neurons and axons.

A pathologically similar disease results from biallelic mutations in BORCS5 (Jia et al. 2017; De Pace et al. 2024; Greenberg et al. in press) BORC (Bloc1-Related Complex) is a protein complex necessary for the coupling of lysosomes to kinesins, transport of lysosomes to the distal axons, and fusion of lysosomes with autophagosomes. In BORC Subunit 5-related disease, the phenotype can be a severe fetal neuroaxonal dystrophy with aqueduct stenosis and numerous periventricular heterotopias (Fig. 13.1g, h, i) and lysosomal accumulations in axons (Fig. 13.1j) and congenital osteopetrosis with giant osteoclasts (Greenbeg et al. in press). Mutations in another proteins of the complex, in particular BORCS8 have been linked to early onset human disease as well, but the pathology is obscure.

Perinatal onset neuroaxonal dystrophies without obvious lysosomal pathology typically present as fetal akinesia or hypokinesia or profound neonatal hypotonia; there may be associated cerebral cortical maldevelopment with polygyria, polymicrogyria, and agenesis or hypogenesis of long tracts. The principal histopathology is that of enlarged glassy axonal spheroids, which are prominent in the spinal cord and deep axonal tracts and can be in the peripheral nervous sys-

P. Shannon et al., *Atlas of Neurodevelopmental Pathology*, https://doi.org/10.1007/978-3-032-14148-4_13

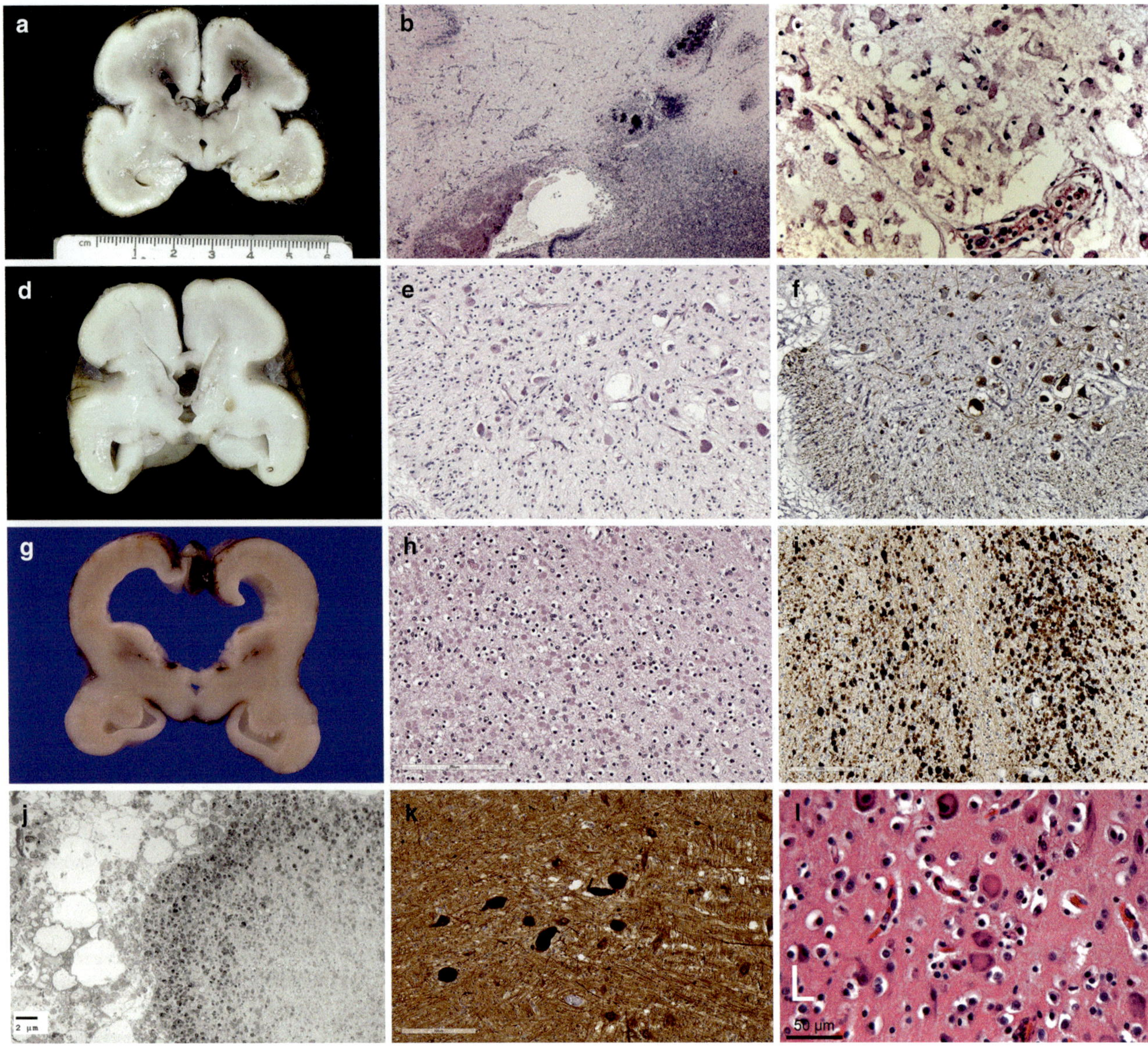

Fig. 13.1 (**a**) A 27-week gestation fetus with Gaucher disease, demonstrating delayed cortical sulcation, mild ventricular dilation, and periventricular hemorrhagic infarction. (**b**) Subcortical calcification and hemorrhage with prominent microvasculature cuffed with macrophages. (**c**) Spinal cord of case (**a**), demonstrating numerous swollen Gaucher cells and loss of neurons. (**d**) Coronal section at 21 weeks' gestation, ATP6V0A1 mutation, with mild ventricular dilation and hypoplastic hippocampal formations. (**e**) Spinal cord demonstrating numerous enlarged neuronal somas containing granular PAS (+) material. (**f**) Immunohistochemistry for neurofilament light chain, demonstrating neuronal somas distended by negative staining material. (**g**) A 23-week-gestation BORCS5 mutation with ventriculomegaly, hypoplastic and thin corpus callosum, and irregular ventricular lining with multiple small periventricular heterotopias and large nodular excrescences. (**h**) Internal capsule demonstrating innumerable flocculent eosinophilic spheroids, which stain strongly for amyloid beta A4 precursor protein (**i**). (**j**) On electron microscopy, numerous axonal swellings with polymorphic electron-dense lysosomes. (**k**) Neonatal axonal dystrophy with swollen axons in deep cerebral hemispheres and brainstem, here in the oculomotor nerve nuclear complex. (**l**) Cortical neurons of layer 5 show Lewy body-like histology

tem as well (Fig. 13.1k). In neonates, there may be an accompanying chromatolytic and even Lewy body-like change in the soma of cortical pyramidal neurons (Fig. 13.1l). Similar pathology has been described in cases accompanying mutations in kinesin genes impairing axonal transport (Priya et al. 2024).

13.2 Glycogen Storage Disease

Type 4 glycogen storage disease (OMIM #232500) results from a homozygous deficiency in glycogen branching enzyme (GBE1), resulting in insoluble glycogen polymers deposited as polyglucosan bodies, often easily found in the

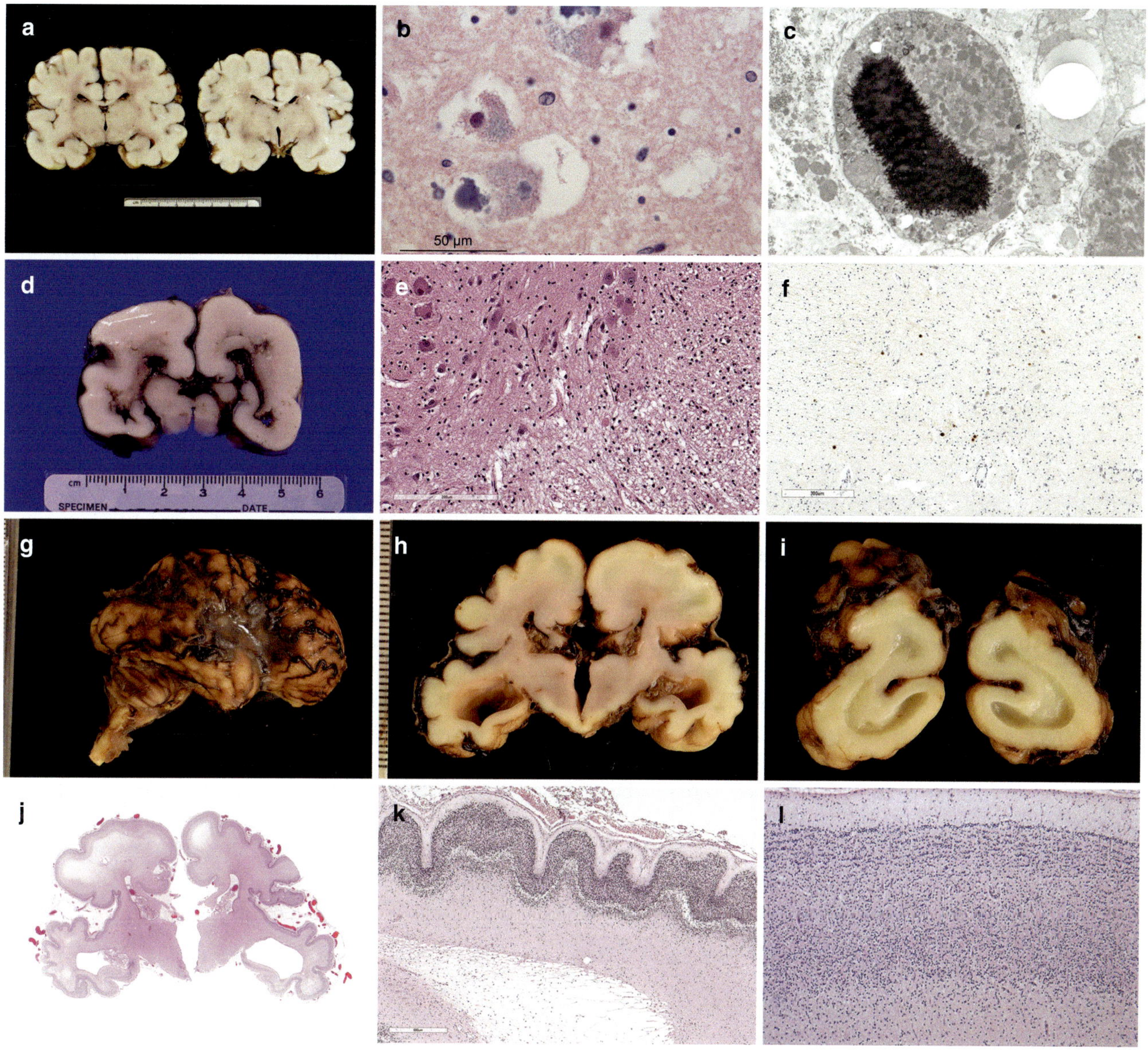

Fig. 13.2 (**a**) Andersen (Type 4 glycogen storage disease) disease in term infant with mild cortical atrophy and otherwise appropriate development. (**b**) Motor neurons of the brainstem and cortex, demonstrating perikaryal basophilic polyglucosan bodies. (**c**) Electron microscopy of the skeletal muscle with delayed maturation and massive non-membrane-bound cytoplasmic accumulation of electron-dense staining glycogen. (**d**) A 28-week gestation fetus, adenylate lyase deficiency with hypoplastic shortened corpus callosum and delayed cortical sulcation. (**e**) Thalamic, brainstem, and spinal cord neuronal groups with normal architecture and occasional axonal spheroids. (**f**) Immunohistochemistry for amyloid beta A4 precursor protein demonstrating numerous scattered axonal spheroids. (**g**) A 39-week gestation, Neu–Laxova syndrome, demonstrating dramatic global micrencephaly and irregular shallow cerebral sulci. (**h**) Relative ventriculomegaly with absent corpus callosum and germinal matrix cystic change. (**i**) Occipital pole demonstrating marked deep white matter rarefaction. (J) Whole mount of section showing dramatic rarefied subcortical white matter and thinned cortical structures. (**k**) Widespread posterior polygyria but retaining six layers with rarefaction of layer 5. (**l**) Frontal cortex with hypocellularity, rhythmic lamination, and poorly defined deep layers

liver and skeletal muscle. There are four clinical variants, and GBE1 deficiency with less than 1% of normal activity presents as fetal akinesia, hydrops fetalis, or neonatal hypotonia and respiratory insufficiency. Polyglucosan bodies in this neuropathic form can be readily found in the motor neurons of the spinal cord and brainstem (Fig. 13.2a, b) and in the skeletal muscle (Fig. 13.2c) and liver (Tay et al. 2004).

13.3 Metabolic Disorders

This is a diverse group of diseases wherein a principal defect in synthesis or degradation of metabolites results in malformation and/or an early neurodegenerative process. The prominent features are often delayed or arrested brain maturation, cortical simplification, or a spongiform or microcystic change predominantly in the white matter. In fetal life however, the microscopic features may be subtle.

13.4 Purine Synthesis Defects

Adenylosuccinate lyase (ADSL) is active in both the de novo and salvage pathways of purine synthesis, and loss of activity (adenylosuccinate lyase deficiency (OMIM #13050)) results in a very wide range of clinical presentations. In its most severe form (type 1) it can present with neonatal encephalopathy, severe hypotonia, microcephaly, and seizures; neonatal histopathology has demonstrated widespread cerebral cortical and cerebellar neuronal loss with spongiosis and poor myelination (Mierzewska et al. 2009). We have seen one family in which the siblings demonstrated short thin corpus callosum and delayed cortical development as well as a widespread albeit subtle axonal dystrophy with hypoplasia of the gray matter tracts and dentato-olivary dysplasia, as well as thinned cerebral deep tracts (Fig. 13.2d–f).

13.5 Defects of Amino Acid Synthesis

Defects in serine biosynthesis pathways lead to the Neu–Laxova syndromes NLS1 and NLS2 (OMIM #26250 and 616038), due to the deficiency in the activity of phosphoglycerate dehydrogenase or phosphoserine aminotransferase, respectively (Acuna-Hidalgo et al. 2014). NSL1 and NSL2 present with widespread abnormalities, including growth restriction, ichthyosis, proptosis, and ectropion, although NSL2 tended toward the more severe end (Manning et al. 2004). The brain (Fig. 13.2g–l) demonstrates micrencephaly with marked simplification of the cerebral cortical convolutions. One striking feature is the widespread hypoplasia and immaturity of neurons, affecting the cerebral cortex, thalamus, basal ganglia, cerebellar cortex, deep nuclei, and inferior olives accompanied by hypoplasia of the deep tracts and agenesis of long tracts, including the corpus callosum and pyramidal tracts (Ostrovskaya and Lazjuk 1988; Abdelfatteh et al. 2020.)

Glutamine synthetase deficiency (OMIM 610015) due to a deficiency in glutamate–ammonia lyase (GLUL) activity presents with an early-onset encephalopathy accompanied by cerebral cortical simplification (Haberle et al. 2005). Pathological descriptions are uncommon, but in a fetal case of homozygous GLUL deletion (Roifman et al. 2020), there was micrencephaly with global developmental delay and long tract hypoplasia, agenesis of the corpus callosum, dentato-olivary dysplasia, perivascular amphophilic globules, cerebellar cortical thinning and cyst formation, and premature germinal matrix depletion (Fig. 13.3a–d).

Fig. 13.3 (**a**) Glutamine synthetase deficiency: 29 weeks' gestation, demonstrating micrencephaly, ventriculomegaly, agenesis of the corpus callosum, and delayed cortical sulcation. (**b**) Occipital pole with periventricular rarefaction and (**c**) periventricular gliosis (immunohistochemistry for glial acid fibrillary protein). (**d**) The same case with poorly formed and hypoplastic cerebellar dentate nuclei. (**e**) Brain of a term infant with Zellweger syndrome, PEX12 compound heterozygous mutation with agenesis of the corpus callosum, irregular polygyria, and dilated temporal horns. (**f**) Simplified microgyric cortex with four layers and innumerable small subcortical heterotopias, which are often perivascular. (**g**) Cerebellar cortex, immunohistochemistry for calbindin, with numerous heterotopic Purkinje cells in the internal granular cell layer. (**h**) Cerebellar dentate nucleus with fragmentation and decreased crenation

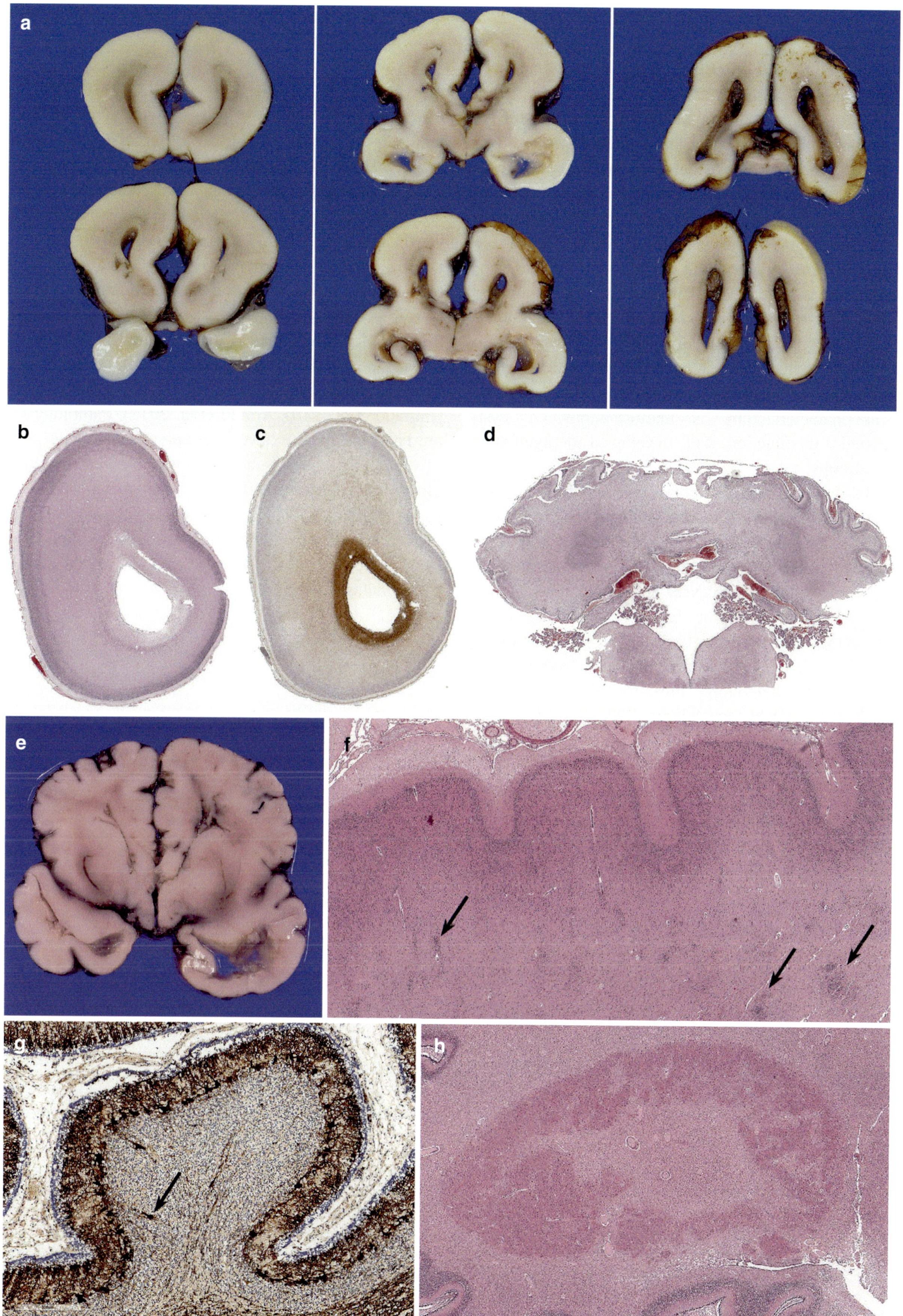
a
b
c
d
e
f
g
h

13.6 Zellweger Spectrum Disorder

Zellweger syndrome is a group of typically autosomal recessive genetic diseases characterized by defects in the formation of peroxisomes, the organelles responsible for the degradation of very long chain and branched fatty acids as well as the synthesis of plasmalogens and bile acids. The genetic basis is heterogeneous, with mutations or deletions in pexin (PEX) genes, which encode proteins required to generate peroxisomes, with currently 13 different PEX genes implicated. Approximately 90% of Zellweger disease arises from alterations in PEX1, PEX6, PEX12, PEX26, and PEX10, with over 60% arising from mutation or deletion of PEX1 (Steinberg et al. 2020). Patients tend to present as neonates with abnormal facies, hypotonia, and difficulty feeding, but there is a wide spectrum of severity. The most severe forms are characterized by CNS malformations, renal cysts, and hepatic dysfunction and develop a demyelinating leukodystrophy.

In fetal imaging, periventricular cysts may be prominent, although these may be difficult to appreciate on postmortem examination in fetal remains. In the cerebrum, the severe forms may demonstrate subcortical and periventricular heterotopias as well as pachygyria and predominantly peri-Sylvian polygyria, overlying an increase in heterotopic neurons in the corona radiata (Evrard et al. 1978), as well as cerebellar dysplasia, most prominent in the nodulus, with large numbers of heterotopic Purkinje cells, and dentato-olivary dysplasia (Volpe and Adams 1972) (Fig. 13.3e–h).

13.7 X-Linked Dominant Chondrodysplasia Punctata

Mutations in the X-linked gene emopamil-binding protein may produce a deficiency in cholesterol synthesis due to a reduced or absent 3-b-hydroxysteroid-D8,D7-isomerase activity. Severely affected females display rhizomelic dwarfism, stippled epiphyses, ichthyosis, cataracts, and growth failure, while in males, severe deficiency is usually lethal in utero. Surviving affected males may display a distinct phenotype (MEND syndrome, OMIM 300960) arising from post-zygotic mosaicism with diffuse ichthyosis, abnormal facies, polydactyly or syndactyly, cataracts, and developmental delay, which may be accompanied by seizures, hypotonia, cerebellar hypoplasia, hydrocephalus, gyral simplification, and hypoplasia of the corpus callosum (Furtado et al. 2010; Arnold et al. 2012). Pathology reports are be scant, but we have seen one affected male in which severe ichthyosis was accompanied by ventriculomegaly, innumerable periventricular nodular heterotopias (Fig. 13.4a, b), cerebellar hypoplasia with microcystic degeneration of the cerebellum around the fourth ventricle, hypoplasia of the basis pontis and inferior olivary complex, and agenesis of the pyramidal tracts (Fig. 13.4c–e).

Fig. 13.4 (**a**) Deficient 3-b-hydroxysteroid-D8,D7-isomerase activity: a 23-week gestation with ventriculomegaly and innumerable periventricular nodular heterotopias. (**b**) Perivascular dilated spaces are numerous near the peduncles, and the hippocampal formations are abnormal. (**c**) Hypoplastic cerebellum with large opening to the fourth ventricle and some cortical irregularity caudally. (**d**) Whole mount of the cerebellum and pons at the level of abducens nucleus showing finely trabeculated and cystic degeneration surrounding the fourth ventricle (arrow). The basis pontis is small. (**e**) Whole mount of rostral medulla demonstrating minute dentate nuclei (this was their greatest extent at any level) without pyramidal tract formation. (**f**) Glutamyl-tRNA synthetase deficiency: a 29-week gestation showing marked micrencephaly, maturational delay with dilation particularly of the dorsal lateral ventricle and with thinning and collapse of the cerebral mantle. (**g**) Immunohistochemistry for vimentin demonstrating dense gliosis of the mantle with subcortical and germinal matrix cysts as well as a hypoplastic poorly formed hippocampus. (**h**) Staining for Collagen IV demonstrates the trabeculae in the subcortical cavities with a microvessel at the center of many trabeculae. (**i**) The collapsed gliotic cortex shows macrophages (arrow) surrounding mineralized processes, suggesting local ischemia and cell death. (**j**) Elsewhere the cortex is thin, hypocellular, and poorly layered with a coarse, sparse microvasculature. (**k**) Term infant with mitochondrial complex IV deficiency, demonstrating marked loss of volume, cortical simplification, and both subcortical and periventricular cysts

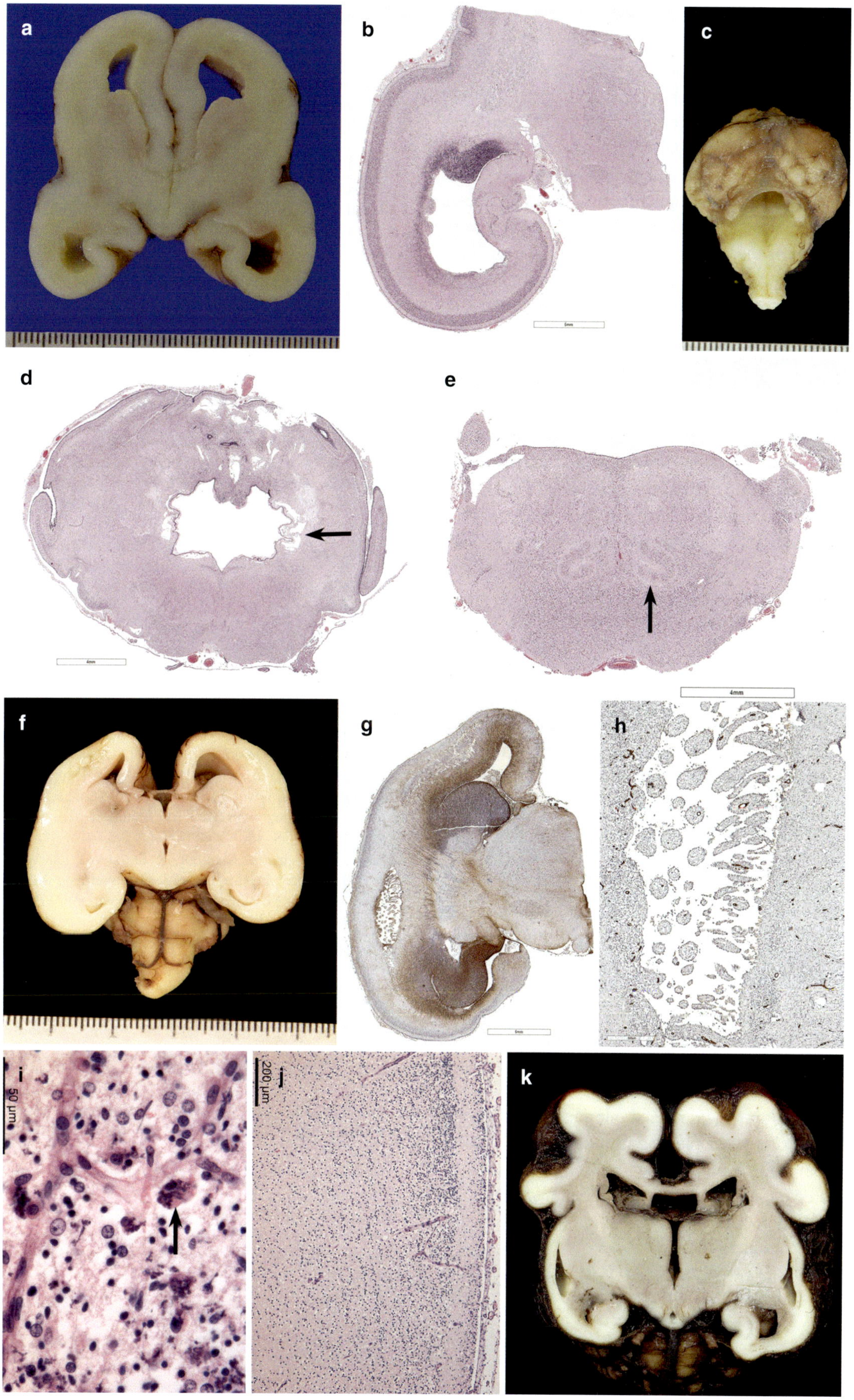
a
b
c
d
e
4mm
f
g
h
i
50 µm
j
200 µm
k

13.8 Mitochondrial Disease

Mitochondrial diseases are disorders characterized by primary deficits in mitochondrial numbers or function, leading to defective tissue oxidative phosphorylation. There are a plethora of clinical syndromes and several dozen genes, carried in the mitochondrial and the nuclear genome. Most such defects affect children or neonates (Pizzamiglio et al. 2024), and in the brain, these often manifest as cystic change or hypomyelination of the white matter, with or without frank necrosis. On occasion, some present with structural abnormalities or arthrogryposis due to fetal immobility or imaging abnormalities in the brain (Tulinius and Oldfors 2011), but reports of fetal pathology are unusual.

Mitochondrial DNA polymerase gamma is a DNA polymerase necessary for mitochondrial genomic replication carried in the nuclear genome. Genotype–phenotype correlations are complex; individuals affected by missense mutations can present in infancy with Alpers–Huttenlocher or Leigh syndrome (Kasiviswanathan et al. 2009). We have seen one family with recurrent homozygous missense mutations (G848S) who demonstrated one fetus with dorsal column hypoplasia, a widespread subtle neuroaxonal pathology, rarefaction of several deep nuclear groups, and dentato-olivary and cerebellar hypoplasia at 22 weeks' gestation in fetal life (Inbar-Feigenberg et al. 2018).

Mitochondrial tRNA synthetase deficiencies have been recorded as affecting the central nervous system in infancy (Konovalova and Tyynismaa 2013), particularly with deficiencies in glutamyl-tRNA synthetase (EARS2 deficiency, OMIM #614924 (Pelayo et al. 2024)), which may present in early infancy with agenesis or dysgenesis of the corpus callosum, white matter abnormalities, and in one report agenesis of the thalamus on imaging. We have seen one family with a compound heterozygous mutation in EARS2l; one allele was a truncating mutation and the other a missense—the affected fetus at 22 weeks' gestation demonstrated micrencephaly (Fig. 13.4f, g) and agenesis of the corpus callosum with a bland, trabeculated cavitation of the convexity subcortical white matter (Fig. 13.4h), as well as areas of necrosis, calcification, and hypocellularity of the overlying cortex (Fig. 13.4i, j).

We have in addition encountered one family with global micrencephaly, cortical atrophy and simplification, and bilateral subcortical white matter cavitation (Fig. 13.4k); on muscle oxidative enzyme testing, a severe defect in complex IV activity was detected, but genetic analyses were unrewarding.

References

Abdelfattah F, Kariminejad A, Kahlert AK, Morrison PJ, Gumus E, Mathews KD, et al. Expanding the genotypic and phenotypic spectrum of severe serine biosynthesis disorders. Hum Mutat. 2020;41(9):1615–28.

Acuna-Hidalgo R, Schanze D, Kariminejad A, Nordgren A, Kariminejad MH, Conner P, et al. Neu-Laxova syndrome is a heterogeneous metabolic disorder caused by defects in enzymes of the L-serine biosynthesis pathway. Am J Hum Genet. 2014;95:285–93.

Arnold AW, Bruckner-Tuderman L, Has C, Happle R. Conradi–Hunermann–Happle syndrome in males vs. MEND syndrome (male EBP disorder with neurological defects). Br J Dermatol. 2012;166:1309–13.

Bhola PT, Mishra R, Posey JE, Hamilton LE, Graham GE, Punetha J, Care4Rare Canada Consortium, Lupski JR, Boycott KM, D'Amours D, Kristin D. Kernohan KD. Phenotypic heterogeneity associated with KIF21A: two new cases and review of the literature. Am J Med Genet A. 2024;194(3):e63455. https://doi.org/10.1002/ajmg.a.63455.

Bott LC, Forouhan M, Lieto M, Sala AJ, Ellerington R, Johnson JO, et al. Variants in ATP6V0A1 cause progressive myoclonus epilepsy and developmental and epileptic encephalopathy. Brain Commun. 2021;3(4):fcab245. https://doi.org/10.1093/braincomms/fcab245. eCollection 2021

De Pace R, Maroofian R, Paimboeuf A, Zamani M, Zaki MS, Sadeghian S, et al. Biallelic BORCS8 variants cause an infantile-onset neurodegenerative disorder with altered lysosome dynamics. Brain. 2024;147(5):1751–67.

Eblan MJ, Goker-Alpan O, Sidransky E. Perinatal lethal Gaucher disease: a distinct phenotype along the neuronopathic continuum. Fetal Pediatr Pathol. 2005;24(4–5):205–22.

Evrard P, Caviness VS, Prats-Vinasl J, Lyon G. The mechanism of arrest of neuronal migration in the Zellweger malformation: an hypothesis based upon cytoarchitectonic analysis. Acta neuropath (Berl.). 1978;41:109–17.

Furtado LV, Bayrak-Toydemir P, Hulinsky B, Damjanovich K, Carey JC, Rope AF. A novel X-linked multiple congenital anomaly syndrome associated with an EBP mutation. Am J Med Genet A. 2010;152A:2838–44.

Greenberg O, Fisher Y, Shannon P, Staines A, Napier M, Chitayat D. Neuroaxonal Dystrophy with Osteopetrosis Associated with a Novel Biallelic Missense Homozygous Variant in BORCS5 in prep. Am J Med Genet. In press;

Haberle J, Gorg B, Rutsch F, Schmidt E, Toutain A, Benoist J-F, Gelot A, Suc A-L, Hohne W, Schliess F, Haussinger D, Koch HG. Congenital glutamine deficiency with glutamine synthetase mutations. New Eng J Med. 2005;353:1926–33.

Hughes DA, Pastores GM. Gaucher disease 2023 gene reviews (Internet). 2023

Inbar-Feigenberg M, Blaser S, Hawkins C, Shannon P, Hewson S, Chitayat D. Mitochondrial POLG related disorder presenting prenatally with fetal cerebellar growth arrest. Metab Brain Dis. 2018;33:1369–73.

Jia R, Guardia CM, Pu J, Chen Y, Bonifacino JS. BORC coordinates encounter and fusion of lysosomes with autophagosomes. Autophagy. 2017;13(10):1648–63.

Kasiviswanathan R, Longley MJ, Chan SSL. Copeland WC mutations in the human mitochondrial DNA polymerase thumb subdomain impart severe defects in mitochondrial DNA replication. J Biol Chem. 2009;284(29):19501–10.

Konovalova S, Tyynismaa H. Mitochondrial aminoacyl-tRNA synthetases in human disease. Mol Genet Metab. 2013;108(4):206–11.

Manning MA, Cunniff CM, Colby CE, El-Sayed YY, Hoyme HE. Neu-Laxova syndrome: detailed prenatal diagnostic and post-mortem findings and literature review. Am J Med Genet. 2004;125A:240–9.

Mierzewska H, Schmidt-Sidor B, Jurkiewicz E, Bogdańska A, Kuśmierska K, Stepień T. Severe encephalopathy with brain atrophy and hypomyelination due to adenylosuccinate lyase deficiency—MRI, clinical, biochemical and neuropathological findings of Polish patients. Folia Neuropathol. 2009;47(4):314–20.

Mignot C, Doummar D, Maire I, De Villemeur TB. Type 2 Gaucher disease: 15 new cases and review of the literature. Brain Dev. 2006;28(1):39–48.

Ostrovskaya TI. Lazjuk GI cerebral abnormalities in the Neu-Laxova syndrome. Am J Med Genet. 1988;30:747–56.

Pelayo G, Coelho MP, Correia J, Bandeir A, Nogueira C, Vilarinho L, Martins E. Phenotyping mitochondrial glutamyl-tRNA synthetase deficiency (EARS2): a case series and systematic literature review. Neurobiol Dis. 2024;200:106644. Epub 2024 Aug 22

Pizzamiglio C, Hanna MG, Robert DS. Primary mitochondrial diseases. Handb Clin Neurol. 2024;204:53–76.

Pollanen MS, Brody BA. Fetal globoid cell leukodystrophy. Arch Pathol Lab Med. 1990;114(2):213–6.

Roifman M, Niles KM, MacNeil L, Blaser S, Noor A, Godoy R, et al. Homozygous GLUL deletion is embryonically viable and leads to glutamine synthetase deficiency. Clin Genet. 2020;98(6):613–9. https://doi.org/10.1111/cge.13844. Epub 2020 Oct 1

Steinberg SJ, Raymond GV, Braverman NE, Moser AB, 2020 Zellweger spectrum disorder, gene reviews (Internet)

Stone DL, Tayebi N, Orvisky E, Stubblefield B, Madike V, Sidransky E. Glucocerebrosidase gene mutations in patients with type 2 Gaucher disease. Hum Mutat. 2000;15(2):181–8.

Tay SKH, Akman HO, Chung WK, Pike MG, Muntoni F, Hays AP, Shanske S, Valberg SJ, Mickelson R, Tanji K, Di Mauro S. Fatal infantile neuromuscular presentation of glycogen storage disease type IV. Neuromuscul Disord. 2004;14(4):253–60.

Tulinius M, Oldfors A. Neonatal muscular manifestations in mitochondrial disorders. Semin Fetal Neonatal Med. 2011;16:229235.

Volpe JJ, Adams RD. Cerebro-Hepato-renal syndrome of Zellweger: an inherited disorder of neuronal migration. Acta neuropath (Berl). 1972;20:175–98.

14 Amniotic Band Syndrome/Amniotic Rupture Sequence

Amniotic rupture syndrome (ARS) is a group of fetal malformations and disruptions associated with in utero rupture of the amnion, with consequent formation of fibrous amniotic strands and membranes. Most often, it is associated with limb or digit reduction and atypical facial clefting, but central nervous system abnormalities may be the prominent or presenting abnormality on ultrasound or autopsy (Cignini et al. 2012; Orioli et al. 2003). There are scattered single reports and a few series describing central nervous system abnormalities, but few systematic examinations, possibly due to the difficulty in assembling a uniformly described series and the continuing obscurity as to the fundamental pathophysiology of the disorder (Shannon 2020).

Common to all cases of amniotic rupture sequence with malformation is the presence of amniotic membrane strands, often detectable by ultrasound in the first or early second trimesters, accompanied by chronic amniotic separation in the placenta, or the replacement of part of the skin or body wall by amniotic membrane. Where there are major body wall or cranial defects, the fetal part involved may be extra-amniotic with amniotic membrane growing in continuity with the fetal skin and replacing portions of the fetal body wall, extremity, or head (Torpin 1965, 1968). While the amniotic fibrous strands can theoretically act to disrupt lines of embryonic body wall fusion or mucosal tract development and can clearly act as constricting bands, leading to digital or limb hypoplasia or amputation, constricting bands do not readily explain the numerous visceral and bony abnormalities that are well understood to accompany amniotic rupture (Opitz et al. 2015; Streeter 1930).

14.1 Associated Neuropathology

When the brain is abnormal in ARS, there is typically accompanying craniofacial malformation, and the brain may display highly variable combinations of any or all of malformation, distortion, and post-encephaloclastic pathologies.

Acrania/acalvaria: Acalvaria can be partial or complete and may be associated with cranioplacental adhesion (Chanran et al. 2000; Menekse et al. 2015; Shannon 2020; da Silva 2020; Merrimen et al. 2006; Urich and Herrick 1985). In most cases of acalvaria, the calvarium and dura as well as the skin are at least partially replaced by amniotic membrane. The underlying brain can display mechanical distortion, secondary injury due to hemorrhage or necrosis, malformation, and histological abnormalities of unclear pathogenesis. The degree of malformation and secondary injury may be so extensive that the gross pathology resembles anencephaly. In some cases of acalvaria, the brain is adherent to the chorionic plate (a cranioplacental adhesion, Fig. 14.1a–c), but in general, acalvaria results when the brain develops in the extra-amniotic space, while the rest of the body is effectively intra-amniotic (Fig. 14.1e, f).

Holoprosencephaly: Holoprosencephaly (Fig. 14.1d) has been reported as a recurrent association both in case reports and case series. In a series compiled by one of us, holoprosencephaly was present in two of the eight cases of ARS with affected central nervous system: since then, we have encountered a third case (Shannon 2020).

Aqueductal lesions: Aqueductal stenosis, aqueductal atresia, neuronal heterotopias (Fig. 14.1g), and mesencephalosynapsis may be present. Obstructive hydrocephalus may be present, but there may not be ventriculomegaly, especially when accompanied by broad-based encephaloceles or acalvaria (Shannon 2020; Fisher et al. 2024).

Encephalocele: Both broad- and narrow-based encephaloceles can be present, with variable placement (da Silva 2019; da Silva et al. 2020). Occasionally, with careful examination, small amniotic adhesions may be present adherent to the overlying scalp. The tissue contained within the encephaloceles of ARS may undergo the same degenerative changes present in other encephaloceles (Fig. 14.1h, i).

Other brain lesions: Polymicrogyria, porencephaly, old or recent hemorrhage, ventricular diverticula or ventricular compression and fusion at the frontal or occipital poles, periventricular nodular heterotopias, absent septum pellucidum,

P. Shannon et al., *Atlas of Neurodevelopmental Pathology*, https://doi.org/10.1007/978-3-032-14148-4_14

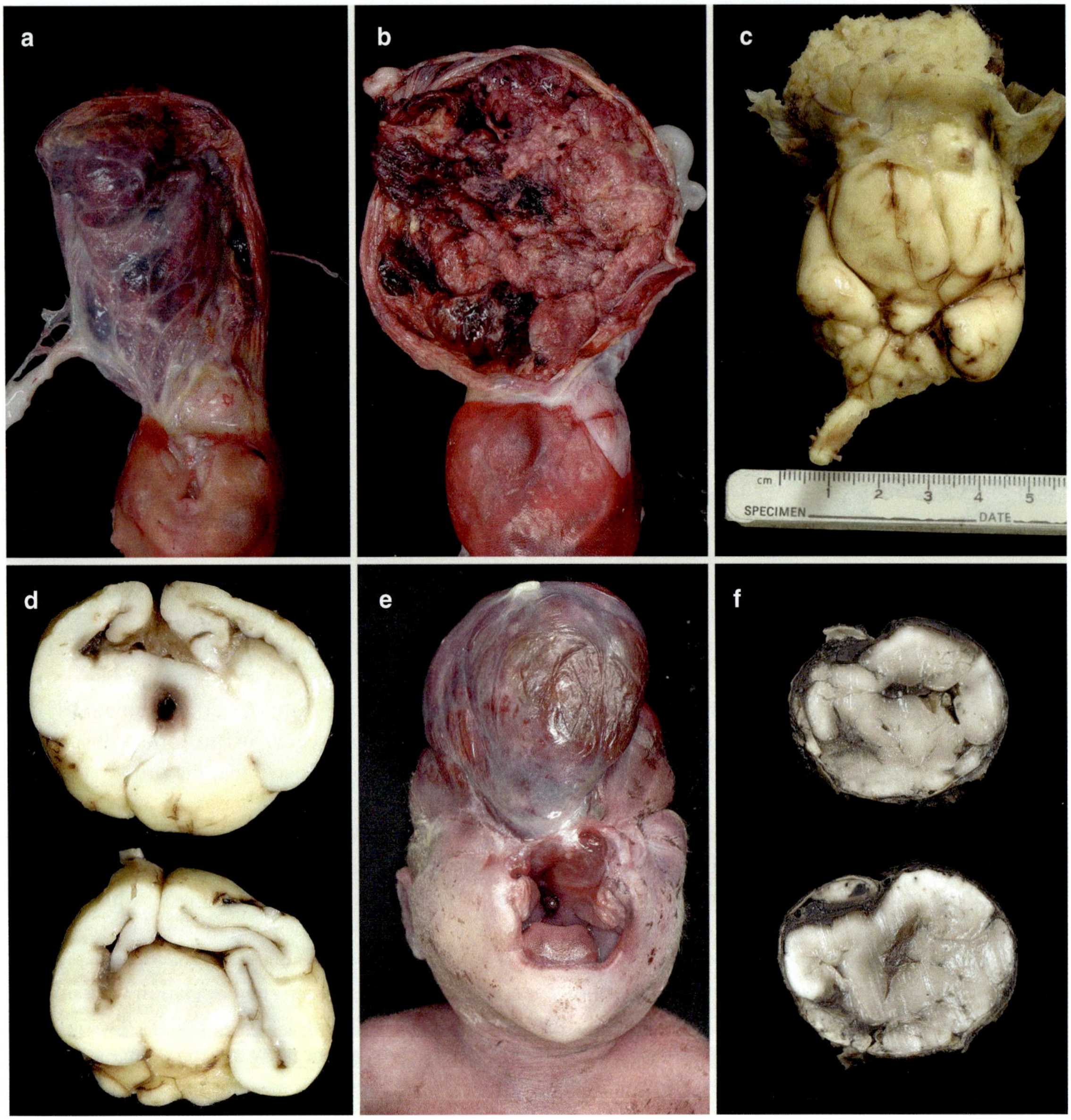

Fig. 14.1 (**a**) Anterior view of cranioplacental adhesion. Only the left eye is present, and the mouth is small and distorted by a large median cleft directly continuous with the amniotic surface. The umbilical cord is emerging from the right of the placental cake, which has the fetal surface turned toward the viewer. The brain can be seen through the amnion immediately above the left junction of the amnion with the skin over the remaining brow line. (**b**) Posterior view, demonstrating the maternal surface of the placenta. (**c**) The ventral surface of the dissected brain shown in (**a**): the surface of the brain is in contact with the chorionic plate, demonstrating an extra-amniotic location. Note that there are no olfactory bulbs or tracts and the interhemispheric fissure is poorly delineated. (**d**) Coronal section through the brain rostrally (top) and caudally (bottom). The dark focus rostrally is acute hematoma. The central gray mass is fused and hypoplastic, and there is a single U-shaped holoventricle. (**e**) Third-trimester case, where the scalp and calvarium have been replaced by amnion, with the amniotic epithelium in continuity with the surface of the skin. (**f**) Coronal cross sections demonstrating a chaotically distorted and fractured brain in which normal architecture is difficult to evaluate. (**g**) Axial sections through two different midbrains, demonstrating irregular heterotopias distorting a simplified tube (top) or non-separated dorsal colliculi with an atretic aqueduct (bottom). (**h**) Calvarium replaced by elongated, twisting tube of amnion (an 18-week-gestation fetus). (**i**) Careful axial sectioning demonstrates amnion surrounding a thin layer of arachnoid lined with chaotically arranged neural elements, including a developing brain and fragments of calcified or necrotic brain tissue

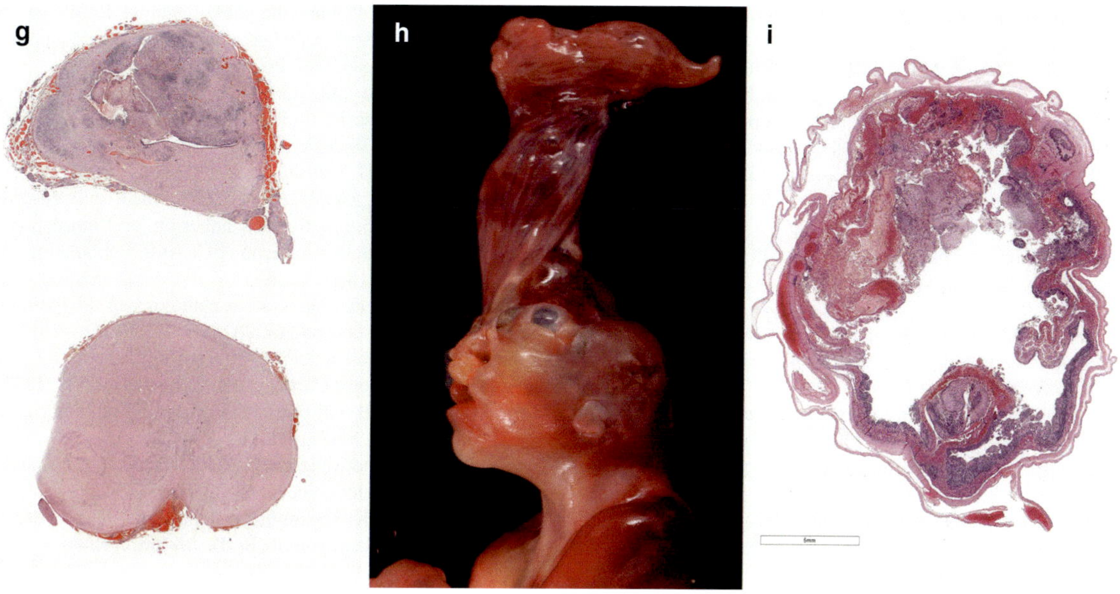

Fig. 14.1 (continued)

hypoplastic thalami and/or basal ganglia, septo-optic dysplasia, brainstem tegmental dysplasia, and absent descending tracts have all been observed (Shannon 2020; Amiji et al. 2019).

Other craniofacial anomalies: Complex or irregular craniofacial clefting or webs; large, small, or abnormally shaped palpebral fissures; eyelid or ocular globe coloboma; facial asymmetry; anophthalmia; microphthalmia; unilateral optic nerve hypoplasia; and hypoplastic pituitary stalk can all be present (Becerra-Solano et al. 2018).

14.2 Pathogenesis

Consistent genetic abnormalities are not documented. Although, in our experience, array cytogenetics is consistently normal, there is a report of a microdeletion at chromosome 2p15 (Mallett et al. 2018) in one case. Occasional cases of familial occurrence are recorded, but no consistent genetic basis for amniotic rupture sequence has been demonstrated.

Amniotic bands have been proposed to form due to either rupture or dysgenesis of the amnion (Torpin 1965, 1968), with subsequent generation of fibrous bands, which act to constrict the fetal or embryonic body or interfere with body folding and closure of clefts. While fibrous constricting bands certainly can explain constriction and amputation of limbs, the brain anomalies (holoprosencephaly, mesencephalosynapsis) are difficult to explain on this basis (Opitz et al. 2015).

Vascular pathology: Amniotic rupture has also been hypothesized to be due to an embryonic vascular event, with consequent injury to the developing fetus. Vascular instability in the post-embryonic period also seems to be a feature of the central nervous system pathology. However, the presence of features like holoprosencephaly and mesencephalosynapsis and the distribution of lesions are less readily explained by primary vascular anomalies or transient malperfusion (Shannon 2020).

Abnormal induction events: Abnormalities in ectodermal differentiation, whether secondary to displacement of amniotic epithelium due to rupture, heterotopic amniotic differentiation, or a primary abnormality in ectodermal development, could explain abnormalities in developing viscera, soft tissue, and body wall by a failure of local induction events (Shannon 2020).

References

Amiji IA, Mohamed UH, Rutashobya AG, et al. Septo-optic dysplasia with amniotic band syndrome sequence: a case report. J Med Case Rep. 2019;13(1):370.

Becerra-Solano LE, Castañeda-Cisneros G, Corona-Rivera JR, et al. Severe craniofacial involvement due to amniotic band sequence. Fetal Pediatr Pathol. 2018;37(1):27–37.

Chanran S, Lim MK, Yu VY. Fetal acalvaria with amniotic band syndrome. Arch Dis Child Fetal Neonatal Ed. 2000;82(1):F11–3.

Cignini P, Giorlandino C, Padula F, Dugo N, Cafà EV, Spata A. Epidemiology and risk factors of amniotic band syndrome, or ADAM sequence. J Prenat Med. 2012;6(4):59–63.

da Silva AJF, Silva CSME, Mariano SCR. Amniotic band syndrome with double encephalocele: a case report. Surg Neurol Int. 2020;11:448. https://doi.org/10.25259/SNI_454_2020. eCollection 2020.

da Silva AJF. Amniotic band syndrome associated with Exencephaly: a case report and literature review. J Pediatr Neurosci. 2019;14(2):94–6.

da Silva AJF. Amniotic band syndrome with placenta-Encephalocele adhesion: an uncommon case. J Pediatr Neurosci. 2020;15(2):160–1.

Mallett T, McElroy M, Swift K, Reuter S, et al. Chromosome 2 microdeletion syndrome in a newborn with amniotic band sequence. SD Med. 2018;71(4):154–7.

Menekse G, Mert MK, Olmaz B, et al. Placento-cranial adhesions in amniotic band syndrome and the role of surgery in their management: an unusual case presentation and systematic literature review. Pediatr Neurosurg. 2015;50(4):204–9.

Merrimen J, McNeely PD, Bendor-Samuel RL, et al. Congenital placental-cerebral adhesion: an unusual case of amniotic band sequence. J Neurosurg. 2006;104(5):3352–5.

Fisher Y, Shannon P, Greenberg O, Chitayat D, Chong K, Blaser S, Shinar S. Mesencephalosynapsis and aqueductal stenosis. J Neuropathol Exp Neurol. 2024.

Opitz JM, Johnson DR, Gilbert-Barness EF. ADAM "sequence" part II: hypothesis and speculation. Am J Med Genet A. 2015;167A(3):478–503. https://doi.org/10.1002/ajmg.a.36937. Epub 2015 Jan 21. PMID: 25604972.

Orioli IM, Ribeiro MG, Castilla EE. Clinical and epidemiological studies of amniotic deformity, adhesion, and mutilation (ADAM) sequence in a South American (ECLAMC) population. Am J Med Genet A. 2003;118A(2):135–45.

Shannon P. Central nervous system pathology in the amniotic rupture sequence. Clin Neuropathol. 2020;39(6):288–99.

Streeter GL. Focal deficiencies in fetal tissues and their relation to intrauterine amputations. Carnegie Inst Contrib Embryol. 1930;22:1–44.

Torpin R. 1968 Fetal malformations caused by amnion rupture during gestation. 1st ed. Springfield: CC Thomas.

Torpin R. Amniochorionic mesoblastic fibrous strings and amniotic bands. Am J Obstet Gynecol. 1965;91:65–75.

Urich H, Herrick MK. The amniotic band syndrome as a cause of anencephaly. Actal Neuropathol (Berl). 1985;67:190–4.

Index

P. Shannon et al., *Atlas of Neurodevelopmental Pathology*, https://doi.org/10.1007/978-3-032-14148-4

MIX
Papier aus verantwortungsvollen Quellen
Paper from responsible sources
FSC® C105338

FSC
www.fsc.org

If you have any concerns about our products,
you can contact us on
ProductSafety@springernature.com

In case Publisher is established outside the EU,
the EU authorized representative is:
Springer Nature Customer Service Center GmbH
Europaplatz 3, 69115 Heidelberg, Germany

Printed by Libri Plureos GmbH
in Hamburg, Germany